METHODS IN MOLECULAR BIOLOGY™

Series Editor
John M. Walker
School of Life Sciences
University of Hertfordshire
Hatfield, Hertfordshire, AL10 9AB, UK

For further volumes:
http://www.springer.com/series/7651

Retinal Degeneration

Methods and Protocols

Edited by

Bernhard H.F. Weber and Thomas Langmann

Institute of Human Genetics, University of Regensburg, Regensburg, Germany

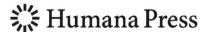 Humana Press

Editors
Bernhard H.F. Weber
Institute of Human Genetics
University of Regensburg
Regensburg, Germany

Thomas Langmann
Institute of Human Genetics
University of Regensburg
Regensburg, Germany

ALISTAIR MACKENZIE LIBRARY
Barcode: 3690289963
Class no: WW 270 WEB

ISSN 1064-3745   ISSN 1940-6029 (electronic)
ISBN 978-1-62703-079-3   ISBN 978-1-62703-080-9 (eBook)
DOI 10.1007/978-1-62703-080-9
Springer New York Heidelberg Dordrecht London

Library of Congress Control Number: 2012948131

© Springer Science+Business Media, LLC 2013
This work is subject to copyright. All rights are reserved by the Publisher, whether the whole or part of the material is concerned, specifically the rights of translation, reprinting, reuse of illustrations, recitation, broadcasting, reproduction on microfilms or in any other physical way, and transmission or information storage and retrieval, electronic adaptation, computer software, or by similar or dissimilar methodology now known or hereafter developed. Exempted from this legal reservation are brief excerpts in connection with reviews or scholarly analysis or material supplied specifically for the purpose of being entered and executed on a computer system, for exclusive use by the purchaser of the work. Duplication of this publication or parts thereof is permitted only under the provisions of the Copyright Law of the Publisher's location, in its current version, and permission for use must always be obtained from Springer. Permissions for use may be obtained through RightsLink at the Copyright Clearance Center. Violations are liable to prosecution under the respective Copyright Law.
The use of general descriptive names, registered names, trademarks, service marks, etc. in this publication does not imply, even in the absence of a specific statement, that such names are exempt from the relevant protective laws and regulations and therefore free for general use.
While the advice and information in this book are believed to be true and accurate at the date of publication, neither the authors nor the editors nor the publisher can accept any legal responsibility for any errors or omissions that may be made. The publisher makes no warranty, express or implied, with respect to the material contained herein.

Printed on acid-free paper

Humana Press is a brand of Springer
Springer is part of Springer Science+Business Media (www.springer.com)

Preface

Vision is crucial to allow for reliable orientation in the three-dimensional space and an immediate response to changing situations of the surrounding environment. In higher life forms, the ability of the visual system is intriguing in terms of resolution and the utilization of a wide range of ambient light conditions as well as the speed with which information is generated and transmitted to the brain where it triggers a direct reaction. To accomplish such remarkable tasks, highly complex networks of neuronal and auxiliary cells have evolved which are required to convey the physical energy of a light quantum via a molecular cascade to an electrical signal in the nervous system.

Over the past decades, our knowledge about the cellular and molecular basis underlying the visual process has remarkably increased. Hereby, a most fruitful approach included the study of the causes of visual impairment, in particular the analysis of degenerative diseases of the retina. Elucidating photoreceptor degeneration in animal model species such as *Drosophila melanogaster*, zebrafish, *Xenopus laevis*, or the mouse greatly advanced the field of eye research and has also fueled progress in delineating retinal degeneration in humans.

In accordance with the general objectives of the *Methods in Molecular Biology* series, the aim of the current volume *Retinal Degeneration: Methods and Protocols* is to provide a comprehensive step-by-step guide of relevant and state-of-the-art methods for studying retinal homeostasis and disease. Consequently, this book covers a broad range of techniques addressing cell culture systems and animal models of disease, their generation, their phenotypic and molecular characterization as well as their use in therapeutic approaches to the retina.

This volume is divided into seven parts. In an introductory chapter, Part I provides an overview of successfully applied approaches in human gene identification and characterization of retinal disease. Part II describes the mouse as a suitable animal model for monitoring and functionally analyzing retinal degeneration in vivo while Part III addresses specific technical aspects of vision research in non-rodent animal models such as frog, zebrafish, and the fruitfly *D. melanogaster*. In Part IV techniques for the analysis of retinal tissue and specific cell types in situ are described. Part V details some methods for tissue culturing and the use of cellular models to study homoeostatic processes in specific retinal cell types. Part VI addresses transcription and gene regulation in the healthy and diseased retina. Finally, Part VII is devoted to crucial aspects of therapy to treat retinal degeneration. Specifically, this part addresses the technique of subretinal injection, the adeno-associated viral vectors as vehicle to deliver gene constructs, and an innovative approach to barrier modulation to efficiently deliver drugs to the retina. These topics are most relevant as part of proof-of-concept approaches in animal models and also to advance treatment options in human patients.

The current volume *Retinal Degeneration: Methods and Protocols* should be helpful to all those researchers from academia, biotech, and industry interested in cutting-edge techniques to study retinal cell biology in health and disease. We would like to thank all authors of this volume for their excellent contributions. It is their expertise and willingness to share bits and pieces of valuable information which is usually not readily available in the scientific literature but makes all the difference between a successful and a useless experiment. We are also deeply grateful to John Walker for inviting us to contribute this volume to the *Methods in Molecular Biology* series and for his expert editorial assistance during the preparation of this book.

Regensburg, Germany   *Bernhard H.F. Weber*
                                                                    Thomas Langmann

Contents

Alistair Mackenzie Library
Wishaw General Hospital
50 Netherton Street
Wishaw
ML2 0DP

Preface... *v*

Contributors... *xi*

PART I   HUMAN GENETICS

1   Identification and Analysis of Inherited Retinal Disease Genes............. 3
    Kornelia Neveling, Anneke I. den Hollander, Frans P.M. Cremers,
    and Rob W.J. Collin

PART II   MOUSE MODELS

2   Mouse Models for Studies of Retinal Degeneration and Diseases........... 27
    Bo Chang

3   Retinal Fundus Imaging in Mouse Models of Retinal Diseases............. 41
    Anne F. Alex, Peter Heiduschka, and Nicole Eter

4   Functional Phenotyping of Mouse Models with ERG 69
    Naoyuki Tanimoto, Vithiyanjali Sothilingam, and Mathias W. Seeliger

5   Phenotyping of Mouse Models with OCT......................... 79
    M. Dominik Fischer, Ahmad Zhour, and Christoph J. Kernstock

6   Light Damage as a Model of Retinal Degeneration 87
    Christian Grimm and Charlotte E. Remé

7   N-Methyl-D-Aspartate (NMDA)-Mediated Excitotoxic Damage:
    A Mouse Model of Acute Retinal Ganglion Cell Damage 99
    Roswitha Seitz and Ernst R. Tamm

PART III   OTHER ANIMAL MODELS

8   Generation of Transgenic *X. laevis* Models of Retinal Degeneration 113
    Beatrice M. Tam, Christine C.-L. Lai, Zusheng Zong,
    and Orson L. Moritz

9   Analysis of Photoreceptor Degeneration in the Zebrafish *Danio rerio* 127
    Holger Dill, Bastian Linder, Anja Hirmer, and Utz Fischer

10   Analysis of Optokinetic Response in Zebrafish
     by Computer-Based Eye Tracking 139
     Sabina P. Huber-Reggi, Kaspar P. Mueller, and Stephan C.F. Neuhauss

11   Analysis of the *Drosophila* Compound Eye with Light
     and Electron Microscopy 161
     Monalisa Mishra and Elisabeth Knust

Part IV   In Situ Analyses

12 Cell-Specific Markers for the Identification of Retinal Cells
by Immunofluorescence Microscopy   185
Christiana L. Cheng, Hidayat Djajadi, and Robert S. Molday

13 A Method of Horizontally Sliced Preparation of the Retina   201
Ryosuke Enoki and Amane Koizumi

14 Detection of DNA Fragmentation in Retinal Apoptosis by TUNEL   207
Francesca Doonan and Thomas G. Cotter

15 High-Throughput RNA In Situ Hybridization in Mouse Retina   215
Seth Blackshaw

16 Assessment of Mitochondrial Damage in Retinal Cells and Tissues
Using Quantitative Polymerase Chain Reaction for Mitochondrial
DNA Damage and Extracellular Flux Assay for Mitochondrial
Respiration Activity   227
Stuart G. Jarrett, Bärbel Rohrer, Nathan R. Perron,
Craig Beeson, and Michael E. Boulton

17 Analysis of Photoreceptor Rod Outer Segment Phagocytosis
by RPE Cells In Situ   245
Saumil Sethna and Silvia C. Finnemann

Part V   Tissue Culture and Cell Models

18 Ca^{2+} Microfluorimetry in Retinal Müller Glial Cells   257
Antje Wurm, Thomas Pannicke, and Andreas Reichenbach

19 Functional Analysis of Retinal Microglia and Their Effects
on Progenitors   271
Debra A. Carter, Balini Balasubramaniam, and Andrew D. Dick

20 Analysis of Photoreceptor Outer Segment Phagocytosis
by RPE Cells in Culture   285
Yingyu Mao and Silvia C. Finnemann

21 Ca^{2+}-Imaging Techniques to Analyze Ca^{2+} Signaling in Cells
and to Monitor Neuronal Activity in the Retina   297
Olaf Strauß

Part VI   Gene Regulation

22 Double Chromatin Immunoprecipitation: Analysis of Target
Co-occupancy of Retinal Transcription Factors   311
Guang-Hua Peng and Shiming Chen

23 Quantifying the Activity of *cis*-Regulatory Elements in the Mouse Retina
by Explant Electroporation   329
Cynthia L. Montana, Connie A. Myers, and Joseph C. Corbo

PART VII   THERAPY

24 Optimized Technique for Subretinal Injections in Mice   343
    Regine Mühlfriedel, Stylianos Michalakis, Marina Garcia Garrido,
    Martin Biel, and Mathias W. Seeliger

25 Adeno-Associated Viral Vectors for Gene Therapy of Inherited
    Retinal Degenerations   351
    John G. Flannery and Meike Visel

26 Barrier Modulation in Drug Delivery to the Retina   371
    Matthew Campbell, Marian M. Humphries, and Peter Humphries

Index *381*

Contributors

ANNE F. ALEX • *Department of Ophthalmology, Westfaelische Wilhelms-University Münster, Münster, Germany*

BALINI BALASUBRAMANIAM • *Bristol Eye Hospital, School of Clinical Sciences, University of Bristol, Bristol, UK*

CRAIG BEESON • *Division of Research, Pharmaceutical Sciences, Medical University of South Carolina, Charleston, SC, USA*

MARTIN BIEL • *Center for Integrated Protein Science Munich (CIPSM), Department of Pharmacy–Center for Drug Research, Ludwig-Maximilians-Universität, Munich, Germany*

SETH BLACKSHAW • *The Salomon H. Snyder Department of Neuroscience, John Hopkins University School of Medicine, Baltimore, MD, USA*

MICHAEL E. BOULTON • *Department of Anatomy and Cell Biology, College of Medicine, University of Florida, Gainesville, FL, USA*

MATTHEW CAMPBELL • *Ocular Genetics Unit, Department of Genetics, Trinity College, Dublin, Ireland*

DEBRA A. CARTER • *Bristol Eye Hospital, School of Clinical Sciences, University of Bristol, Bristol, UK*

BO CHANG • *The Jackson Laboratory, Bar Harbor, ME, USA*

SHIMING CHEN • *Department of Ophthalmology and Visual Sciences, Washington University School of Medicine, St. Louis, MO, USA; Department of Developmental Biology, Washington University School of Medicine, St. Louis, MO, USA*

CHRISTIANA L. CHENG • *Department of Biochemistry and Molecular Biology, University of British Columbia, Vancouver, BC, Canada*

ROB W.J. COLLIN • *Department of Human Genetics, Radboud University Nijmegen Medical Centre, Nijmegen, The Netherlands*

JOSEPH C. CORBO • *Department of Pathology and Immunology, Washington University School of Medicine, St. Louis, MO, USA*

THOMAS G. COTTER • *Tumour Biology Laboratory, Biochemistry Department, Bioscience Research Institute, University College Cork, Cork, Ireland*

FRANS P.M. CREMERS • *Department of Human Genetics, Radboud University Nijmegen Medical Centre, Nijmegen, The Netherlands*

ANNEKE I. DEN HOLLANDER • *Department of Human Genetics, Radboud University Nijmegen Medical Centre, Nijmegen, The Netherlands*

ANDREW D. DICK • *Bristol Eye Hospital, School of Clinical Sciences, University of Bristol, Bristol, UK*

HOLGER DILL • *Department of Biochemistry, Biocenter, University of Würzburg, Würzburg, Germany*

HIDAYAT DJAJADI • *Department of Biochemistry and Molecular Biology, University of British Columbia, Vancouver, BC, Canada*

FRANCESCA DOONAN • *Tumour Biology Laboratory, Biochemistry Department, Bioscience Research Institute, University College Cork, Cork, Ireland*

RYOSUKE ENOKI • *Photonic Bioimaging Center, Hokkaido University Graduate School of Medicine, Sapporo, Japan*

NICOLE ETER • *Department of Ophthalmology, Westfaelische Wilhelms-University Münster, Münster, Germany*

SILVIA C. FINNEMANN • *Department of Biological Sciences, Larkin Hall, Fordham University, Bronx, NY, USA*

M. DOMINIK FISCHER • *Centre for Ophthalmology, University Eye Hospital, University of Tuebingen, Tuebingen, Germany*

UTZ FISCHER • *Department of Biochemistry, Biocenter, University of Würzburg, Würzburg, Germany*

JOHN G. FLANNERY • *Neuroscience Division, Department of Molecular and Cell Biology, Helen Wills Neuroscience Institute, University of California, Berkeley, CA, USA*

MARINA GARCIA GARRIDO • *Division of Ocular Neurodegeneration, Centre for Ophthalmology, Institute for Ophthalmic Research, University of Tuebingen, Tuebingen, Germany*

CHRISTIAN GRIMM • *Lab for Retinal Cell Biology, Department Ophthalmology, University of Zürich, Schlieren, Switzerland*

PETER HEIDUSCHKA • *Department of Ophthalmology, Westfaelische Wilhelms-University Münster, Münster, Germany*

ANJA HIRMER • *Department of Biochemistry, Biocenter, University of Würzburg, Würzburg, Germany*

SABINA P. HUBER-REGGI • *Institute of Molecular Life Sciences, University of Zurich, Zurich, Switzerland*

MARIAN M. HUMPHRIES • *Ocular Genetics Unit, Department of Genetics, Trinity College, Dublin, Ireland*

PETER HUMPHRIES • *Ocular Genetics Unit, Department of Genetics, Trinity College, Dublin, Ireland*

STUART G. JARRETT • *Department of Molecular and Biomedical Pharmacology, College of Medicine, University of Kentucky, Lexington, KY, USA*

CHRISTOPH J. KERNSTOCK • *Centre for Ophthalmology, University Eye Hospital, University of Tuebingen, Tuebingen, Germany*

ELISABETH KNUST • *Max-Planck-Institute of Molecular Cell Biology and Genetics, Dresden, Germany*

AMANE KOIZUMI • *Photonic Bioimaging Center, Hokkaido University Graduate School of Medicine, Sapporo, Japan*

CHRISTINE C.-L. LAI • *Department of Ophthalmology & Visual Sciences, University of British Columbia, Vancouver, BC, Canada*

THOMAS LANGMANN • *University of Regensburg, Institute of Human Genetics, Regensburg, Germany*

BASTIAN LINDER • *Department of Biochemistry, Biocenter, University of Würzburg, Würzburg, Germany*

YINGYU MAO • *Department of Biological Sciences, Fordham University, Bronx, NY, USA*

STYLIANOS MICHALAKIS • *Center for Integrated Protein Science Munich (CIPSM), Department of Pharmacy–Center for Drug Research, Ludwig-Maximilians-Universität, Munich, Germany*

MONALISA MISHRA • *Max-Planck-Institute of Molecular Cell Biology and Genetics, Dresden, Germany*

ROBERT S. MOLDAY • *Department of Biochemistry and Molecular Biology, Health Sciences Mall, University of British Columbia, Vancouver, BC, Canada*

CYNTHIA L. MONTANA • *Department of Pathology and Immunology, Washington University School of Medicine, St. Louis, MO, USA*

ORSON L. MORITZ • *Department of Ophthalmology & Visual Sciences, University of British Columbia, Vancouver, BC, Canada*

KASPAR P. MUELLER • *Institute of Molecular Life Sciences, University of Zurich, Zurich, Switzerland*

REGINE MÜHLFRIEDEL • *Division of Ocular Neurodegeneration, Centre for Ophthalmology, Institute for Ophthalmic Research, University of Tuebingen, Tuebingen, Germany*

CONNIE A. MYERS • *Department of Pathology and Immunology, Washington University School of Medicine, St. Louis, MO, USA*

STEPHAN C.F. NEUHAUSS • *Institute of Molecular Life Sciences, University of Zurich, Zurich, Switzerland*

KORNELIA NEVELING • *Department of Human Genetics, Radboud University Nijmegen Medical Centre, Nijmegen, The Netherlands*

THOMAS PANNICKE • *Paul Flechsig Institute for Brain Research, Department of Pathophysiology of Neuroglia, University of Leipzig, Leipzig, Germany*

GUANG-HUA PENG • *Department of Ophthalmology and Visual Sciences, Washington University School of Medicine, St. Louis, MO, USA*

NATHAN R. PERRON • *Division of Research, Departments of Ophthalmology, Medical University of South Carolina, Charleston, SC, USA*

CHARLOTTE E. REMÉ • *University Zürich, Zürich, Switzerland*

ANDREAS REICHENBACH • *Paul Flechsig Institute for Brain Research, Department of Pathophysiology of Neuroglia, University of Leipzig, Leipzig, Germany*

BÄRBEL ROHRER • *Division of Research, Departments of Ophthalmology, and Neurosciences, Medical University of South Carolina, Charleston, SC, USA*

MATHIAS W. SEELIGER • *Division of Ocular Neurodegeneration, Centre for Ophthalmology, Institute for Ophthalmic Research, University of Tuebingen, Tuebingen, Germany*

ROSWITHA SEITZ • *Institute for Human Anatomy and Embryology, University of Regensburg, Regensburg, Germany*

SAUMIL SETHNA • *Department of Biological Sciences, Fordham University, Bronx, NY, USA*

VITHIYANJALI SOTHILINGAM • *Division of Ocular Neurodegeneration, Centre for Ophthalmology, Institute for Ophthalmic Research, University of Tuebingen, Tuebingen, Germany*

OLAF STRAUß • *Experimental Ophthalmology, Eye Hospital, University Medical Center Regensburg, Regensburg, Germany*

BEATRICE M. TAM • *Department of Ophthalmology & Visual Sciences, University of British Columbia, Vancouver, BC, Canada*

ERNST R. TAMM • *Institute for Human Anatomy and Embryology, University of Regensburg, Regensburg, Germany*

NAOYUKI TANIMOTO • *Division of Ocular Neurodegeneration, Centre for Ophthalmology, Institute for Ophthalmic Research, University of Tuebingen, Tuebingen, Germany*

MEIKE VISEL • *Neuroscience Division, Department of Molecular and Cell Biology, Helen Wills Neuroscience Institute, University of California, Berkeley, CA, USA*

BERNHARD H.F. WEBER • *University of Regensburg, Institute of Human Genetics, Regensburg, Germany*

ANTJE WURM • *Paul Flechsig Institute for Brain Research, Department of Pathophysiology of Neuroglia, University of Leipzig, Leipzig, Germany*

AHMAD ZHOUR • *Centre for Ophthalmology, University Eye Hospital, University of Tuebingen, Tuebingen, Germany*

ZUSHENG ZONG • *Department of Ophthalmology & Visual Sciences, University of British Columbia, Vancouver, BC, Canada*

Part I

Human Genetics

Chapter 1

Identification and Analysis of Inherited Retinal Disease Genes

Kornelia Neveling, Anneke I. den Hollander, Frans P.M. Cremers, and Rob W.J. Collin

Abstract

Inherited retinal diseases display a very high degree of clinical and genetic heterogeneity, which poses challenges in identifying the underlying defects in known genes and in identifying novel retinal disease genes. Here, we outline the state-of-the-art techniques to find the causative DNA variants, with special attention for next-generation sequencing which can combine molecular diagnostics and retinal disease gene identification.

Key words: Sanger sequencing, Microarrays, Linkage analysis, Homozygosity mapping, Next-generation sequencing

1. Introduction

1.1. Spectrum of Retinal Diseases

Inherited retinal diseases represent a heterogeneous group of disorders affecting the retina. These diseases can be classified based on whether they predominantly affect the rods (e.g., retinitis pigmentosa) and the cones (e.g., cone and cone–rod dystrophies (CRDs)), or cause a more generalized photoreceptor disease (e.g., Leber congenital amaurosis) (1, 2). Most retinal dystrophies are associated with a gradual deterioration over time, but some are nonprogressive (e.g., congenital stationary night blindness, achromatopsia, some forms of Leber congenital amaurosis). The distinction between various retinal dystrophies can sometimes be difficult, as the clinical features of some diseases can be overlapping, both at early and late stages (Fig. 1).

Retinal dystrophies can be inherited in an autosomal recessive, autosomal dominant, and X-linked fashion. Some diseases are caused by mutations in a relatively small number of genes, but

Bernhard H.F. Weber and Thomas Langmann (eds.), *Retinal Degeneration: Methods and Protocols*, Methods in Molecular Biology, vol. 935, DOI 10.1007/978-1-62703-080-9_1, © Springer Science+Business Media, LLC 2013

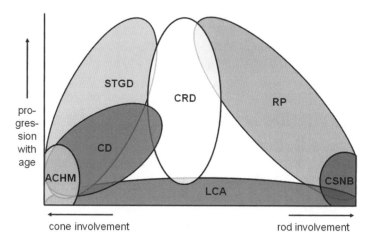

Fig. 1. Phenotypic overlap between autosomal recessive retinal diseases. Patients with achromatopsia (ACHM) display a virtually stationary cone defect in which cones are principally defective. At end stages, cone dystrophy (CD) can hardly be distinguished from cone–rod dystrophy (CRD). Patients with Stargardt disease (STGD1) later in life show mid-peripheral defects similar to CRD patients. Patients with retinitis pigmentosa (RP) initially display night blindness, followed by tunnel vision due to rod defects which very often progresses to complete blindness when the cones are also afflicted. In patients with Leber congenital amaurosis (LCA), the defects can occur in both types of photoreceptors, or in Müller or RPE cells, and therefore both clinical and molecular genetic overlap with CD, CRD, or RP can be expected. Patients with congenital stationary night blindness (CSNB) show a rod-specific defect.

others are genetically heterogeneous. The most extreme example is retinitis pigmentosa (RP), which has been associated with mutations in more than 50 different genes. The genetic heterogeneity has hampered the identification of retinal dystrophy genes, as most genes affect only a small number of cases. To date, mutations in more than 165 genes have been identified in patients with inherited non-syndromic and syndromic retinal diseases, and it is estimated that approximately one-third of the causative genes remains to be identified (3). All known retinal disease genes and the corresponding modes of inheritance can be found at http://www.sph.uth.tmc.edu/RetNet/.

1.2. The Changing Landscape of Retinal Disease Gene Identification

The methods and tools available for gene identification studies have evolved dramatically during the last two decades. The first retinal disease gene identified was the ornithine aminotransferase (*OAT*) gene involved in gyrate atrophy. An enzymatic defect of OAT activity was measured in patient's cells in 1977 (4), and 11 years later the *OAT* gene was cloned and the first mutation identified (5). In 1990, mutations in the rhodopsin gene were identified in patients with autosomal dominant retinitis pigmentosa using a candidate gene approach (6), after linkage analysis in a large Irish adRP family had pointed towards a genomic region encompassing this gene (7). In 1990, the choroideremia (*CHM*) gene was identified using a positional cloning approach by mapping deletions in patients with syndromic and non-syndromic chroideremia (8).

The candidate gene approach has been successfully used to identify a large number of retinal disease genes, and mainly focused on genes specifically expressed in the retina and those encoding components of the phototransduction cascade and visual cycle. Positional cloning by linkage analysis has been used effectively to localize retinal disease genes, though this generally requires the availability of large families. In the early years linkage analysis using polymorphic microsatellite markers was a labor-intensive and tedious method, but was lifted to a fast and genome-wide approach with the development of microarray technology allowing rapid genotyping of thousands of single-nucleotide polymorphisms (SNPs) spread across the genome. SNP microarrays have also proven very valuable for identity-by-descent (IBD)-mapping of recessive disease genes not only in consanguineous families but also in small families and single patients of non-consanguineous marriages (9).

We are witnessing a new era in disease gene identification with the introduction of next-generation sequencing (NGS), allowing the analysis of all genes in a defined linkage interval, all exons in the genome (the "exome"), or even the entire genomic sequence. This also brings new challenges, such as data analysis and interpretation of genomic variants. Given the huge number of variants present in a patient's genome, positional information on where the causative gene may be localized (e.g., by linkage analysis and/or homozygosity mapping) remains very helpful to pinpoint the genetic defect.

1.3. Importance of Molecular Diagnostics

Receiving a molecular diagnosis becomes increasingly important with the development of (gene) therapy for retinal dystrophies (3). Up to 4 years ago, it was not possible to slow down, stabilize, or treat the vision impairment in patients with retinal dystrophies. This changed for a small group of patients with *RPE65* mutations, as gene augmentation was successfully and safely applied through subretinal injections of recombinant adeno-associated viruses (rAAVs) (10–12). rAAVs transduce the retinal pigment epithelium (RPE) cells, upon which the viruses are shuttled to the nucleus, and the rAAV vector remains a stable extrachromosomal element. In the meantime, 18 patients have been treated in three centers in Philadelphia and London. Vision improvement was variable and in general modest and appears to be more effective in younger patients. In addition, oral 9-*cis* retinoid supplementation therapy seems highly effective in patients with *RPE65* and *LRAT* mutations. Several therapies that will be developed in the next years will be gene or even mutation specific, emphasizing the importance for patients to receive a molecular diagnosis.

To provide a more accurate prognosis, and to determine which forms of retinal dystrophy would most likely benefit from (gene) therapy, patients should be thoroughly clinically examined using standardized protocols. Ocular coherence tomography (OCT) studies have shown that some forms of retinal dystrophies are likely less suitable for therapy, while in other forms photoreceptors remain viable for a prolonged period (13).

Retinal dystrophies are sometimes the first sign of a syndromic disease, such as Senior–Loken syndrome that involves renal failure. Since the ocular phenotype precedes the manifestation of kidney abnormalities, there is often a delay in the diagnosis of nephronophthisis. This causes a risk for sudden death from fluid and electrolyte imbalance. Nephronophthisis patients that receive kidney transplants have excellent outcomes that are shown to be better compared with the general pediatric transplant population. Determining an early molecular diagnosis may therefore allow physicians to monitor patients carrying mutations in syndromic genes more closely for kidney disease and other systemic features.

2. Techniques

2.1. Sanger Sequencing

Sanger sequencing is based on the incorporation of deoxynucleotides and fluorochrome-labeled dideoxynucleotides using DNA polymerase, the latter of which abrogate the replication of a DNA fragment at random positions. In this way, a mixture of DNA fragments is synthesized and size-separated through capillary electrophoresis. The most widely used apparatus (Applied Biosystems) can analyze up to 96 samples in parallel. Sanger sequencing is preceded by PCR amplification of a DNA fragment of interest, and is the most widely used sequencing technique for a limited number of exons or amplicons. Its advantages are its accuracy, flexibility, speed, and relatively low costs.

2.2. Allele-Specific Primer Extension

The analysis of a large number of known DNA variants can be performed using the Allele-Specific Primer Extension (APEX) technique, which in essence is a mini-sequencing method. Allele-specific primers are designed up to, but not including, the sequence variants that are to be tested. DNA fragments amplified from patients' genomic DNA samples are hybridized to these primers, and the allele-specific primers are elongated with one of the four fluorochrome-labeled dideoxynucleotides depending on the variant present in the patient's DNA. Currently, several hundreds of variants are being tested using APEX technology by Asper Ophthalmics (http://www.asperbio.com/asper-ophthalmics) for each of the genetically heterogeneous retinal diseases. The most important disadvantage of APEX is that it only tests for the presence of known variants, the occurrence of which may vary tremendously between patients of different ethnic origins.

2.3. Single-Nucleotide Polymorphism Microarrays

Genome-wide SNP arrays have become a commonly used tool in medical genetics over the past decade, and allow a rapid and cost-effective simultaneous genotyping analysis of SNPs evenly distributed over the genome. SNP array analysis is based on the specificity of hybridization of patient-derived DNA fragments with the oligonucleotides (25-mers) bound to the array. One-nucleotide mismatches distinguish fully matching from incomplete matching DNA fragments. SNP arrays are used for genome-wide linkage studies, including homozygosity mapping, and copy number variant (CNV) detection in Mendelian diseases, and for association studies in multifactorial diseases.

Depending on the characteristics of the family or patient that is being studied, one can either opt for a low-resolution or a high-resolution array that varies in the amount of SNPs that are genotyped. "Low-resolution SNP arrays" generally contain up to 10,000 SNPs and can be used to perform classical linkage analysis in autosomal dominant or recessive families, or for homozygosity mapping purposes in families with a high degree of consanguinity. The amount of SNPs present on higher resolution arrays varies from 50,000 to even 2.7 million sequence variants, allowing a very accurate analysis of relatively small IBD regions, genomic deletions or duplications, or genomic regions segregating with the disease in a family.

2.4. Linkage Analysis

Linkage analysis, following genome-wide SNP genotyping, is performed to determine the chromosomal region that segregates with a trait. The *logarithm of the odds* (LOD)-score is the $\log_{10}$-ratio of the likelihood that the disease locus and a given genomic marker (e.g., SNP) are linked versus the likelihood that they are unlinked, and is generally used as an outcome measure in linkage calculations. In order to reach statistical significant locus assignment by genome-wide genotyping, a minimum LOD score of 3.3 has to be obtained, whereas an LOD-score of 1.86 is suggestive for linkage (14). The more individuals (both affected and unaffected) are genotyped in the linkage analysis, the higher the final LOD-score will be. Generally, linkage analysis is only performed if an LOD-score of >2 can be obtained with the available relatives, which can be calculated by a linkage simulation prior to the actual genotyping.

Issues that occasionally can interfere with linkage analysis are the occurrence of phenocopies (e.g., affected relatives with the same phenotype but a different (genetic) cause), or non-penetrance (e.g., the occurrence of individuals that carry the same causative mutation but do not, or hardly, display the clinical phenotype). Especially in some dominant retinal diseases, like for instance familial exudative vitreoretinopathy (15) and adRP caused by mutations in *PRPF31* (16), non-penetrance is frequently observed. The actual linkage calculations can be performed by freely available software programs, like LINKAGE, Allegro, Genehunter, or SimWalk2. Graphical user interfaces for linkage analysis software on Microsoft Windows-based operating systems like easyLINKAGE (17) or Alohamora (18) allow to use each of these programs, with manually adjustable settings for the mode of inheritance, ethnic origin of the family, disease prevalence, and penetrance, amongst others. A more detailed description on linkage analysis is provided in several textbooks (19, 20).

2.5. Identity-by-Descent-Mapping

For recessively inherited retinal dystrophies, the genotyping data resulting from the SNP array analyses can also be used for IBD-mapping. IBD regions are genomic regions where two identical haplotypes (i.e., parts of a chromosome) are inherited from both parents. Since the ancestral haplotypes are the same, also the SNP alleles on these haplotypes will be identical and hence appear in a homozygous state upon SNP genotyping. Several software programs including HomozygosityMapper (21), PLINK, or Beagle (22) are available to extract IBD regions that subsequently can be scrutinized for the gene causative for the phenotype. In families with a high degree of consanguinity, the causative mutation underlying recessive disease almost exclusively appears in a homozygous state. Hence, such families are extremely suitable for IBD-mapping. In families without a history of consanguinity, not all causative mutations will appear in a homozygous state, and IBD-mapping will not always point towards the genomic region harboring the genetic defect. However, we and others have previously shown that in a substantial percentage of cases, IBD mapping appeared to be a powerful method to identify homozygous mutations, also in non-consanguineous patients (9, 23–28). And although this is not true for all autosomal recessive diseases, in general, homozygous mutations are more frequently detected in diseases that are rare in the population.

The amount and size of the homozygous regions that are detected mainly depend on the degree of relatedness between patients' parents. For patients whose parents are first cousins, the total percentage of homozygosity in the genome can range up to 10%, with numerous homozygous regions that individually can cover up to 90 Mb of genomic DNA (9, 29). In non-consanguineous patients, the amount and the size of the IBD regions are smaller, although regions of 30 Mb or more are occasionally detected in this group of patients. However, the majority of IBD regions are smaller, and range from 1 to 10 Mb, but still potentially harbor the causative genetic defect, exemplified by the detection of a *PDE6A* mutation in an IBD region of only 1.5 Mb of genomic DNA (9).

2.6. Copy Number Variant-Detection

High-resolution SNP genotyping data can also be used to detect genomic copy number aberrations that might be causative for the disease. Copy number variations, or CNVs, are defined as deletions or duplications that range from 1 kb up to several Mb of genomic DNA, and hence can contain only a part of a single gene or multiple genes on one chromosome (30). Variations in copy number are detected by comparing the intensity of the signal that is derived from each probe (e.g., the SNP or a non-polymorphic probe for copy number detection) represented on the SNP array. The more consecutive probes that show an aberrant intensity, the more likely it is that the region represents a true CNV, and the easier it is to define the size and boundaries. Depending on the type of array that is used, CNV analysis can be performed with software programs such as CNAG (31), Affymetrix Genotype Console, or Partek Genomic Suite software.

The role of CNVs in human disease has mainly been studied in the context of complex genomic disorders, where gene dosage aberrations in one or more adjacent genes are causative for the phenotype (30). For retinal disease, there are only a few reports on causal CNVs (32, 33). However, the increased density of the SNP arrays that are nowadays used will allow a more reliable detection of CNVs that span only (a part of) a single gene, and most likely identify more CNVs underlying retinal disease in the near future.

2.7. Next-Generation Sequencing

NGS (also called "massive parallel sequencing" (MPS) or "second-generation sequencing") describes a new era of sequencing that will become increasingly important for retinal diseases not only for the identification of new disease genes but also for molecular diagnostics. The term NGS thereby comprises many different new sequencing technologies (34, 35) all having a much higher throughput than the previously used gold standard technology "Sanger sequencing." Nowadays, more than 20 different NGS platforms from different companies are available, including the widely used Roche 454 systems (GS FLX Titanium and GS Junior), Life Technologies systems (e.g., SOLiD 4, 5500XL), and the Illumina platforms (e.g., HiSeq, MiSeq, Genome Analyzer IIx). Although all these platforms have a much higher throughput than conventional Sanger sequencing, they still differ significantly in the used sequencing technologies and/or chemistries, leading to different capacities, false-positive rates, and read lengths (e.g., 454 GS FLX Titanium: up to 500 bp reads; SOLiD 5500XL: up to 75 bp (+35 bp) reads; HiSeq2000: up to 2×100 bp reads). As conventional Sanger sequencing is preceded by PCR amplification of the DNA fragments of interest, NGS also requires an enrichment of the region(s) of interest. Several options are available, like for example amplicon-based enrichment strategies or gene capturing on array or in liquid using baits (36). One can enrich for complete genomic regions (including promoter regions, introns, etc.), for only the coding regions of certain genes, or even for all exons of all human genes (the so-called exome) or the entire genome. Whole genome sequencing is still very expensive, but whole exome sequencing is becoming increasingly the method of choice for research and diagnostics (37). Recently upcoming new machines (third-generation sequencers) now also enable single molecule (real-time) sequencing (e.g., Pacific Bioscience, Helicos), making the enrichment strategies unnecessary for future approaches. Others make use of H^+ detection instead of fluorescent dyes (post-light sequencing, Ion Torrent), enabling low-cost manufacturing by using commercial microchip design standards and not needing cameras, lasers, and fluorescent dyes (35).

2.8. Targeted Resequencing Versus Whole Exome Sequencing

For inherited retinal diseases, like for many other inherited disorders, NGS is already a very powerful tool for the identification of new disease genes and also for clinical molecular diagnostics. For disease gene identification, a good approach is to combine the positional information gained from linkage or homozygosity mapping with a targeted resequencing or exome sequencing approach, as exemplified by the identification of the autosomal dominant exudative vitreo-retinopathy gene *TSPAN12* (38), and the autosomal recessive retinitis pigmentosa gene *C8ORF37* Mutations in *C8orf37*, encoding a ciliary protein, are associated with autosomal-recessive retinal dystrophies with early macular involvement (39). Positional information of the culprit mutation(s) however is generally lacking in small non-consanguineous families with inherited retinal diseases, and therefore whole exome sequencing would be the method of choice. In a diagnostic setting, however, one might argue that whole exome sequencing could be problematic due to the huge number of variants identified and the additional risk of incidental findings. In contrast, whole exome sequencing is a generic approach that can be performed for any kind of disorder, meaning that every diagnostic lab would need to do only one approach instead of many different assays for the different diseases. The problem of incidental findings can be reduced by analyzing only the known disease genes instead of the whole exome. Only in cases where there is no mutation found in a known gene there would be a need to scrutinize the exome to analyze the remaining genes as well. Another advantage of whole exome sequencing in contrast to a targeted resequencing approach is that the assay does not need to be changed with each discovery of a new gene, as the whole exome is already sequenced, and only the data analysis needs to be adapted. In contrast to other diagnostic approaches, whole exome sequencing by NGS therefore will likely soon result in performing relatively cheap and efficient molecular diagnostics.

2.9. Technical Challenges

A big challenge in NGS-based sequencing is to select the one detrimental mutation(s) among the huge number of detected sequence variants. The number of variants varies from several hundred in targeted resequencing up to more than 20,000 variants for a whole exome. Data analysis and variant filtering therefore belong to the most crucial steps after the sequencing has been performed. For data analysis, several different software packages are available, either belonging to the respective NGS platforms, open source, or offered by different independent suppliers (40). Most of these software tools concentrate on the detection of single nucleotide variants and smaller indels, while the detection of larger CNVs still remains difficult. Platforms working with the long-read technology have the clear advantage of the possibility of using the so-called split reads, which are reads that are split into parts and are then mapped to the reference genome independently. By this, even heterozygous deletions can be detected efficiently Next-generation genetic testing for retinitis pigmentosa (41). For the short read technology such an approach is not possible, and therefore several programs try to overcome this problem by using coverage information for the detection of CNVs. Also paired-end sequencing (sequencing from both ends of a DNA template) and mate-pair sequencing (sequencing from the ends of DNA templates that have been circularized to physically ligate originally distinct sequences) can give useful information for the investigation of CNVs (35).

Variant filtering is another crucial step that should be considered carefully. Variants detected by the NGS software include in first instance differences between the sequenced sample and a given reference sample (for example NCBI build 37, hg19). To determine the disease-causing variant(s) among those, it is crucial to reduce the number of variants as much as possible, without too much risk of losing the disease-causing variant during these prioritization steps. Most laboratories in first instance select for exonic, non-synonymous variants and canonical splice site variants that have not been reported as SNPs. For rare monogenic diseases in which all causative mutations are likely to be found in a single gene, this is usually a very good approach as it reduces the number of potential candidates (42, 43). For more frequent autosomal and X-linked recessive disorders, like the inherited retinal diseases, this approach is not recommendable. Due to the high prevalence of recessive disease-causing variants in the healthy population, a relatively high number of known pathogenic mutations have ended up in databases like dbSNP. Based on the prevalence of mutations in the 34 known arRP genes, we estimate that ~1 in 6 normal individuals is a heterozygous carrier of an arRP variant F.P.M. Cremers, unpublished data). Filtering against all variants in dbSNP therefore has a high risk of filtering out one or more of these disease-causing variants. An alternative for filtering against known SNPs would be to consider the frequency of a given variant: a variant that is seen in more than 5% of the general population will probably not be a disease-causing variant, and thus can be filtered out. If known, the inheritance pattern of a given gene or of the investigated sample might also be used as a prioritization tool: if a variant is for example found in a gene that has been implicated in autosomal recessive disease, without a second variant being present in that gene, this variant is not very likely to be disease-causing in the investigated sample. In contrast, if the inheritance pattern of a given sample is known, for example in a pedigree with a dominant inherited phenotype, the search for the disease-causing variant might be restricted to heterozygous changes only. The more information is available about a phenotype and its segregation in a given family, the more this will facilitate finding the disease-causing variant in a fast and efficient way. In our hands, filtering for exonic, non-synonymous variants and splice site variants that are seen with a frequency of less than 5% in a control cohort, in combination with given inheritance information, was able to reduce the amount of possible candidate disease variants more than 99% Next-generation genetic testing for retinitis pigmentosa (41).

2.10. Data Interpretation, Determination of Pathogenicity

After having reduced the number of variants dramatically, one usually still has to discriminate the pathologic from several nonpathologic variant(s), in particular with regard to missense variants. Therefore, interpretation of variants is another very important aspect in NGS. Several different tools for variant interpretation, including prediction programs like PolyPhen (http://www.bork. embl-heidelberg.de/PolyPhen), SIFT (http://www.blocks.fhcrc. org/sift/SIFT.html), or MutPred (http://mutpred.mutdb.org/) for missense variants, and SpliceSiteFinder (http://www.genet.sick-kids.on.ca/~ali/splicesitefinder.html), MaxEntSplice (http:// genes.mit.edu/burgelab/maxent/Xmaxentscan_scoreseq.html), and NNSplice (http://www.fruitfly.org/seq_tools/splice.html) for splice site variants, are publically available. Since there are often discrepancies in the output of different programs, a more integrated and systematic approach to get an idea of the effect of a mutation is to use at least three different prediction programs, use a majority vote on their results, and combine the outcome with frequency data and evolutionary conservation of the respective nucleotide or amino acid that is mutated, as further illustrated in Fig. 2.

The interpretation of candidate disease-associated variants is greatly facilitated by segregation analysis and therefore it is of utmost importance to ascertain as many first-degree relatives of a patient as possible, especially in genetically heterogeneous disorders such as RP. Targeted resequencing studies (of 111 inherited retinal disease genes) on 100 RP samples have led to the recommendation that in the future the availability of DNAs from the parents of an affected person will become a prerequisite for a proper validation and interpretation of variants in NGS Next-generation genetic testing for retinitis pigmentosa (41).

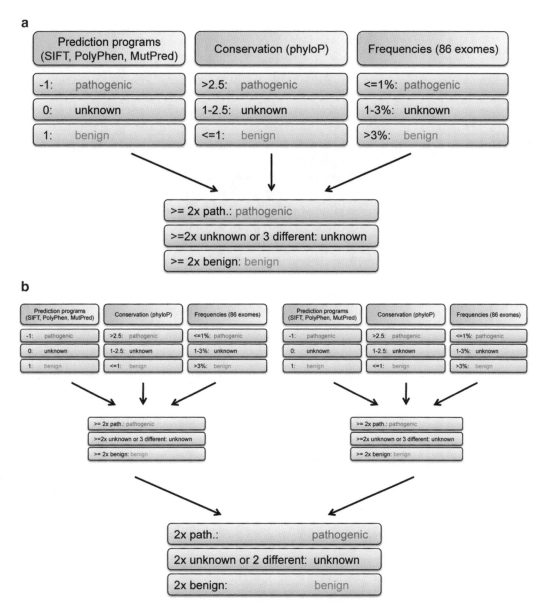

Fig. 2. Bioinformatic assessment of the pathogenicity of missense variants. (**a**) A systematic pipeline for the determination of pathogenicity should include in silico analyses of variants by different prediction programs, in combination with conservation and frequency data. Due to the possibility of different output, the usage of at least three different prediction programs is recommended. Using a majority vote, the scores for the different tools can be combined resulting in a single classification of "probably pathogenic," "unknown," or "probably benign." Evolutionary conservation can be based on phyloP values (44 vertebrate species), with a score ≤1 as considered "benign," >2.5 as considered to be "pathogenic," and everything in between as "unknown" (76). Concerning population frequencies, variants found at a population frequency of >3% can be classified as "benign," variants with a frequency between 1 and 3% can be classified as "unknown," and the remaining variants can be classified as "pathogenic." (**b**) The final classification for recessive genes can then be established by accounting for combinations of variants (K.N., R.W.J.C., A.I.d.H., F.P.M.C., unpublished data).

2.11. The Advantage of NGS for Inherited Retinal Diseases

Inherited retinal diseases not only display a high degree of locus heterogeneity but are also clinically and genetically overlapping. As exemplified by patients with different mutations in the *RDS/ peripherin* gene (44), or different combinations of mutations in *ABCA4* (45, 46), variants in the same gene can be associated with several distinct retinal phenotypes. In diseases such as RP, ophthalmologic features rarely predict which of the currently known 52 RP genes carries the causative mutation(s). This makes conventional Sanger sequencing too cost- and time-intensive. The possibility of sequencing the whole exome is now offering completely new perspectives. First results have now shown why in some cases it was so difficult to find the disease-causing mutations. The clinical diagnosis in many cases is not accurate as it is very difficult to assign a specific clinical diagnosis in young or old patients. When syndromic retinal disease genes are implicated, young patients may not yet display extraocular features that arise later in life. At older age, a clinical diagnosis is very difficult as the rod–cone dystrophies (RP) and CRDs will converge to the same end stage in which both rods and cones are severely affected (Fig. 1). In other cases, the predicted inheritance pattern was not correct. A significant fraction of isolated cases turned out to carry mutations in X-linked and autosomal dominant genes. In the latter group, several mutations were de novo, explaining why the disease-causing mutations were not found before, since a recessive inheritance model was expected Next-generation genetic testing for retinitis pigmentosa (41). This latter finding will have important implications for the patients, as a de novo mutation in a dominant gene has nearly no recurrence risk, but a transmission risk of 50%. For a recessive inheritance in contrast, the recurrence risk is 25% but the transmission risk is nearly zero.

In conclusion, exome NGS will improve the diagnostic yield for retinal diseases, as sequencing all genes at once enables a hypothesis-free approach, independent of a given clinical phenotype and a presumed inheritance pattern.

3. Strategies for Mutation and Gene Identification

3.1. Criteria to Select the Most Promising Molecular Approach

The best method of choice to determine an individual's genetic defect largely depends on two aspects, e.g., the clinical diagnosis and the presumed mode of inheritance within a family. As previously stated, the different genetic subtypes of retinal dystrophy often show clinical overlap (Fig. 1), and hence do not always directly point towards a clear candidate gene to be analyzed first. In other retinal diseases, however, like Bietti crystalline corneoretinal dystrophy or CHM, specific clinical hallmarks suggest a single causative gene to be mutated. As such, based on a detailed

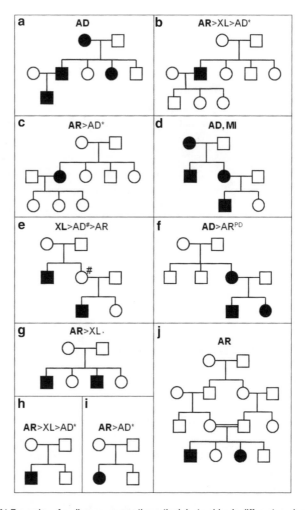

Fig. 3. (**a-h**) Examples of pedigrees segregating retinal dystrophies in different modes of inheritance. Illustration of inheritance models based on the occurrence and gender of affected individuals and their position in the pedigree. In *bold* above the pedigrees, the most likely modes of inheritance are given, followed by the less likely modes of inheritance. *AD* autosomal dominant, *AR* autosomal recessive, *MI* mitochondrial inheritance, *PD* pseudodominant (=autosomal recessive) inheritance, *XL* X-linked recessive, *de novo mutation, #non-penetrant individual.

description of the phenotype, one could decide to perform Sanger sequencing on one or only a few genes, or to opt for genome-wide approaches such as SNP genotyping and/or NGS. The second aspect is the structure of the family, and the presumed mode of inheritance. If a disease manifests in multiple affected relatives, one can easily determine the most likely mode of inheritance, e.g., autosomal dominant, autosomal recessive, X-linked, or, occasionally, mitochondrial. However, if little family information is available, or only one or two family members are affected, determining the mode of inheritance might be more difficult (Fig. 3). Below, we give an overview on the different genetic subtypes of retinal dystrophies, clustered by the different modes of inheritance, and provide tools to determine the molecular cause in an efficient way.

3.2. X-Linked Retinal Diseases

X-linked inheritance is most likely in pedigrees with multiple affected males in more than one generation, and displaying maternal transmission of the genetic defect (Fig. 3e). For some genetic subtypes of X-linked retinal dystrophy, female carriers of the genetic defect may also display (mild) clinical symptoms. The X-chromosome contains several retinal disease genes, such as the *CHM* gene (8), the Norrie disease pseudoglioma (*NDP*) gene (47), and the retinoschisis (*RS1*) gene (48). Patients with X-linked CSNB carry mutations in *NYX* or *CACNA1F* (49, 50). Patients with X-linked CRD carry mutations in *RPGR* (51) or *CACNA1F* (52). The majority of patients with X-linked RP carry mutations in the *RPGR* gene (53, 54), in particular in exon 15, also termed ORF15 (55). Due to its repetitive nature, PCR and sequence analysis of ORF15 require a specific protocol. Its sequences are not enriched using standard exome enrichment protocols. A smaller percentage of X-linked RP mutations are located in *RP2* (56), and there are also still four unsolved loci on the X-chromosome (http://www.sph.uth.tmc.edu/RetNet/sum-dis.htm#A-genes).

3.3. Autosomal Dominant Retinal Diseases

Families segregating autosomal dominant retinal dystrophy are easily recognizable by the presence of affected individuals in each branch of the pedigree and a clear parent-to-child transmission of the disease (Fig. 3a, f), although non-penetrance might occasionally perturb a clear establishment of the mode of inheritance (Fig. 3e). Thus far 22 autosomal dominant RP genes have been identified (http://www.sph.uth.tmc.edu/RetNet/sum-dis.htm#A-genes) that collectively explain more than 65% of the cases (57). As the rhodopsin gene carries mutations in 28.7% of patients with adRP (57), it is cost-effective to analyze this gene first by conventional Sanger sequencing. The low prevalence of mutations in the remaining known adRP genes warrants exome NGS to identify the pathologic variants. Furthermore, autosomal dominant cone and CRDs display considerable genetic heterogeneity in which there are no genes that carry a significant fraction of the mutations.

3.4. Autosomal Recessive Retinal Diseases

For autosomal recessive retinal diseases, locus heterogeneity is even higher, with more than 100 different causative genes known to date (http://www.sph.uth.tmc.edu/Retnet/). For some subtypes of autosomal recessive retinal diseases, the majority of patients are explained by mutations in a single or only a few genes, for instance in Stargardt disease (*ABCA4*) (45), or achromatopsia (*CNGA3*, *CNGB3*, *GNAT2*, and *PDE6C*) (58–61). Sanger sequencing of the causative genes or an APEX analysis (detecting known *ABCA4* mutations in Stargardt disease) (62) will likely resolve the genetic defect in the majority of patients. For other subtypes, however, like arRP (34 genes, excluding syndromic RP genes), the genetic heterogeneity is enormous, often hampering a fast molecular diagnosis. Sanger sequencing of all arRP genes is not cost-effective and APEX analysis has a reduced diagnostic yield since variants are found in 11–30% of patients F.P.M. Cremers & A.I. den Hollander, unpublished data) (63). In addition, Sanger sequencing is still required to confirm the APEX results and, in approximately half of the cases in which variants are found, to screen the relevant patient for a new mutation on the second allele.

Families segregating autosomal recessive disease are usually characterized by the presence of multiple affected siblings in one generation of the pedigree (Fig. 3g, j). In almost all consanguineous families, the affected individuals carry the mutation in a homozygous state (Fig. 3j). In these individuals' genomes, not only the causative mutation but also chromosomal segments flanking the mutation are present in a homozygous state. Such homozygous or IBD regions can be detected by performing genome-wide SNP analysis, which facilitates the identification of the underlying genetic defects. In non-consanguineous families, affected individuals can carry their genetic defect either in a compound heterozygous state or in a homozygous state. The latter can be explained by the occurrence of founder mutations (e.g., a single change frequently present in a certain ethnic group) like for instance a nonsense mutation in Finnish Usher syndrome type III patients (64), an intronic mutation in *CEP290* in LCA patients of European descent (65), or a recently identified frameshift mutation in *FAM161A*, present in Ashkenazi Jewish RP patients (66). Alternatively, parents of affected individuals unknowingly share a common ancestor many generations up in the pedigree. Although many meiotic recombinations throughout the generations have shortened the ancestral allele, the homozygous regions surrounding the causative mutation still outstand genomic segments that are identical by state, e.g., blocks of apparent homozygosity caused by consecutive homozygous SNP calls for which the major allele is frequently present in the population. Hence, applying high-resolution homozygosity mapping may also aid in the identification of genetic defects underlying recessive disease in non-consanguineous patients not only to detect mutations in known retinal dystrophy genes (9) but also to find novel genes causative for autosomal recessive retinal diseases (24, 25, 67, 68).

With the rapidly evolving technology of NGS, the possibilities to determine genetic defects underlying recessive diseases are growing at an unprecedented rate. Especially for diseases like arRP, for which many genes are known to date, and a substantial number still awaits discovery, a simultaneous analysis of multiple genes is both time- and cost-effective. Ideally, potential pathogenic variants remaining after NGS data filtering can be further evaluated by performing segregation analysis in available relatives and/or by cross-comparing them with positional information resulting from genome-wide SNP analysis, as was illustrated by the recent identification of *DHDDS* as a novel arRP gene after combining exome sequencing in three siblings with high-resolution homozygosity mapping (69).

3.5. Mitochondrial Inheritance

Mitochondrial DNA is transmitted from mother to child. Pedigrees segregating mitochondrial inheritance are characterized by transmission of the genetic defect from mother to child, but often, at a first glance, they appear as autosomal dominant pedigrees (Fig. 3d). Although mitochondrial inheritance is not frequently observed in retinal dystrophies, mutations in a few mitochondrial genes can cause Leber hereditary optic neuropathy (LHON), Kearns–Sayre syndrome (that includes retinal pigmentary degeneration), or combinations of retinal dystrophy and sensineural deafness (http://www.sph.uth.tmc.edu/Retnet/).

3.6. Isolated Cases

In general, identifying the genetic defect in a patient is alleviated by having an a priori knowledge on the mode of inheritance, based on pedigree information. In many western countries, however, families are increasingly getting smaller, and often display only one affected individual. For instance in isolated male cases, a mutation in an autosomal recessive as well as in an X-linked recessive gene may underlie the disease (Fig. 3h). Again, taking RP as an example, many isolated males could carry a mutation in the X-linked *RPGR* gene, which is one of the most frequently mutated RP genes. However, percentage-wise, isolated cases are more likely to carry a mutation in a recessive gene rather than in an X-linked gene. In addition, although the mechanism has been known for decades, we recently identified an unexpectedly high number of seven de novo mutations in a targeted NGS study analyzing all known retinal dystrophy genes in a large cohort that included 78 isolated RP patients Next-generation genetic testing for retinitis pigmentosa (41), indicating that autosomal dominant genes also need to be considered in the molecular diagnosis of isolated cases. Together, this example shows the extreme complexity in assessing a molecular diagnosis in isolated cases.

4. Discussion and Future Outlook

Gene identification studies have changed dramatically over the past decades. The major challenge of current technologies involves the interpretation of genomic variants to identify the causative mutation. Though several programs are available that can predict pathogenicity of missense variants, e.g., based on phylogenetic conservation, this can still leave one with a considerable number of variants with pathogenic potential. One can get a clue of which of the variants in the remaining genes is the causative one by for example determining its expression in retina. Also the number of CRX-binding sites in genes can aid in the selection of the causative gene, a method that has been recently used to successfully prioritize candidate genes from a genomic interval (70) or from exome data (71). Depending on the type of protein, it may be possible to design functional assays to determine the pathogenic nature of genetic variants, e.g., the measurement of enzymatic activity in mutant versions of the MAK protein (71) or RDH12 (72). To determine the effect of reduced activity of a certain gene on photoreceptor function and retinal morphology, one can perform morpholino knockdown experiments in zebrafish embryos. Fish injected with morpholinos targeting the *DHDDS* gene did not respond to light on–off switches and the photoreceptor outer segments were very short or completely missing (69). Alternatively, induced pluripotent stem (iPS) cells derived from skin of affected individuals were successfully used to prove aberrant splicing of a novel arRP gene, *MAK*. Upon differentiation of these iPS cells to retinal precursor cells, the insertion of an Alu element in *MAK* prevented the switch to a retina-specific isoform, showing the value of using patient's skin cells to study the regulation of genes that are only expressed in inaccessible tissues like retina (73). All these examples show that functional assays can be very effective to determine the pathogenic effect of mutations in a gene, although it is often not feasible to perform such studies on a large scale.

Microarrays and NGS allow the analysis of all retinal dystrophy genes in individual patients Next-generation genetic testing for retinitis pigmentosa (41, 57, 74, 75). Such analyses show that a considerable number of retinal dystrophy patients carry potential pathogenic variants in more than one gene Next-generation genetic testing for retinitis pigmentosa (41). This may make it difficult to establish the causative gene in certain patients, which may hamper gene therapeutic approaches in these individuals. Variants in other retinal dystrophy genes may also influence the severity of the disease by acting as modifiers, thereby making it more difficult to establish an accurate prognosis.

NGS technology will rapidly move from exome sequencing towards whole genome sequencing. This will increase the number of variants identified in a certain individual, and interpretation of variants may even become more complex involving regulatory components rather than coding variants alone. Although the new genetic era has enabled us to determine the letters of personal genomes, we are now facing challenges to interpret the sequence and understand the genetic language.

Acknowledgments

This work was supported by the European Community's Seventh Framework Program FP7/2007-2013, grant nr. 223143-TECHGENE, and by the Netherlands Organization for Health Research and Development, ZonMW grant 912-09-047.

References

1. Saiki RK, Scharf S, Faloona F, Mullis KB, Horn GT, Erlich HA et al (1985) Enzymatic amplification of beta-globin genomic sequences and restriction site analysis for diagnosis of sickle cell anemia. Science 230:1350–1354

2. Berger W, Kloeckener-Gruissem B, Neidhardt J (2010) The molecular basis of human retinal and vitreoretinal diseases. Prog Retin Eye Res 29:335–375

3. den Hollander AI, Black A, Bennett J, Cremers FPM (2010) Lighting a candle in the dark: advances in genetics and gene therapy of recessive retinal dystrophies. J Clin Invest 120:3042–3053

4. Valle D, Kaiser-Kupfer MI, Del Valle LA (1977) Gyrate atrophy of the choroid and retina: deficiency of ornithine aminotransferase in transformed lymphocytes. Proc Natl Acad Sci U S A 74:5159–5161

5. Mitchell GA, Brody LC, Looney J, Steel G, Suchanek M, Dowling C et al (1988) An initiator codon mutation in ornithine-delta-aminotransferase causing gyrate atrophy of the choroid and retina. J Clin Invest 81:630–633

6. Dryja TP, McGee TL, Reichel E, Hahn LB, Cowley GS, Yandell DW et al (1990) A point mutation of the rhodopsin gene in one form of retinitis pigmentosa. Nature 343:364–366

7. McWilliam P, Farrar GJ, Kenna P, Bradley DG, Humphries MM, Sharp EM et al (1989) Autosomal dominant retinitis pigmentosa (ADRP): localization of an ADRP gene to the long arm of chromosome 3. Genomics 5:619–622

8. Cremers FPM, van de Pol TJR, van Kerkhoff EPM, Wieringa B, Ropers HH (1990) Cloning of a gene that is rearranged in patients with choroideraemia. Nature 347:674–677

9. Collin RWJ, van den Born LI, Klevering BJ, de Castro Miro M, Littink KW, Arimadyo K et al (2011) High-resolution homozygosity mapping is a powerful tool to detect novel mutations causative of autosomal recessive RP in the Dutch population. Invest Ophthalmol Vis Sci 52:2227–2239

10. Bainbridge JWB, Smith AJ, Barker SS, Robbie S, Henderson R, Balaggan K et al (2008) Effect of gene therapy on visual function in Leber's congenital amaurosis. N Engl J Med 358:2231–2239

11. Hauswirth WW, Aleman TS, Kaushal S, Cideciyan AV, Schwartz SB, Wang L et al (2008) Treatment of leber congenital amaurosis due to RPE65 mutations by ocular subretinal injection of adeno-associated virus gene vector: short-term results of a phase I trial. Hum Gene Ther 19:979–990

12. Maguire AM, Simonelli F, Pierce EA, Pugh EN Jr, Mingozzi F, Bennicelli J et al (2008) Safety and efficacy of gene transfer for Leber's congenital amaurosis. N Engl J Med 358:2240–2248

13. Pasadhika S, Fishman GA, Stone EM, Lindeman M, Zelkha R, Lopez I et al (2010) Differential macular morphology in patients with RPE65-, CEP290-, GUCY2D-, and AIPL1-related Leber congenital amaurosis. Invest Ophthalmol Vis Sci 51:2608–2614

14. Lander E, Kruglyak L (1995) Genetic dissection of complex traits: guidelines for interpreting and reporting linkage results. Nat Genet 11:241–247

15. Boonstra NF, van Nouhuys CE, Schuil J, de Wijs I, van der Donk KP, Nikopoulos K et al (2009) Clinical and molecular evaluation of probands and family members with familial exudative vitreoretinopathy (FEVR). Invest Ophthalmol Vis Sci 50:4379–4385

16. Al-Maghtheh M, Vithana E, Tarttelin E, Jay M, Evans K, Moore T et al (1996) Evidence for a major retinitis pigmentosa locus on 19q13.4 (RP11) and association with a unique bimodal expressivity phenotype. Am J Hum Genet 59:864–871

17. Hoffmann K, Lindner TH (2005) easyLINKAGE-Plus–automated linkage analyses using large-scale SNP data. Bioinformatics 21:3565–3567

18. Ruschendorf F, Nurnberg P (2005) ALOHOMORA: a tool for linkage analysis using 10 K SNP array data. Bioinformatics 21:2123–2125

19. Terwillinger DJ, Ott J (1994) Handbook for human genetic linkage. Johns Hopkins University Press, Baltimore

20. Nyholt DR (2008) In: Neale BM, Ferreira MAR, Medland SE, Posthuma D (eds) Principles of linkage analysis. Statistical genetics: gene mapping through linkage and association. Taylor & Francis Group, New York, pp 113–134

21. Seelow D, Schuelke M, Hildebrandt F, Nurnberg P (2009) HomozygosityMapper–an interactive approach to homozygosity mapping. Nucleic Acids Res 37:W593–W599

22. Browning BL, Browning SR (2011) A fast, powerful method for detecting identity by descent. Am J Hum Genet 88:173–182

23. Littink KW, Koenekoop RK, van den Born LI, Collin RWJ, Moruz L, Veltman JA et al (2010) Homozygosity mapping in patients with cone–rod dystrophy: novel mutations and clinical characterizations. Invest Ophthalmol Vis Sci 51:5943–5951

24. Collin RWJ, Littink KW, Klevering BJ, van den Born LI, Koenekoop RK, Zonneveld-Vrieling MN et al (2008) Identification of a 2 Mb human ortholog of *Drosophila eyes shut/spacemaker* that is mutated in patients with retinitis pigmentosa. Am J Hum Genet 83:594–603

25. Collin RWJ, Safieh C, Littink KW, Shalev SA, Garzozi HJ, Rizel L et al (2010) Mutations in *C2ORF71* cause autosomal-recessive retinitis pigmentosa. Am J Hum Genet 86:783–788

26. Hildebrandt F, Heeringa SF, Ruschendorf F, Attanasio M, Nurnberg G, Becker C et al (2009) A systematic approach to mapping recessive disease genes in individuals from outbred populations. PLoS Genet 5:e1000353

27. den Hollander AI, Koenekoop RK, Mohamed MD, Arts HH, Boldt K, Towns KV et al (2007) Mutations in *LCA5*, encoding the ciliary protein lebercilin, cause Leber congenital amaurosis. Nat Genet 39:889–895

28. Harville HM, Held S, Diaz-Font A, Davis EE, Diplas BH, Lewis RA et al (2010) Identification of 11 novel mutations in eight BBS genes by high-resolution homozygosity mapping. J Med Genet 47:262–267

29. Woods CG, Cox J, Springell K, Hampshire DJ, Mohamed MD, McKibbin M et al (2006) Quantification of homozygosity in consanguineous individuals with autosomal recessive disease. Am J Hum Genet 78:889–896

30. Stankiewicz P, Lupski JR (2010) Structural variation in the human genome and its role in disease. Annu Rev Med 61:437–455

31. Nannya Y, Sanada M, Nakazaki K, Hosoya N, Wang L, Hangaishi A et al (2005) A robust algorithm for copy number detection using high-density oligonucleotide single nucleotide polymorphism genotyping arrays. Cancer Res 65:6071–6079

32. Abd El-Aziz MM, Barragan I, O'Driscoll C, Borrego S, Abu-Safieh L, Pieras JI et al (2008) Large-scale molecular analysis of a 34 Mb interval on chromosome 6q: major refinement of the RP25 interval. Ann Hum Genet 72:463–477

33. Humbert G, Delettre C, Senechal A, Bazalgette C, Barakat A, Bazalgette C et al (2006) Homozygous deletion related to Alu repeats in RLBP1 causes retinitis punctata albescens. Invest Ophthalmol Vis Sci 47:4719–4724

34. Metzker ML (2010) Sequencing technologies: the next generation. Nat Rev Genet 11:31–46

35. Glenn TC (2011) Field guide to next-generation DNA sequencers. Mol Ecol Resour 11(5):759–769

36. Mamanova L, Coffey AJ, Scott CE, Kozarewa I, Turner EH, Kumar A et al (2010) Target-enrichment strategies for next-generation sequencing. Nat Methods 7:111–118

37. Gilissen C, Hoischen A, Brunner HG, Veltman JA (2011) Unlocking mendelian disease using exome sequencing. Genome Biol 12(9):228

38. Nikopoulos K, Gilissen C, Hoischen A, van Nouhuys CE, Boonstra FN, Blokland EAW et al (2010) Next-generation sequencing of a 40 Mb linkage interval reveals *TSPAN12* mutations in patients with familial exudative vitreoretinopathy. Am J Hum Genet 86:240–247

39. Estrada-Cuzcano A, Neveling K, Kohl S, Banin E, Rotenstreich Y, Sharon D, Falik-Zaccai TC, Hipp S, Roepman R, Wissinger B, Letteboer SJ, Mans DA, Blokland EA, Kwint MP, Gijsen SJ, van Huet RA, Collin RWJ, Scheffer H, Veltman JA, Zrenner E; European Retinal Disease Consortium, den Hollander AI, Klevering BJ, Cremers FPM. Am J Hum Genet. 2012 Jan 13;90(1):102–109.

40. Bao S, Jiang R, Kwan W, Wang B, Ma X, Song YQ (2011) Evaluation of next-generation sequencing software in mapping and assembly. J Hum Genet 56:406–414

41. Neveling K, Collin RWJ, Gilissen C, van Huet RA, Visser L, Kwint MP, Gijsen SJ, Zonneveld MN, Wieskamp N, de Ligt J, Siemiatkowska AM, Hoefsloot LH, Buckley MF, Kellner U, Branham KE, den Hollander AI, Hoischen A, Hoyng C, Klevering BJ, van den Born LI, Veltman JA, Cremers FPM, Scheffer H. Hum Mutat. 2012 Jun;33(6):963–972.

42. Gilissen C, Arts HH, Hoischen A, Spruijt L, Mans DA, Arts P et al (2010) Exome sequencing identifies WDR35 variants involved in Sensenbrenner syndrome. Am J Hum Genet 87:418–423

43. Hoischen A, van Bon BW, Gilissen C, Arts P, van Lier B, Steehouwer M et al (2010) De

novo mutations of SETBP1 cause Schinzel-Giedion syndrome. Nat Genet 42:483–485

44. Keen TJ, Inglehearn CF (1996) Mutations and polymorphisms in the human peripherin-*RDS* gene and their involvement in inherited retinal degeneration. Hum Mutat 8:297–303

45. Allikmets R, Singh N, Sun H, Shroyer NF, Hutchinson A, Chidambaram A et al (1997) A photoreceptor cell-specific ATP-binding transporter gene (*ABCR*) is mutated in recessive Stargardt macular dystrophy. Nat Genet 15:236–246

46. Cremers FPM, van de Pol TJR, van Driel M, den Hollander AI, van Haren FJJ, Knoers NVAM et al (1998) Autosomal recessive retinitis pigmentosa and cone–rod dystrophy caused by splice site mutations in the Stargardt's disease gene *ABCR*. Hum Mol Genet 7:355–362

47. Berger W, van de Pol TJR, Warburg M, Gal A, Bleeker-Wagemakers EM, de Silva H et al (1992) Mutations in the candidate gene for Norrie disease. Hum Mol Genet 1:461–465

48. Grayson C, Reid SN, Ellis JA, Rutherford A, Sowden JC, Yates JR et al (2000) Retinoschisin, the X-linked retinoschisis protein, is a secreted photoreceptor protein, and is expressed and released by Weri-Rb1 cells. Hum Mol Genet 9:1873–1879

49. Bech-Hansen NT, Naylor MJ, Maybaum TA, Pearce WG, Koop B, Fishman GA et al (1998) Loss-of-function mutations in a calcium-channel α1-subunit gene in Xp11.23 cause incomplete X-linked congenital stationary night blindness. Nat Genet 19:264–267

50. Bech-Hansen NT, Naylor MJ, Maybaum TA, Sparkes RL, Koop B, Birch DG et al (2000) Mutations in *NYX*, encoding the leucine-rich proteoglycan nyctalopin, cause X-linked complete congenital stationary night blindness. Nat Genet 26:319–323

51. Yang Z, Peachey NS, Moshfeghi DM, Thirumalaichary S, Chorich L, Shugart YY et al (2002) Mutations in the RPGR gene cause X-linked cone dystrophy. Hum Mol Genet 11:605–611

52. Jalkanen R, Mantyjarvi M, Tobias R, Isosomppi J, Sankila EM, Alitalo T et al (2006) X linked cone–rod dystrophy, CORDX3, is caused by a mutation in the CACNA1F gene. J Med Genet 43:699–704

53. Roepman R, van Duynhoven G, Rosenberg T, Pinckers AJLG, Bleeker-Wagemakers EM, Bergen AAB et al (1996) Positional cloning of the gene for X-linked retinitis pigmentosa: homology with the guanine-nucleotide-exchange factor RCC1. Hum Mol Genet 5:1035–1041

54. Meindl A, Dry K, Herrmann K, Manson F, Ciccodicola A, Edgar A et al (1996) A gene (*RPGR*) with homology to the *RCC1* guanine nucleotide exchange factor is mutated in X-linked retinitis pigmentosa (RP3). Nat Genet 13:35–42

55. Vervoort R, Lennon A, Bird AC, Tulloch B, Axton R, Miano MG et al (2000) Mutational hot spot within a new *RPGR* exon in X-linked retinitis pigmentosa. Nat Genet 25:462–466

56. Schwahn U, Lenzner S, Dong J, Feil S, Hinzmann B, van Duijnhoven G et al (1998) Positional cloning of the gene for X-linked retinitis pigmentosa 2. Nat Genet 19:327–332

57. Bowne SJ, Sullivan LS, Koboldt DC, Ding L, Fulton R, Abbott RM et al (2011) Identification of disease-causing mutations in autosomal dominant retinitis pigmentosa (adRP) using next-generation DNA sequencing. Invest Ophthalmol Vis Sci 52:494–503

58. Kohl S, Marx T, Giddings I, Jägle H, Jacobson SG, Apfelstedt-Sylla E et al (1998) Total colourblindness is caused by mutations in the gene encoding the α-subunit of the cone photoreceptor cGMP-gated cation channel. Nat Genet 19:257–259

59. Kohl S, Baumann B, Broghammer M, Jägle H, Sieving P, Kellner U et al (2000) Mutations in the *CNGB3* gene encoding the β-subunit of the cone photoreceptor cGMP-gated channel are responsible for achromatopsia (*ACHM3*) linked to chromosome 8q21. Hum Mol Genet 9:2107–2116

60. Kohl S, Baumann B, Rosenberg T, Kellner U, Lorenz B, Vadala M et al (2002) Mutations in the cone photoreceptor G-protein alpha-subunit gene GNAT2 in patients with achromatopsia. Am J Hum Genet 71:422–425

61. Thiadens AAHJ, den Hollander AI, Roosing S, Nabuurs SB, Zekveld-Vroon RC, Collin RWJ et al (2009) Homozygosity mapping reveals *PDE6C* mutations in patients with early-onset cone photoreceptor disorders. Am J Hum Genet 85:240–247

62. Jaakson K, Zernant J, Kulm M, Hutchinson A, Tonisson N, Hawlina M et al (2003) Genotyping microarray (gene chip) for the *ABCR* (*ABCA4*) gene. Hum Mutat 22:395–403

63. Avila-Fernandez A, Cantalapiedra D, Aller E, Vallespin E, Aguirre-Lamban J, Blanco-Kelly F et al (2010) Mutation analysis of 272 Spanish families affected by autosomal recessive retinitis pigmentosa using a genotyping microarray. Mol Vis 16:2550–2558

64. Joensuu T, Hamalainen R, Yuan B, Johnson C, Tegelberg S, Gasparini P et al (2001) Mutations in a novel gene with transmembrane domains

underlie Usher syndrome type 3. Am J Hum Genet 69:673–684

65. den Hollander AI, Koenekoop RK, Yzer S, Lopez I, Arends ML, Voesenek KEJ et al (2006) Mutations in the *CEP290* (*NPHP6*) gene are a frequent cause of Leber congenital amaurosis. Am J Hum Genet 79:556–561

66. Zelinger L, Banin E, Obolensky A, Mizrahi-Meissonnier L, Beryozkin A, Bandah-Rozenfeld D et al (2011) A missense mutation in DHDDS, encoding dehydrodolichyl diphosphate synthase, is associated with autosomal-recessive retinitis pigmentosa in Ashkenazi Jews. Am J Hum Genet 88:207–215

67. den Hollander AI, Lopez I, Yzer S, Zonneveld MN, Janssen IM, Strom TM et al (2007) Identification of novel mutations in patients with Leber congenital amaurosis and juvenile RP by genome-wide homozygosity mapping with SNP microarrays. Invest Ophthalmol Vis Sci 48:5690–5698

68. Bandah-Rozenfeld D, Collin RWJ, Banin E, van den Born LI, Coene KLM, Siemiatkowska AM et al (2010) Mutations in *IMPG2*, encoding interphotoreceptor matrix proteoglycan 2, cause autosomal-recessive retinitis pigmentosa. Am J Hum Genet 87:199–208

69. Zuchner S, Dallman J, Wen R, Beecham G, Naj A, Farooq A et al (2011) Whole-exome sequencing links a variant in DHDDS to retinitis pigmentosa. Am J Hum Genet 88:201–206

70. Langmann T, Di Gioia SA, Rau I, Stohr H, Maksimovic NS, Corbo JC et al (2010) Nonsense mutations in FAM161A cause RP28-associated recessive retinitis pigmentosa. Am J Hum Genet 87:376–381

71. Ozgul RK, Siemiatkowska AM, Yucel D, Myers CA, Collin RWJ, Zonneveld MN et al (2011) Exome sequencing and cis-regulatory mapping identify mutations in MAK, a gene encoding a regulator of ciliary length, as a cause of retinitis pigmentosa. Am J Hum Genet 89:253–264

72. Thompson DA, Janecke AR, Lange J, Feathers KL, Hubner CA, McHenry CL et al (2005) Retinal degeneration associated with RDH12 mutations results from decreased 11-cis retinal synthesis due to disruption of the visual cycle. Hum Mol Genet 14:3865–3875

73. Tucker BA, Scheetz TE, Mullins RF, Deluca AP, Hoffmann JM, Johnston RM et al (2011) Exome sequencing and analysis of induced pluripotent stem cells identify the cilia-related gene male germ cell-associated kinase (MAK) as a cause of retinitis pigmentosa. Proc Natl Acad Sci U S A 108(34):E569–E576

74. Booij JC, Bakker A, Kulumbetova J, Moutaoukil Y, Smeets B, Verheij J et al (2011) Simultaneous mutation detection in 90 retinal disease genes in multiple patients using a custom-designed 300-kb retinal resequencing chip. Ophthalmology 118:160–167

75. Coppieters F, De Baere E, Leroy B (2011) Development of a next-generation sequencing platform for retinal dystrophies, with LCA and RP as proof of concept. Bull Soc Belge Ophtalmol 317:59–60

76. Vissers LELM, de Ligt J, Gilissen C, Janssen I, Steehouwer M, de Vries P et al (2010) A *de novo* paradigm for mental retardation. Nat Genet 42:1109–1112

Part II

Mouse Models

Chapter 2

Mouse Models for Studies of Retinal Degeneration and Diseases

Bo Chang

Abstract

Mouse models, with their well-developed genetics and similarity to human physiology and anatomy, serve as powerful tools with which to investigate the etiology of human retinal degeneration. Mutant mice also provide reproducible, experimental systems for elucidating pathways of normal development and function. Here, I describe the tools used in the discoveries of many retinal degeneration models, including indirect ophthalmoscopy (to look at the fundus appearance), fundus photography and fluorescein angiography (to document the fundus appearance), electroretinography (to check retinal function), as well as the heritability test (for genetic characterization).

Key words: Mouse models, Retinal degeneration, Indirect ophthalmoscopy, Fundus, Electroretinography

1. Introduction

The number of known serious or disabling eye diseases in humans is large and affects millions of individuals worldwide. Yet research on these diseases frequently is limited by the obvious restrictions on studying pathophysiologic processes in the human eye. Mouse models of inherited ocular disease provide powerful tools for genetic analysis and characterization and intervention assessment. Studies of mouse models of human retinal degeneration are important to understanding the pathophysiology, as well as the etiology, of these diseases. Using these mouse models much progress has been made in elucidating gene defects underlying retinal disease, understanding mechanisms leading to disease, and designing molecules for translational research and gene-based therapy to interfere with the progression of disease.

Discovery of human retinal degenerations is not particularly difficult when patients visit their ophthalmologist for eye examinations,

Bernhard H.F. Weber and Thomas Langmann (eds.), *Retinal Degeneration: Methods and Protocols*, Methods in Molecular Biology, vol. 935, DOI 10.1007/978-1-62703-080-9_2, © Springer Science+Business Media, LLC 2013

but research on human retinal degenerations is impeded by the lack of availability of human eye tissues and the impossibility of doing genetic manipulation for research. Human eye tissue (including biopsies) for most human ocular diseases is seldom available because it is difficult to obtain tissue samples from the eye without the risk of damage to the patient's vision. Compared with diagnosis in humans, animal models of human retinal degeneration are not easy to find, but animal models make research advances feasible not only through developmental and invasive studies but also through rapid genetic analysis. By screening mice using indirect ophthalmoscopy and electroretinography at The Jackson Laboratory (TJL), many mouse models of retinal degeneration and diseases have been discovered (1, 2). A major advantage in using the mouse as a model system is the depth of well-developed techniques available for manipulating the genome. The ability to target and alter a specific gene(s) is an important and necessary tool to produce mouse models with mutations in genes of choice. Inducing mutations in genes of choice (known as knockout or transgenic) is termed "reverse genetics," as it is the opposite of "forward genetics" approaches whereby spontaneous/induced mutations are discovered as a result of the overt phenotypes and the underlying mutation is subsequently identified. Through the "forward" and "reverse" genetic approaches, mouse models in 100 genes that underlie human retinal diseases have been studied (3). In some cases there are multiple models available for the same mutated gene. For example, of the mouse models for human Leber Congenital Amaurosis 2 (LCA2) caused by mutation in the retinal pigment epithelium 65 ($Rpe65$) gene, there is a knockout model $Rpe65^{tm1Tmr}$ (4), a transgenic (knockin) model $Rpe65^{tm1Lrcb}$ (5), an induced model $Rpe65^{tvrm148}$ (2), as well as a spontaneous model $Rpe65^{rd12}$ (6, 7). The mouse eye is remarkably similar in structure to the human eye, and both species have many similar ocular disorders. Not only are developmental and invasive studies possible in mice, but also the mouse's accelerated life span and generation time (one mouse year = about 30 human years) make it possible to follow the natural progression of eye diseases in a relatively brief length of time. Because mouse mutations can be maintained on controlled genetic backgrounds, mutant and control mice can differ only by the mutated gene being studied. Thus, it is possible to analyze the effects of a mutant gene in same-sex, same-age littermates that differ only by whether they carry a specific mutation.

Models of retinal degeneration in mice have been known for many years. The first retinal degeneration, discovered by Dr. Clyde E. Keeler more than 80 years ago, is $Pde6b^{rd1}$ (formerly $rd1$, rd, identical with Keeler rodless retina, r) (8–10). Fifty years later, the second retinal degeneration was discovered and it was named retinal degeneration-slow (Rds) (11). The third retinal degeneration was discovered in 1993 and it was named $rd3$ in sequence allowing rd to be equivalent to $rd1$ and Rds to be equivalent to $Rd2$ (12).

During the last 20 years, many mouse models of retinal degeneration have been found because common methods used in human clinical eye examinations have been adapted for use with mouse eyes to screen for mouse retinal degeneration (1, 2, 12–14). These methods, including indirect ophthalmoscopy, fundus photography, fluorescein angiography, electroretinography, as well as histology, are broadly used in identifying and characterizing mouse models of retinal degeneration and diseases.

2. Materials

TJL, having the world's largest collection of mouse mutant stocks and genetically diverse inbred strains (http://jaxmice.jax.org/index.html), is an ideal place to discover and characterize genetically determined retinal disorders.

2.1. Mice

The mice were bred and maintained in standardized conditions in the Research Animal Facility at TJL. They were maintained on NIH31 6% fat chow and acidified water, with a 14-h light/10-h dark cycle in conventional facilities that were monitored regularly to maintain a pathogen-free environment. All experiments were approved by the Institutional Animal Care and Use Committee and conducted in accordance with the ARVO Statement for the Use of Animals in Ophthalmic and Vision Research.

2.2. Drugs and Chemicals

1. 1% Atropine Sulfate Ophthalmic Solution (sterile), Alcon Laboratories, INC. Fort Worth, TX 76134, USA.

2. 1% Cyclopentolate Hydrochloride Ophthalmic Solution USP (sterile), Bausch & Lomb Incorporated Tampa, FL 33637, USA.

3. Cyclomydril® (0.2% cyclopentolate hydrochloride, 1% phenylephrine hydrochloride ophthalmic solution, sterile), Alcon Laboratories, INC. Fort Worth, TX 76134, USA.

4. 2.5% Gonioscopic Prism Solution (Hypromellose Ophthalmic Demulcent Solution, sterile), Wilson Ophthalmic, Mustang, OK 73064, USA.

5. 25% Fluorescein Sodium Injection (250 mg/ml, for intravenous injection only), Altaire Pharmaceuticals, Inc., Aquebogue, NY 11931, USA.

6. Ketathesia (ketamine HCL injection USP, 100 mg/ml), Dublin, OH 43017, USA.

7. AnaSed® Injection (Xylazine sterile solution, 20 mg/ml), Shenandoah, IA, 51601, USA.

8. 0.9% Sodium Chloride, Injection, USP (for use as sterile diluents), Hospira, INC., Lake Forest, IL 60045, USA.

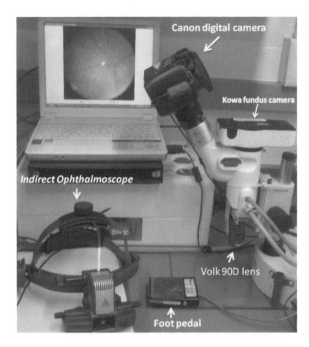

Fig. 1. Ophthalmic instruments used for mouse fundus examination.

2.3. Ophthalmic Instruments and Equipment

1. Heine Omega 500® Binocular Indirect Ophthalmoscope (Fig. 1), Heine USA Ltd., 10 Innovation Way, Dover, NH 03820.

2. Classic 78D, Classic 90D, SuperField NC Volk Optical Lenses, Volk Optical, Inc., 7893 Enterprise Drive, Mentor, OH 44060, USA.

3. Kowa Genesis small animal fundus camera (Fig. 1) (Tokyo, Japan) (15).

4. Canon digital camera (Canon EOS Rebel Xsi) (Fig. 1) (Canon USA., Inc., headquartered in Lake Success, New York, USA).

5. Electroretinogram (ERG) system (Fig. 2) (16).

3. Methods

Retinal vessel attenuation and retinal pigment epithelial disturbance are easily detected signs that are often associated with retinal degenerations and diseases. However if the retina looks normal (normal fundus), it is still possible that retinal functional abnormalities exist. A quick screening ERG test is needed to detect any retinal functional defects, such as retinal cone photoreceptor function loss (achromatopsia) (17, 18) and no b-wave (nob) mutations (19, 20). Heritability is subsequently established by genetic characterization (1, 2).

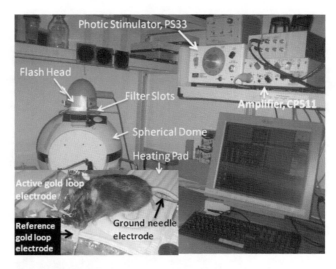

Fig. 2. The major components of the electroretinogram system used in our laboratory.

3.1. Mouse Fundus Examination

For indirect ophthalmoscopy the examiner wears a light attached to a headband and uses a small handheld lens to see inside the fundus of the mouse eye. The fundus of a mouse eye is the interior surface of the eye and includes the retina and optic disc. The color of the mouse fundus varies between pigmented (black) and albino (red). Dilated fundus examination is a diagnostic procedure that employs the use of mydriatic eye drops (such as 1% atropine) to dilate or enlarge the pupil in order to obtain a better view of the fundus of the eye. Once the pupil is dilated, examiners often use specialized equipment such as an indirect ophthalmoscope or fundus camera to view the inner surfaces of the eye. Abnormal signs that can be detected from observation of mouse fundus include hemorrhages, exudates, cotton wool spots, blood vessel abnormalities (tortuosity, pulsation, and new vessels), and pigmentation. Mouse fundus examination is a more effective method for the evaluation of internal ocular health and is routinely used to screen whether a mouse presents with abnormalities of the fundus such as retinal degeneration, optic disc coloboma, or vascular problems (see Note 1).

3.1.1. Routine Fundus Examination

1. Pupil dilation: Remove the screw top from the vial containing the mydriatic (1% atropine). Restrain and hold the mouse firmly in one hand, pick up the vial containing the mydriatic, and squeeze directly above an eye of the mouse allowing a drop to cover the surface of the eye. Repeat the procedure for the second eye. Return the mouse to its cage and allow at least 5 min for the effect of the mydriatic to take place.

2. Fundus examination 1: Place the Heine Omega 500® Binocular Indirect Ophthalmoscope onto your head and adjust the binoculars accordingly. Adjust the light being emitted from the ophthalmoscope. Hold and restrain the mouse firmly in one

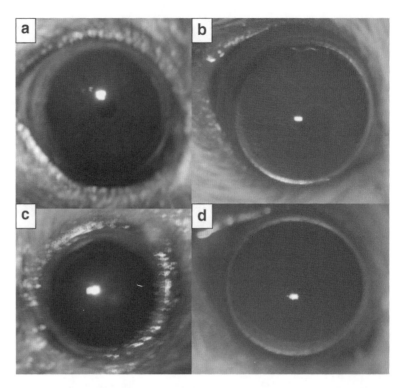

Fig. 3. An eye prior to dilation in pigmented mice (**a**) and albino mice (**b**) and the pupil of the same eye in its dilated state (**c, d**).

hand and shine the light into the mouse eye to see if the pupil has fully dilated (Fig. 3).

3. Fundus examination 2: Pick up the Volk 90D or 78D lens and place it between the mouse eye and the beam of light. Pass (or focus) the beam of light through the Volk lens and you should see the mouse eye through the lens. Adjust the lens in and out until the back of the retina can be visualized. Orientate the field of view by visualizing the optic disc and then moving the lens around the eye (or twist the mouse head) to alter the view so that the whole fundus can be examined.

4. Repeat the above for the second eye examination.

5. Record the fundus appearance, such as retinal spots, retinal pigment patch, or retinal vessel changes. If any fundus abnormalities are observed, fundus photography is taken. If no fundus abnormalities are observed, this mouse will go through the simple screening ERG test.

3.1.2. Fundus Photography and Fluorescein Angiography

Mouse fundus photography and fluorescein angiography are used to document the new phenotypes discovered by fundus examination. In the past, we used the Kowa Genesis small animal fundus camera fitted to a dissection microscope base (15) to take fundus pictures with special films, but have improved the efficiency and reduced the cost of this system by adapting a digital camera (Canon EOS Rebel Xsi) to focus through the eyepiece view (Fig. 1). This Canon digital camera can be directly connected to a personal computer (through the USB port) and the fundus view is displayed on the computer monitor. Fundus pictures are then captured and saved on the computer by using the Canon EOS utility software.

1. Pupil dilation, same as in step 1 in Subheading 3.1.1 above.

2. Plug the Canon camera USB cable to the computer's USB port and turn on the computer (the Canon EOS utility software should be installed first).

3. Switch the Canon camera power on and wait for the Canon EOS utility software to start. Once the Canon EOS utility software is running, select the "Camera Setting/Remote Shooting," and then select "Remote Live View Shooting" from the software menu.

4. Turn on the power (light) from the powerpack and the "Remote Live View Shooting" window lights up on the computer monitor.

5. Hold and restrain the mouse firmly in one hand and place the mouse eye under the light beneath the Volk lens to see on the computer monitor if the pupil has fully dilated (Fig. 3). Retract the mouse eyelids with two fingers from your other hand, orientate the field of view by visualizing the optic disc, and then move the mouse eye around until you get the best fundus view (the most focused).

6. Capture the fundus images by a foot pedal (to operate the shutter) when the best fundus view occurs on the computer monitor. Figure 4 shows the normal mouse fundus in pigmented mice (C57BL/6J) as well as albino mice (BALB/cJ) and abnormal fundus in pigmented mice (C3H/HeJ) as well as albino mice (FVB/NJ) (see Note 2).

7. For retinal angiography the same general fundus photography procedure is used except one must push a button on the powerpack to select the fluorescein filter for angiography.

8. Intraperitoneally inject the mouse with 25% sodium fluorescein at a dose of 0.01 ml per 5–6 g body weight. The retinal vessels began filling about 30 s after fluorescein administration. Single photographs are then taken at appropriate intervals. Although timing varies due to variable rates of intraperitoneal absorption, capillary washout usually occurs 5 min after dye administration. Figure 5 shows the mouse fundus as well as fluorescein angiogram.

3.2. Simple Screening Electroretinograpy

The basic method of recording the electrical response, known as the global or full-field ERG, is to stimulate the eye with a bright light source such as a flash produced by LEDs or a strobe lamp.

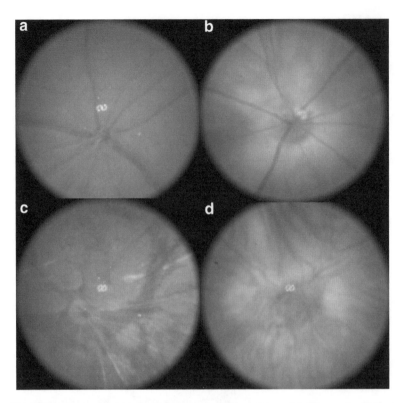

Fig. 4. Normal mouse fundus in pigmented mice (**a**) and albino mice (**b**) as well as retinal degeneration fundus in pigmented mice (**c**) and albino mice (**d**).

The flash of light elicits a biphasic waveform recordable at the cornea. The two components that are most often measured are the *a*- and *b*-waves. The *a*-wave is the first large negative component, followed by the *b*-wave which is corneal positive and usually larger in amplitude. Two principal measures of the ERG waveform are taken: (1) the amplitude (*a*) from the baseline to the negative trough of the *a*-wave, and the amplitude of the *b*-wave measured from the trough of the *a*-wave to the following peak of the *b*-wave, and (2) the time (*t*) from flash onset to the trough of the *a*-wave and the time (*t*) from flash onset to the peak of the *b*-wave. These times, reflecting peak latency, are referred to as "implicit times" in the jargon of electroretinography. Scotopic ERGs (also called dark-adapted) are used to evaluate responses starting from rod photoreceptors exposed to flush light in darkness, and photopic ERGs (also called light-adapted) are used to evaluate responses starting from cone photoreceptors exposed to flush light under constant light exposure. Because regular ERG testing is time consuming (about 30–60 min per mouse without the time used for dark adaption), we have developed a simple screening ERG test. Our simple screening ERG testing does not need dark or light adaption and one simple ERG test takes less than 10 min (see Note 3). Most of the simple screening ERGs are normal and only a few of them are

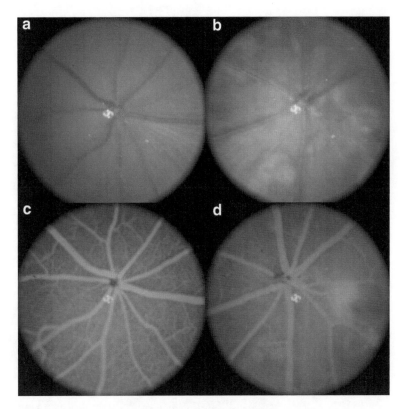

Fig. 5. Normal mouse fundus prior to the fluorescein injection (**a**) and the same eye after the fluorescein injection (**c**). Mouse fundus with neovascular depigmented spots (**b**) prior to the fluorescein injection and the same eye after the fluorescein injection (**d**).

abnormal, but once a mouse shows an abnormal ERG, it is tested again through our regular ERG test (21, 22).

1. Pupil dilation: Restrain and hold the mouse firmly in one hand, pick up the vial containing 1% Cyclopentolate (1% Cyclopentolate Hydrochloride Ophthalmic Solution), and squeeze directly above the right eye of the mouse allowing a drop to cover the surface of the eye (we test only one eye and usually the right eye). A group of 5–10 mice can be dilated in one time.

2. Anesthetize the mouse with an intraperitoneal injection. Weigh the mouse and record the weight. Restrain and hold the mouse firmly in one hand, pick up the second vial containing Cyclomydril (0.2% cyclopentolate hydrochloride, 1% phenylephrine hydrochloride ophthalmic solution, sterile), and squeeze directly above the right eye a drop to cover the surface of the eye; then inject the mouse with the anesthetic mixture solution (5 ml mixture containing 0.8 ml Katamine, 0.8 ml Xylazine, and 3.4 ml 0.9% Sodium Chloride) at a dosage of 0.1 ml per 20 g of body weight.

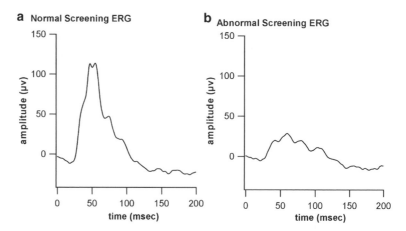

Fig. 6. Representative ERG responses to a bright flash obtained from a mouse with normal retinal function (**a**) and a mouse with abnormal retinal function (**b**).

3. Prepare the test: Place the sufficiently sedated mouse on the heated pad. Insert a needle probe just under the skin at the base of the tail, place the gold loop electrode between the gum and cheek, position the mouse near the far end of the heating pad, and place the active gold loop electrode on the cornea slightly below the middle of the eye. Pick up the third vial containing 2.5% Gonioscopic Prism Solution and squeeze directly above the cornea and electrode a drop to assure a good contact.

4. The simple ERG test: Set the photic Stimulator to 1-s flash, the flash intensity to 16 (the highest), and then set the "Sweeps" to 10 (average 10 flashes) from the ERG software menu. Click the "Aver" from the software menu, and then turn on the photic Stimulator to start the test.

5. Save the test data and analyze the results: Press the "Save" button to save the ERG data to the computer and print a copy for instant view. If a mouse has a, b-wave amplitude at or above 100 µV and the implicit times at about 50 ms, this mouse has a normal simple ERG response (Fig. 6a). If a mouse has b-wave amplitude at or below 50 µV and implicit times longer than 50 ms, this mouse has an abnormal simple ERG response (Fig. 6b).

6. Regular ERG test: Once we discover a mouse with an abnormal simple ERG response, we test the same mouse with our regular ERG protocol to determine if the mouse has the abnormal rod response (dark-adapted ERG), abnormal cone ERG response (light-adapted ERG), or abnormal rod and cone ERG. Then we mate this mouse to a normal mouse to produce the next generation for the heritability test.

3.3. Heritability Test

Heritability is established by outcrossing a retinal mutant mouse to a normal retinal wild-type mouse to generate F1 progeny, with subsequent intercrossing of the resultant F1 mice to generate F2 progeny. Both F1 and F2 mice are examined by fundus examination and/or simple screening ERG depending on which phenotype occurs first. If F1 mice are affected, the pedigree is designated as a dominant mutation. If F1 mice are not affected but ~25% of F2 mice are affected, the pedigree is designated as a recessive mutation. Once heritability of the observed retinal phenotype is established, retinal mutants are bred and maintained for further characterization leading to gene identification (23, 24).

4. Notes

1. Mouse fundus examination is a very powerful, noninvasive, and high-throughput method for evaluating mouse retinal appearances. It is also very effective in screening for mouse models of human retinal degeneration and diseases, as there are many examples of mouse models of retinal degeneration that were discovered by fundus examination (see refs. 1, 2, 13) such as mouse retinal degeneration 3 ($Rd3^{rd3}$) (see refs. 12, 25) and mouse retinal degeneration 4 ($Gnb1^{Rd4}$) (see refs. 26, 27).

2. It is important for investigators evaluating eyes to be aware of $Pde6b^{rd1}$ and its associated morphological findings, as it is a frequent strain background disease. Since the $Pde6b^{rd1}$ mutation is common in mice, it is important to avoid mouse strains or stocks carrying the $Pde6b^{rd1}$ allele, or to exclude the $Pde6b^{rd1}$ allele contamination in studying new retinal disorders. Mice with the $Pde6b^{rd1}$ mutation can be easily typed by fundus examination (see Fig. 4).

3. The simple screening ERG is another powerful, noninvasive, and high-throughput method to evaluate mouse retinal function. If a mouse has a normal fundus through fundus examination, it is very important to run this mouse through the simple screening ERG test because mouse retinal function loss mutants can have a normal retinal appearance (see refs. 17–20).

Acknowledgments

This work has been supported by the Macula Vision Research Foundation (MVRF) and the National Eye Institute Grant EY19943. I am grateful to Mark Lessard and David Davis for adapting the Canon Digital Camera to our mouse fundus camera, and Melissa Berry and Da Chang for their critical reading and editing of the manuscript.

References

1. Chang B, Hawes NL, Hurd RE, Wang J, Howell D, Davisson MT, Roderick TH, Nusinowitz S, Heckenlively JR (2005) Mouse models of ocular diseases. Vis Neurosci 22:587–593

2. Won J, Shi LY, Hicks W, Wang J, Hurd R, Naggert JK, Chang B, Nishina PM (2011) Mouse model resources for vision research. J Ophthalmol 2011:391384

3. Samardzija M, Neuhauss SCF, Joly S, Kurz-Levin M, Grimm C (2010) Animal models for retinal degeneration. In: Pang I, Clark AF (eds) Animal models for retinal diseases. The Humana Press Inc, New York, pp 51–79

4. Redmond TM, Yu S, Lee E, Bok D, Hamasaki D, Chen N, Goletz P, Ma JX, Crouch RK, Pfeifer K (1998) Rpe65 is necessary for production of 11-cis-vitamin A in the retinal visual cycle. Nat Genet 20(4):344–351

5. Samardzija M, von Lintig J, Tanimoto N, Oberhauser V, Thiersch M, Reme CE, Seeliger M, Grimm C, Wenzel A (2008) R91W mutation in Rpe65 leads to milder early-onset retinal dystrophy due to the generation of low levels of 11-cis-retinal. Hum Mol Genet 17(2):281–292

6. Chang B, Hawes NL, Hurd RE, Davisson MT, Nusinowitz S, Heckenlively JR (2002) A point mutation in the Rpe65 gene causes retinal degeneration (rd12) in mice. Invest Ophthalmol Vis Sci 3670 (abstract)

7. Pang JJ, Chang B, Hawes NL, Hurd RE, Davisson MT, Li J, Noorwez SM, Malhotra R, McDowell JH, Kaushal S, Hauswirth WW, Nusinowitz S, Thompson DA, Heckenlively JR (2005) Retinal degeneration 12 (rd12): a new, spontaneously arising mouse model for human Leber congenital amaurosis (LCA). Mol Vis 11:152–162

8. Keeler C (1924) The inheritance of a retinal abnormality in white mice. Proc Natl Acad Sci U S A 10:329

9. Keeler C (1966) Retinal degeneration in the mouse is rodless retina. J Hered 57(2):47–50

10. Pittler SJ, Keeler CE, Sidman RL, Baehr W (1993) PCR analysis of DNA from 70-year-old sections of rodless retina demonstrates identity with the mouse rd defect. Proc Natl Acad Sci U S A 90(20):9616–9619

11. van Nie R, Ivanyi D, Demant P (1978) A new H-2-linked mutation, rds, causing retinal degeneration in the mouse. Tissue Antigens 12(2):106–108

12. Chang B, Heckenlively JR, Hawes NL, Roderick TH (1993) New mouse primary retinal degeneration (rd-3). Genomics 16(1):45–49

13. Chang B, Hawes NL, Hurd RE, Davisson MT, Nusinowitz S, Heckenlively JR (2002) Retinal degeneration mutants in the mouse. Vision Res 42(4):517–525

14. Chang B, Hawes N, Davisson M, Heckenlively J (2007) Mouse models of RP. In: Tombran-Tink J, Barnstable C (eds) Retinal degenerations: biology, diagnostics, and therapeutics. The Humana Press Inc, New York, pp 149–164

15. Hawes NL, Smith RS, Chang B, Davisson M, Heckenlively JR, John SMM (1999) Mouse fundus photography and angiography: a catalogue of normal and mutant phenotypes. Mol Vis 5:22

16. Nusinowitz S, Ridder WH III, Heckenlively JR (2002) Electrophysiological testing of the mouse visual system. In: Smith RS (ed) Systematic evaluation of the mouse Eye: anatomy, pathology, and biomethods. CRC, Boca Raton, pp 320–344

17. Chang B, Dacey MS, Hawes NL, Hitchcock PF, Milam AH, Atmaca-Sonmez P, Nusinowitz S, Heckenlively JR (2006) Cone photoreceptor function loss-3, a novel mouse model of achromatopsia due to a mutation in Gnat2. Invest Ophthalmol Vis Sci 47(11):5017–5021

18. Chang B, Grau T, Dangel S, Hurd R, Jurklies B, Sener EC, Andreasson S, Dollfus H, Baumann B, Bolz S, Artemyev N, Kohl S, Heckenlively J, Wissinger B (2009) A homologous genetic basis of the murine cpfl1 mutant and human achromatopsia linked to mutations in the PDE6C gene. Proc Natl Acad Sci U S A 106(46):19581–19586

19. Chang B, Heckenlively JR, Bayley PR, Brecha NC, Davisson MT, Hawes NL, Hirano AA, Hurd RE, Ikeda A, Johnson BA, McCall MA, Morgans CW, Nusinowitz S, Peachey NS, Rice DS, Vessey KA, Gregg RG (2006) The nob2 mouse, a null mutation in Cacna1f: anatomical and functional abnormalities in the outer retina and their consequences on ganglion cell visual responses. Vis Neurosci 23(1):11–24

20. Maddox DM, Vessey KA, Yarbrough GL, Invergo BM, Cantrell DR, Inayat S, Balannik V, Hicks WL, Hawes NL, Byers S, Smith RS, Hurd R, Howell D, Gregg RG, Chang B, Naggert JK, Troy JB, Pinto LH, Nishina PM, McCall MA (2008) Allelic variance between GRM6 mutants, Grm6nob3 and Grm6nob4 results in differences in retinal ganglion cell visual responses. J Physiol 586(Pt 18):4409–4424

21. Hawes NL, Chang B, Hageman GS, Nusinowitz S, Nishina PM, Schneider BS, Smith RS, Roderick TH, Davisson MT, Heckenlively JR (2000) Retinal degeneration 6(rd 6): a new mouse model for human retinitis

punctata albescens. Invest Ophthalmol Vis Sci 41(10):3149–3157

22. Chang B, Hawes NL, Pardue MT, German AM, Hurd RE, Davisson MT, Nusinowitz S, Rengarajan K, Boyd AP, Sidney SS, Phillips MJ, Stewart RE, Chaudhury R, Nickerson JM, Heckenlively JR, Boatright JH (2007) Two mouse retinal degenerations caused by missense mutations in the "beta"-subunit of rod cGMP phosphodiesterase gene. Vision Res 47:624–633

23. Friedman JS, Chang B, Krauth DS, Lopez I, Waseem NH, Hurd RE, Feathers KL, Branham KE, Shaw M, Thomas GE, Brooks MJ, Liu C, Bakeri HA, Campos MM, Maubaret C, Webster AR, Rodriguez IR, Thompson DA, Bhattacharya SS, Koenekoop RK, Heckenlively JR, Swaroop A (2010) Loss of lysophosphatidylcholine acyltransferase 1 leads to photoreceptor degeneration in rd11 mice. Proc Natl Acad Sci U S A 107(35):15523–15528

24. Chang B, Khanna H, Hawes N, Jimeno D, He S, Lillo C, Parapuram SK, Cheng H, Scott A, Hurd RE, Sayer JA, Otto EA, Attanasio M, O'toole JF, Jin G, Shou C, Hildebrandt F, Williams DS, Heckenlively JR, Swaroop A (2006) An in-frame deletion in a novel centrosomal/ciliary protein CEP290/NPHP6 perturbs its interaction with RPGR and results in early-onset retinal degeneration in the rd16 mouse. Hum Mol Genet 15(11):1847–1857

25. Friedman JS, Chang B, Kannabiran C, Chakarova C, Singh HP, Jalali S, Hawes NL, Branham K, Othman M, Filippova E, Thompson DA, Webster AR, Andreasson S, Jacobson SG, Bhattacharya SS, Heckenlively JR, Swaroop A (2006) Premature truncation of a novel protein, RD3, exhibiting subnuclear localization is associated with retinal degeneration. Am J Hum Genet 79(6):1059–1070

26. Roderick TH, Chang B, Hawes NL, Heckenlively JR (1997) A new dominant retinal degeneration (Rd4) linked with a chromosome 4 inversion in the mouse. Genomics 42(3):393–396

27. Kitamura E, Danciger M, Yamashita C, Rao NP, Nusinowitz S, Chang B, Farber DB (2006) Disruption of the gene encoding the {beta}1-subunit of transducin in the Rd4/+ mouse. Invest Ophthalmol Vis Sci 47(4):1293–1301

Chapter 3

Retinal Fundus Imaging in Mouse Models of Retinal Diseases

Anne F. Alex, Peter Heiduschka, and Nicole Eter

Abstract

The development of in vivo retinal fundus imaging in mice has opened a new research horizon, not only in ophthalmic research. The ability to monitor the dynamics of vascular and cellular changes in pathological conditions, such as neovascularization or degeneration, longitudinally without the need to sacrifice the mouse, permits longer observation periods in the same animal. With the application of the high-resolution confocal scanning laser ophthalmoscopy in experimental mouse models, access to a large spectrum of imaging modalities in vivo is provided.

Key words: Retinal imaging, Choroidal neovascularization, Retinal neovascularization, Confocal scanning laser ophthalmoscopy, Optical coherence tomography, Fluorescein angiography, Indocyanine green angiography

1. Introduction

In vivo monitoring of physiological and pathological processes has gained increasing interest in experimental settings of diseases. In ophthalmology, we take advantage of the instance that the eye is perfectly suitable for optical imaging due to its transparency, both in the anterior and posterior segment. Therefore, in vivo monitoring of the eye allows longitudinal observations of changes in the same animal, improves the investigation of pathogenesis and/or effects of therapeutic approaches in disease models, and permits combination of in vivo and ex vivo imaging for maximum information. Last but not least, the number of animals needed for investigation can be reduced, and less time for the screening of a large number of animals is demanded with modern imaging techniques.

Examination through the dilated pupil easily enables funduscopic imaging in the living animal. Behavior of cells can be monitored in

Bernhard H.F. Weber and Thomas Langmann (eds.), *Retinal Degeneration: Methods and Protocols*, Methods in Molecular Biology, vol. 935, DOI 10.1007/978-1-62703-080-9_3, © Springer Science+Business Media, LLC 2013

pathologic conditions, as well as vascular changes, which is of particular importance in neovascular diseases of the eye.

In this chapter, we provide an overview of in vivo retinal fundus imaging techniques in mice. Thereby, we explain the procedures in detail and give examples by focusing on different mouse models of neovascular and degenerating diseases as well as on immune cell changes in the eye.

In all neovascular eye diseases, competing factors of inflammation, angiogenesis, and proteolysis modulate the stage of disease.

Choroidal neovascularization (CNV) is a nonspecific and dynamic response in different eye diseases. Age-related macular degeneration (AMD) is the leading cause for severe vision impairment in humans at the age over 50 in the industrialized world (1), and choroidal neovascularization is the hallmark of the wet form of AMD. Reduction in the metabolic activity of the retinal pigment epithelium (RPE) leads to accumulation of subretinal deposits and destruction of Bruch's membrane and the RPE. Macrophages and other immune cells are also known to play an important role in the initiation and/or progression, at least in the formation of CNV. Resident and immigrating immune cells are responsible for disease advancement. A pathologic dynamic process is initiated, and proinflammatory and proangiogenic factors, such as TNF-α, MMPs, MCP-1, IL-8, PEDF, bFGF, and VEGF, are secreted and monocyte and endothelial cell recruitment is modulated (2). A fibrin matrix is generated as a fundament in the area of neovascularization. Neovascularization in the choroid is stimulated, and new vessels are able to penetrate into the neurosensoric retina when disease is advanced.

The leading cause for *retinal neovascularization* is hypoxia. Examples for retinal neovascularization are diabetic retinopathy and retinopathy of prematurity (ROP). Diabetic retinopathy is the leading cause of acquired blindness in young adults and therefore an increasing socioeconomic challenge. Neuronal dysfunction and vascular damage occur (3). When disease proceeds, neovascularization with immature retinal blood vessels develops. These blood vessels can cause complications, such as bleeding, or even retinal detachment. ROP in contrast is a neovascular disease that occurs during the stage of vasculogenesis. A careful differentiation has to be made between vasculogenesis (development of vessels from mesodermal progenitor cells) and angiogenesis (sprouting of newly formed blood vessels out of the existing vessels), as the pathological pathways and consequently the morphological changes may vary (4).

Retinal cell degeneration occurs in many inherited and acquired diseases. In frequent cases, photoreceptors degenerate due to genetic defects, and many of such diseases belong to the group named *Retinopathia pigmentosa*. These patients suffer from a progressive reduction of the field of vision already as young adults, preventing them from pursuing a normal employment.

Mouse models are used to either watch morphological retinal changes or changes in retinal layers due to disease dynamics.

The opportunity to image retinal changes in a time-dependent manner allows the assignment of molecular findings to morphological changes. Clinically, this in reverse can allow early diagnosis of diseases, simply by retinal fundus imaging.

An important imaging device in ophthalmology is based on the principle of the confocal scanning laser ophthalmoscopy (cSLO). This commonly used method for retinal fundus imaging is integrated in new imaging devices, for example in the SPECTRALIS® HRA. The imaging modalities include infrared, red-free, and fluorescence images. Fluorescence angiography with either fluorescein or indocyanine green can be performed.

A more recent technique is the high-resolution optical coherence tomography (OCT) and its introduction into imaging in experimental ophthalmology. In vivo images similar to histological sections can be generated in a very high resolution.

With modern imaging techniques, it is possible to gain information of disease dynamics and time-dependent changes in retinal morphology in vivo. Furthermore, evidence about cellular characteristics in different stages of disease progression can be obtained.

The established ex vivo imaging tools are also of high importance, with histological sections as the most often used technique. Tissue sections can be stained simply with hematoxylin and eosin to visualize cell nuclei and parts of the cytoplasm. For the detection of distinct proteins, antibodies labeled with fluorescent dyes are used (immunohistochemistry), which can be used on sections as well as on retinal and choroidal whole-mounts. These procedures provide two-dimensional images. Confocal microscopy allows a three-dimensional imaging by recording pictures in different z-planes, in particular in whole-mounts.

2. Materials

2.1. Anesthesia

1. Ketamine 10% (WDT, Garbsen, Germany).

2. Xylazine 2% (CEVA Tiergesundheit GmbH, Düsseldorf, Germany).

3. Isoflurane (Forene® 100%, Abbott GmbH & Co, AG, Wiesbaden, Germany).

2.2. Pupil Dilation

1. Tropicamide (Mydriaticum® Stulln; Pharma Stulln GmbH, Stulln, Germany).

2. Phenylephrine hydrochloride (Neosynephrin® 5%, Ursapharm Arzneimittel GmbH, Saarbrücken, Germany).

3. Cyclopentolate hydrochloride (Zyklolat® EDO, Dr. Mann Pharma und Bausch & Lomb GmbH, Berlin, Germany).

2.3. Imaging

1. Contact lens (to avoid dehydration of the cornea; MPG&E Handel und Service GmbH, Bordesholm, Germany).

2. Hydroxypropyl methylcellulose (Methocel 2%; OmniVision, Puchheim, Germany).

3. Contact lens with +35 spherical diopters (radius 5.0 mm, diameter 7.00 mm; MPG&E Handel und Service GmbH, Bordesholm, Germany).

4. Fluorescein-sodium 10% (Alcon Pharma GmbH, Freiburg im Breisgau, Germany).

5. Indocyanine green 25 mg (ICG-Pulsion®, Pulsion Medical Systems AG, München, Germany).

6. Artificial tears (e.g., Hylo Vision; OmniVision® GmbH, Puchheim, Germany).

7. Proxymetacaine hydrochloride 0.5% (Proparakain-POS®, Ursapharm Arzneimittel GmbH, Saarbrücken, Germany).

2.4. SPECTRALIS® HRA+OCT

The principal function of the SPECTRALIS® HRA+OCT (Heidelberg Engineering, Dossenheim, Germany) is based on the confocal scanning laser ophthalmoscopy. Briefly, the retina is illuminated by a focussed laser beam, and the reflected light is captured by a photodetector after passing through a pinhole. The pinhole blocks the light that is not reflected or emitted by the area of interest and in this way blocks scattered light. The intensity of the reflected light or of the emitted fluorescent light at each point is measured by a light-sensitive detector. The light captured by the detector is converted into a digital signal, and a focussed image with high resolution is generated. The position of the confocal aperture determines from which layer in the back of the eye, i.e., the retina, the reflected light is collected, enabling the performance of confocal imaging (Fig. 1) (5).

The SPECTRALIS® HRA+OCT device is the combination of both, fundus imaging with a confocal scanning laser ophthalmoscope and a cross-section imaging by the spectral-domain optical coherence tomography (SD-OCT). It uses a dual-beam simultaneous imaging system to permit a multimodal imaging, the so-called tracking laser tomography. One laser beam serves as a reference, which continuously monitors the position of the eye. The second beam is directed to the position of interest in the fundus. The SPECTRALIS® HRA+OCT device works with five light sources (Table 1).

This SD-OCT can take up to 40,000 A-scans per second, with an optical axial resolution of about 7 μm, a transverse resolution of about 14 μm, and a scan depth of up to 1.9 mm. The interference signal between the sample beam and the reference beam can be analyzed simultaneously, enabling the fast scanning speed and the high resolution in SD-OCT (Fig. 2).

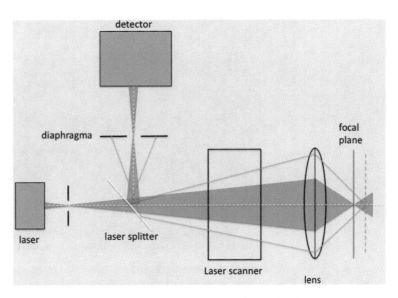

Fig. 1. Scheme of the principle of a confocal scanning laser ophthalmoscope.

Table 1
Light sources of the SPECTRALIS® HRA + OCT device (Heidelberg Engineering, Dossenheim, Germany)

Light source	Effect
486 ± 2 nm blue solid-state laser (barrier filter of 500 nm)	Fluorescein excitation, blue reflectance, autofluorescence
486 ± 2 nm without barrier filter	Red-free images
518 ± 3 nm	Green reflectance
786 ± 2 nm diode laser and barrier filter of 830 nm	Indocyanine green excitation
815 ± 5 nm diode laser	Infrared reflectance images
870 nm (840 to 920 nm) super luminescence diode(SLD) laser	Spectral domain OCT

2.5. Fundus Color Imaging with Visucam® 200

Visucam® 200 (Carl Zeiss AG, Oberkochen, Germany) is a non-mydriatic fundus camera with a 45° and 30° field angle. Color, red-free, blue, red, and anterior segment capture modes are included. The device is described by the manufacturer to require a minimal pupil diameter of 3.3 mm, which is principally suitable for the application with mice. A dilated mouse pupil approximately corresponds to this diameter (6). For compensation of the optical characteristics of the mouse, we used a 20D lens (manufactured, e.g., by Volk).

We built a special tripod system, connected with a planar extent, on which the mouse can be positioned. This extent is also flexibly movable in all directions, so that the mouse position can be varied, which is important because the fundus camera itself is a rigor system (Fig. 3).

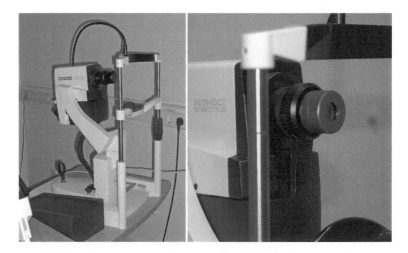

Fig. 2. The SPECTRALIS® HRA + OCT device by Heidelberg Engineering. On the right, the device is shown with the attached additional lens to facilitate imaging of small rodent's eyes.

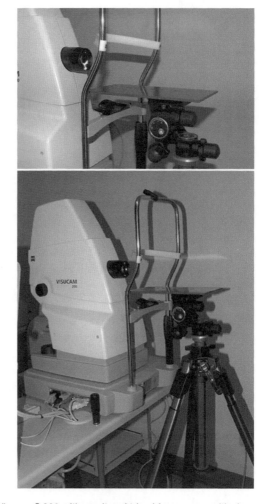

Fig. 3. Zeiss Visucam® 200 with an altered tripod for mouse positioning.

3. Methods

3.1. Anesthesia

To be able to take retinal fundus images of living mice, they have to be anesthetized. Commonly used anesthetics for experimental animals are a mixture of intraperitoneally injected ketamine (120 mg/kg) and xylazine (10 mg/kg). For intraperitoneal injection, the mouse is held tightly discreet overhead so that the inner organs are moving downwards and are not reached by the injection needle. Once the mouse is anesthetized, care has to be taken to maintain the body temperature constant. Besides reduced physiological functions, a reduction of the body temperature leads to the development of a cataract due to the change of lens proteins, which, although being reversible, is not useful for optical imaging (7).

3.2. Pupil Dilation

Pupil dilation is necessary for an optimal insight into the eye. Tropicamide eye drops are commonly used in the clinic. To achieve longer lasting pupil dilation, a combination of neosynephrine 5% and Zyklolat 1% eye drops can be applied. Already after a few minutes, the pupils become dilated (Fig. 4).

3.3. Positioning of the Animal in Front of the Laser/Imaging Device

Anesthetized mice are brought in front of the imaging device. During imaging, it is recommended to maintain the body temperature of the mice constant, because they cool down quickly while being anesthetized, leading to the reversible cataract mentioned before. A possible option is the use of an electronic heating. Special animal heating and monitoring systems are available. We keep the animals on a heated cherry stone filled pad, which proved to be sufficient for the time of examination. This simple auxiliary tool can be easily changed in its shape, and mice can be placed in a stable position (Fig. 5). Regular corneal hydration with commonly used artificial tears is strongly recommended.

3.4. Laser Treatment of the Fundus for CNV Induction

The mouse is brought in front of the laser as described in Subheading 3.3. The cornea is anesthesized with on drop of e.g. Proparakain-POS 0,5% or another local anesthetics. A glass slide

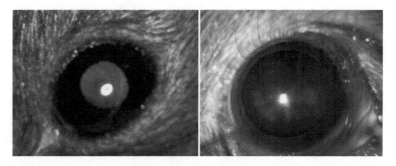

Fig. 4. Mouse pupil in miosis (*left*) and mydriasis (*right*).

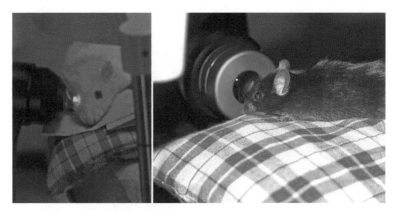

Fig. 5. Examples for rat and mouse positioning in front of the SPECTRALIS® device. Due to the flexibility of the used cherry stone filled pad, rodents of different sizes can be placed stable in various positions.

coated with Methocel® 2% is held carefully against the anesthetized mouse cornea for an optimal sight on the fundus. To evoke CNV, destruction of Bruch's membrane and of the retinal pigment epithelium is achieved by the following laser settings:

In the small mouse eye, small laser spots should be applied, such as 50 µm. In larger rodents, a bigger spot size may be used depending on the size of the required CNV area, using a duration time of 100 ms and an energy of 200 mW (see Note 1).

Successful disruption of Bruch's membrane can be funduscopically evaluated by the formation of a bubble in the laser spot immediately after treatment. Frequently used laser devices are argon laser (argon blue: 488 nm; argon green: 514 nm), frequency-doubled neodym YAG laser (532 nm), and diode laser (810–830 nm wavelength).

After full recovery from anesthesia, the mouse can be returned into the cage.

3.5. Autofluorescence Images

Autofluorescence in the human eye is mainly produced by lipofuscin. Lipofuscin is a poorly defined mixture of nondegradable cross-linked lipids and denatured proteins (8–10). As in most post-mitotic cells, lipofuscin is accumulated during lifetime in the retinal pigment epithelium and exhibits fluorescence over a broad range of excitation (300–600 nm) and emission (480–800 nm) wavelengths (11, 12) due to different fluorophores of distinct excitation and emission spectra, with N-retinylidene-N-retinylethanolamine (A2E) as the major fluorescent component (13). A2E in the RPE cells has an emission maximum at 565–570 nm (14). In various disease models, degeneration of photoreceptors is often accompanied by an accumulation of autofluorescent, retinoid-containing debris material in the subretinal space (15). The retinoids are derived from photoreceptor outer segment breakdown products that contain visual pigment chromophore 11-cis-retinal (16).

Whereas these autofluorescent materials can be excited at any wavelength ranging from UV to yellow light, a wavelength of 488 nm is used in the SPECTRALIS® device.

Less autofluorescence is visible in the human foveal area, because the blue excitation light is attenuated by the macular pigment, i.e., lutein and zeaxanthin. Blood vessels appear nonfluorescent in the autofluorescence mode due to hemoglobin, which absorbs the laser light.

In untreated C57Bl/6 mice, no autofluorescence can be detected. If degenerative changes are elicited, autofluorescent spots can be found, e.g., in the areas of the laser spots in the model of laser-induced CNV 3 weeks after laser treatment.

3.6. Infrared Image

Scanning the back of the eye with a near-infrared laser beam to produce a fundus image is the basic imaging principle of the SPECTRALIS® cSLO device. Infrared (IR) light penetrates the cornea, lens, and vitreous easier than visible light (in particular in the presence of slight opacities), and a lower intensity is needed. Infrared images in mouse models are important, as they give orientation about the localization of the monitored retinal changes and also account for documentation, comparable to color fundus images (Fig. 6).

3.7. Red-Free Image

The red-free image is produced by blocking light of long (red) wavelengths. It is useful for several distinct diagnostic purposes. Filtering of red light can reveal structures in the fundus that are normally hidden by the red light originating from the retina with its blood vessels. As a clinical example, retinal nevi can be distinguished from choroidal nevi. Nerve fibers and subtle changes in their number can also be visualized in red-free images. This is important in animal models of glaucoma and other optic nerve atrophies. In this context, determination of the cup/disk ratio is easier. Optic nerve drusen, hemorrhages, and aneurysms are visible more clearly in red-free images.

3.8. Angiography

The basic principle of angiography is to visualize blood vessels by an intravenous injection of a fluorescent dye (Fig. 7). For this purpose, fluorescein and indocyanine green are the most commonly used dyes in clinical ophthalmology as well as in the majority of animal experiments. In mice, 5 ml/kg of the commercial 2% fluorescein sodium dye solution is intraperitoneally injected (for intraperitoneal injection see Subheading 3.1). To evaluate the status of retinal vasculature and to judge possible pathologies, early angiograms (1–5 min after injection) and late-phase angiograms (5–10 min after injection) are recorded. Distinction is made between hyperfluorescent and hypofluorescent changes (see Note 2). Hyperfluorescent changes can be staining (e.g., scarring, fibrosis), pooling (e.g., edema), and leakage (e.g., neovascularization).

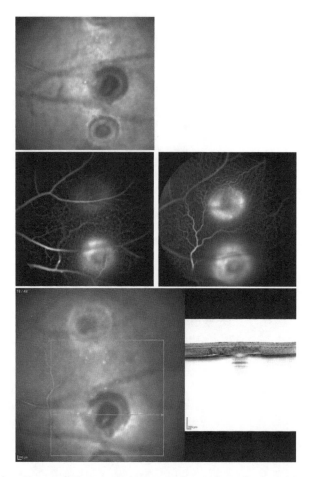

Fig. 6. Infrared image of a laser-treated mouse fundus one hour after laser (*above*); corresponding early and late fluorescein angiographies (*middle*) and OCT volume scan (*below*).

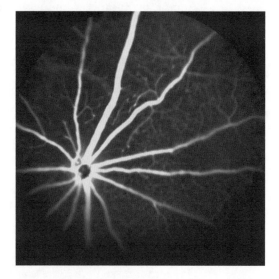

Fig. 7. Typical appearance of a mouse fundus in fluorescein angiography. Note the radial spreading of the large retinal blood vessels, originating at the optic nerve head, which is typical for small rodents that do not have a macula.

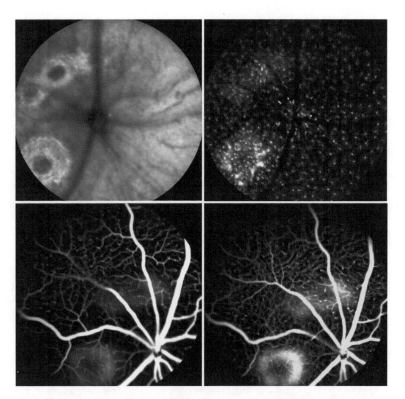

Fig. 8. Fundus imaging of a laser-treated CX3CR1$^{GFP/+}$ mouse. Simultaneous imaging in three modes: Infrared and autofluorescence mode (*above*); early- and late-phase indocyanine green angiographies (*below*).

Hypofluorescence can occur due to blocking phenomenons (e.g., intravitreal bleeding or pigmentation) or perfusion defects (e.g., tumor).

In CX3CR1$^{GFP/+}$ mice, green fluorescent protein (GFP)-positive immune cells fluoresce green in the autofluorescence mode. Obviously, it is not possible to perform a fluorescein angiography parallel to the immune cell imaging. In this case, the ICG angiography is a reasonable alternative (see Note 3). Even though ICG has a strong plasma protein binding and therefore has less visible leakage phenomena, the laser-induced CNV model is strong enough for induction of CNV. Simultaneous imaging of the same fundus area in three different modes, infrared, autofluorescence, and indocyanine green angiography, is possible (Fig. 8).

3.9. Optical Coherence Tomography

OCT was developed on the principle of Michelson interferometry. Basically, low-coherence infrared light is split. One part is traveling to retinal structures, and the second part to a reference mirror. When the reflected light of the reference mirror interacts with the light coming back from the retina, an interference pattern is produced that can be detected and processed into a signal (17). It produces detailed cross-sectional images of the fundus and is

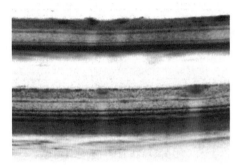

Fig. 9. Examples of OCT images of mouse (*top*) and rat (*bottom*) retinas. Most of the retinal layers can be recognized.

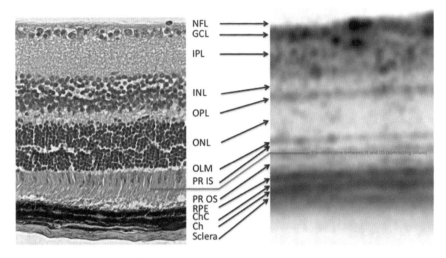

Fig. 10. Comparison between a histological section through a mouse retina (*left*) and an OCT image (*right*). The single layers of the histological section are named and assigned to the layers visible in the OCT image. Additionally, cone photoreceptors are stained with a PNA dye in the histology (*left*).

therefore frequently used for macular imaging in humans. With the SPECTRALIS® OCT device, retinal fundus images of rodents can also be taken through a dilated pupil. Thus, the layered structure of the retina can be visualized in OCT images, and the layers visible in the OCT image can be assigned to the anatomical layers that can be found also in histological sections (Figs. 9 and 10). For the generation of high-resolution OCT images of the mouse fundus, optical aberrations of the mouse eye have to be compensated by an additional lens (see Note 4). The neuroretinal layers, the RPE, and the choriocapillaris are presented in detail (Fig. 10). Pathologies can be attributed to a specific retinal layer by an OCT image. Furthermore, changes in retinal layers point to specific pathologies. Different modes can be adjusted in the OCT. It is possible to generate single sections, star-shaped sections, and, most important, volumetric sections with variable interspaces. Also, follow-up examinations are possible. The system recognizes the corresponding fundus structures and the same area can be reexamined with a pixel-to-pixel acuity (also see Note 2).

It has to be noted explicitly that OCT cannot replace histological sections. Images obtained by OCT are "histology-like" and can be recorded quickly. However, it has to be kept in mind that the gray-scaled images are simply a map of different absorption and reflection characteristics of the retinal layers. No single cells or their phenotypes are displayed, as it is possible in histology.

3.10. Fundus Color Images

Due to the special optical characteristics of the mouse eye, clinically used fundus color cameras do not necessarily fulfil the needs for the application in rodents (see Note 5). Anyway, utilities are available to take accurate images. Contact fundus lenses for the mouse or rat are available to reduce light reflections (Ocular Instruments, Washington, USA). Alternatively, special animal fundus cameras are available, e.g., the Kowa Genesis small animal fundus camera (Tokyo, Japan), which gives satisfactory results of images (18).

A new development is the topical endoscopic fundus imaging (TEFI). An endoscope with an outer diameter of 3 mm is connected on top of a photographic camera objective. The endoscope is placed directly on the cornea. High-resolution images can be obtained in a field of view of 80° (6).

We tested the application of the Zeiss Visucam® 200 nonmydriatic fundus camera. At the beginning, the mouse has to be anesthetized and pupils have to be dilated (see Subheadings 2.1 and 2.2). The anesthetized mouse is positioned on the tripod extension and brought in front of the objective. A 20D Volk lens is held manually directly in front of the objective. The automatic focus of the device should be switched off, as it is calibrated for a human eye. Fundus images should be taken in the 30° angle. The focus can be manually adjusted in the infrared image of the camera. In a C57BL/6 wild-type mouse, the centrally located optic nerve head becomes visible. Veins and arteries are spreading in radial direction from the optic nerve head into the periphery. The fundus has a yellowish-orange ground color. Nerve fibers are also evenly spreading from the optic nerve head parallel to the vessels. They are visible as thin lines and are brighter than the normal fundus color (Fig. 11; see Note 5).

3.11. Mouse Models of Retinal Diseases

Mouse models exist for a large variety of retinal diseases. We will concentrate on retinal fundus imaging in mouse models of neovascular and degenerating fundus diseases, and in immunologically mutated mice.

Neovascularization can occur in the retina and in the choroid. Choroidal and retinal neovascularization mimicking neovascular diseases can be induced in the mouse by laser, surgically, by a special diet, or by hypoxia (2). Intraperitoneally injected streptozotocin

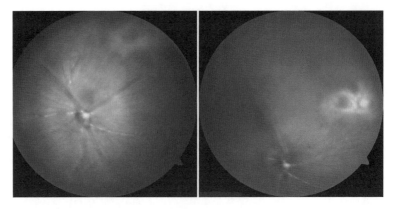

Fig. 11. Color fundus image of a C57Bl/6 mouse, treated with laser 3 weeks before. Vessels are originating from the centrally localized optic nerve head. Laser spots are displayed as lighter spots on the fundus.

induces a diabetic metabolism by selectively killing insulin-producing beta cells in the islets of Langerhans.

Mouse models of retinal degeneration can concern exclusively one cell type, e.g., photoreceptor or ganglion cells. Photoreceptor degeneration in mouse models is usually caused by spontaneous or induced mutations (19) (Table 2).

3.12. Mouse Models of Retinal and Choroidal Neovascularization

3.12.1. Laser-Induced Choroidal Neovascularization

A laser beam destroys Bruch's membrane and initiates a local immunological reaction, which results in a CNV (see Subheading 3.4) (20).

In the infrared image, a crater and a bubble in the area of the laser spots are visible just after the injury. In fluorescence angiography, hyperfluorescent spots appear in the area of laser injury, indicating leakage (Fig. 12). Shortly after the laser injury, diffuse hyperfluorescence occurs, which gets sharper in demarcation over the time. It is even possible to image neovascular vessels in the hyperfluorescent area by focusing through the retinal layer with the cSLO device. Autofluorescent particles can only be detected 3 weeks after laser injury.

The laser-induced destruction of Bruch's membrane and the RPE can be immediately visualized by OCT. After laser treatment, a hyperreflective zone in the neuroretinal layers is visible, reflecting the fundus bubbles (Fig. 13). After 1 week, the RPE becomes hypertrophic in the peripheral rim of the laser spot and over time, the area of laser spot becomes degenerative. CNV induction in this model is described between 60 and 100% (21).

These images can be compared to histological section.

3.12.2. Hypoxia-Induced Retinal Neovascularization

The most commonly investigated disease in a mouse model for retinal neovascularization is the ROP (22). After exposure to 75% oxygen for 5 days in a sealed chamber (BioSpherix, New York, USA) connected to an oxygen controller, mice are brought back to

Table 2
Overview of described mouse models of retinal diseases

Interest of imaging	Mechanism/mouse model	Fundus phenotype	Disease model
Choroidal neovascularization	Laser	Disruption of Bruch's membrane and RPE	Age-related macular degeneration
Choroidal neovascularization	Surgical injection of peptides, microbeads, matrigel, and others	Dependent on the method of injection	Age-related macular degeneration
GFP-positive immune cell imaging	Transgene; CX3CR1$^{GFP/+}$, gene is functional	GFP-positive immune cell imaging	Age-related macular degeneration
GFP-positive immune cell imaging	Transgene; CX3CR1$^{GFP/GFP}$, gene is not functional	GFP-positive immune cell imaging (immune cell receptor knockout)	Age-related macular degeneration
Drusen-like lesions, choroidal neovascularization	Transgene; CCR2$^{-/-}$	Drusen-like lesions develop spontaneously after about 9 months (immune cell receptor knockout)	Age-related macular degeneration
Early choroidal neovascularization	CCR3 visualisation	Early detection of CNV before angiographic changes with antibody-conjugated quantum dots	Age-related macular degeneration
Retinal neovascularization, choroidal anastomosis degeneration	Vldlr−/−	Retinal angiogenesis, subretinal neovascularization, choroidal anastomosis	Macular teleangiectasia
Retinal neovascularization	Hypoxia	Suppression of retinal vasculogenesis	Retinopathy of prematurity
Retinal neovascularization	Intraperitonally injected Streptozotocine	Retinal capillary degeneration (early-stage diabetic fundus changes)	Diabetic retinopathy
Vessel imaging	Flk1:myr-mCherry	Red-fluorescent endothelial cells	Neovascular diseases

(continued)

Table 2
(continued)

Interest of imaging	Mechanism/mouse model	Fundus phenotype	Disease model
Retinal degeneration $Rd1$	Deficiency in the activity of the rod photoreceptor cGMP phosphodiesterase; chromosome 5	Vessel attenuation and pigment patches in the fundus	Rod photoreceptor degeneration; retinopathia pigmentosa
Retinal degeneration $Rd3$	Early-onset photoreceptor degeneration	Early loss of all photoreceptors	Usher syndrome type IIA
Retinal degeneration $Cpfl1$	Autosomal recessive mutation on chromosome 19	Normal fundus (cone cell number diminishes, rod photoreceptors keep their functionality)	Cone photoreceptor degeneration; achromatopsia
Retinal degeneration Rds	$Prph2^{Rd2}$ on chromosome 17	Slow fundus changes; accumulation of photoreceptor outer segments	Rod and cone photoreceptor outer segment degeneration
Retinal degeneration, $RPE65^{-/-}$	Block in the visual cycle	Accumulation of retinyl esters	Leber congenital amourosis

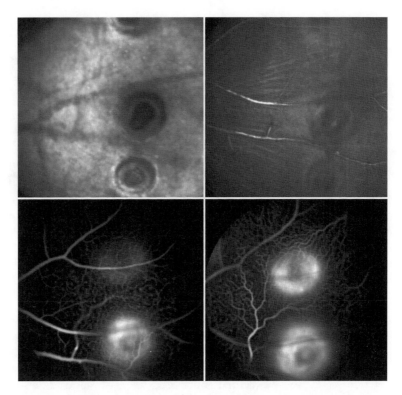

Fig. 12. Appearance of laser spots in the back of the mouse eye in the infrared mode (*top line*) and during fluorescence angiography (*bottom line*). The two columns represent two different focus planes. The areas of the laser spots are clearly visible.

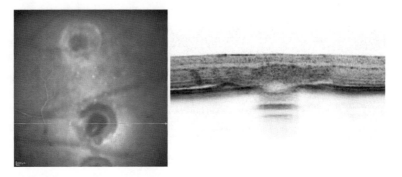

Fig. 13. Infrared (*left*) and OCT (*right*) image of a C56Bl/6 mouse 1 h after laser treatment. Within the laser spot, a hyperreflective area is visible in the OCT.

room air for another 5 days. Central ischemic regions develop, and retinal neovascularization is initiated in the periphery. Vessels become curved and dilated (Fig. 14). The changes are opposite to the fundus changes in a human infant. There, ischemic regions develop in the insufficient oxygenated retinal periphery and neo-vascularization primarily appears in the transition zone between vascularized und non-vascularized retina.

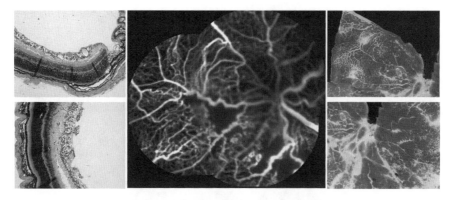

Fig. 14. Fundus images of a mouse with retinopathy of prematurity (ROP): Histological sections show neovascular endothelial cells and large vessel diameter in the neuroretina (*left*), in vivo fluorescein angiographies display central ischemia, curled vessels, and neovascularization in the periphery (*middle*), and ex vivo angiographies in retinal wholemounts of a C57Bl/6 mouse, perfused intracardially with high molecular FITC-dextrane in advance, show similar changes (*right*).

3.12.3. Surgical Induction of Choroidal Neovascularization

CNV in mice can also be induced surgically by injection of proangiogenic or proinflammatory peptides, viral vectors, or cells. Spilsbury and coworkers induced a CNV by subretinal injection of a recombinant adenovirus vector expressing VEGF164 driven by a CMV promoter in rats (23). Schmack et al. induced CNV by subretinal injection of RPE and polystyrene microbeads (24). Unfortunately, the injection itself caused small CNV lesions due to the disruption of Bruch's membrane with injection.

CNV can also be induced by the subretinal injection of matrigel, a mixture of basement membrane proteins, which solidifies after implantation into tissue and stimulates local angiogenesis (25).

3.12.4. Streptozotocin-Induced Diabetic Retinopathy

Diabetic retinopathy can be induced by daily intraperitoneal (IP) injection of 50 mg/kg streptozotocin for 5 days or as a single dose with 150 mg/kg, dissolved in citrate buffer (pH 5.5) (26). Blood glucose levels in the diabetic animals have to be determined on a regular basis in order to ensure their treatment. For inclusion into the study, blood glucose concentrations should exceed 11.1 mmol/l (27).

Fundus changes in the mouse mainly concern characteristics of the early stage of diabetic retinopathy which are retinal capillary degeneration, loss of capillary pericytes and neuroglia, impairment in vessel autoregulation, and deterioration of nonvascular retinal function (28).

3.12.5. Transgene Mouse Models for Neovascularization and for Retinal Cell Imaging

Genetically modified mice can be generated, e.g., by replacing the gene of interest in one of the two alleles by cDNA sequences encoding for a fluorochrome. Cells or cell properties and their dynamics can then be imaged by excitation of the fluorochrome.

A mouse model for endothelial cell imaging is the *Flk1:myr-mCherry* transgenic mouse. This mouse expresses endothelial cell-specific red fluorescent mCherry protein on the cell membranes (excitation wavelength: 532 or 543 nm (optimum: 587 nm);

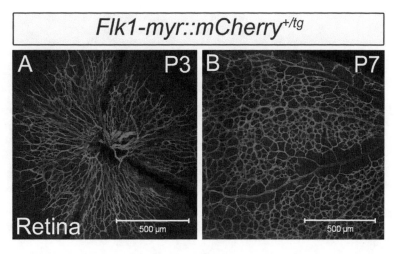

Fig. 15. Retinal wholemounts of a Flk1:myr-mCherry transgenic mouse. Developing retinal vessels at day 3 (**A**) and day 7 (**B**). All endothelial cells express the red fluorescent mCherry protein (images were kindly supplied by Ross A. Poché, Baylor College of Medicine, Department of Molecular Physiology and Biophysics, Houston, TX, USA).

emission wavelength: 610 nm (optimum: 615 nm)) (29, 30). This enables direct monitoring of dynamic vascular changes (Fig. 15).

CX3CR1, named Fractalkine receptor, is a seven-transmembrane receptor, expressed by dendritic cells, macrophages, microglia, and monocytes (31). By substitution of the first 390 base pairs of one allele of the CX3CR1 gene by cDNA which encodes for enhanced green fluorescent protein (EGFP; excitation wavelength: 488 nm; emission wavelength: 514 nm), we were able to monitor the behavior of these immune cells, which are still completely functional, by excitation of the GFP with the cSLO. When both alleles are replaced by EGFP, the immune function is knocked out. Cells lose their chemotactic properties due to the loss of this receptor. Subsequently, no CX3CR1-positive immune cells are immigrating into an area of inflammation. Because of its excitation wavelength, GFP can be monitored in the autofluorescence mode of modern imaging devices, such as the SPECTRALIS® HRA. Cells appear point-shaped with filiform branches and build a network in a regular distribution all over the fundus. When an area of inflammation is induced, e.g., by laser treatment, these immune cells migrate into the area of laser spots (Fig. 16). This is already visible 20 min after laser treatment (20). The cell density declines around the laser spots and increases within them, indicating a migration of resident cells. Over time, also nonresident cells may immigrate into this area.

CCR2 is also known to participate in the progression of AMD. This receptor binds monocyte chemoattractant protein 1 (MCP-1) or Ccl-2 (produced by RPE and choroidal endothelial cells in response to an inflammatory stimulus), and regulates the immigration of macrophages into an inflammation focus. If this receptor or its chemokine is lacking, complement and IgG are

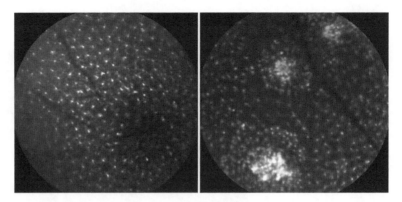

Fig. 16. Autofluorescence fundus imaging in a CX3CR1$^{GFP/+}$ mouse. Non-treated (*left*) and laser-treated (*right*) fundus. CX3CR1$^{GFP/+}$ cells are migrating into the area of laser treatment.

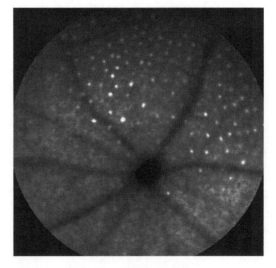

Fig. 17. Autofluorescence of a mouse fundus in a CCR2$^{-/-}$ mouse. Equally distributed autofluorescent dots become visible (here with 9 months of age).

accumulating, leading to increased VEGF production by the RPE. This may initiate CNV (32, 33). Excessive metabolism products similar to drusen are visible in the fundus in the autofluorescence mode in cSLO (Fig. 17).

A combined knockout of the receptor CX3CR1 and the ligand Ccl-2 leads to spontaneously occurring AMD-typical fundus changes like drusen, RPE alteration, and photoreceptor degeneration already around the age of 6 weeks (34). 15% develop CNV.

CCR3, also a chemokine receptor, is known to promote eosinophil and mast cell trafficking. This receptor was recently found to be expressed exclusively on endothelial cells in CNV due to AMD (35). Visualization of this receptor by antibody-conjugated quantum dots enabled the detection of CNV before angiographic changes occurred.

In a mouse model for hypercholesterolemia, AMD-like retinal changes were discovered. ApoE4 overexpression in mice which were additionally fed with a high-fat cholesterol-rich diet developed drusen-like deposits and after over 1 year about one-fifth also developed CNV (36).

Rhodopsin-promotor VEGF overexpression transgenic mice developed intraretinal neovascularization that extended into the subretinal space (37).

In a knockout mouse model for very-low-density lipoprotein receptor (Vldlr; B6;129-*Vldlr^{tm1Her}*), retinal angiogenesis, subretinal neovascularization, and formation of choroidal vascular anastomosis are initiated by 15 days after birth. Homozygous mice have a 100% expression (38).

3.13. Mouse Models of Retinal Degeneration

There are many retinal diseases caused by inherited or acquired degeneration of retinal cells. Many mouse models for retinal degeneration exist. *Retinopathia pigmentosa* is characterized by an inherited degeneration of mainly rod outer segments, which finally leads to a decrease of the visual field to a small central concentric residual, caused by mutations in different genes on variable chromosomes.

Rod dysplasia (*rd*) mouse models contain a group of many different mutations, which all lead to photoreceptor degeneration, differing in both mutation location and degenerative phenotype (39). In the rod dysplasia mouse 1 (*rd1*), the defective gene is located on chromosome five (allele *Pde6b*) and affects photoreceptors, particularly rods, as pathologically occurring in humans suffering from *Retinopathia pigmentosa*. Retinal degeneration is caused by a loss-of-function mutation in the gene encoding for the β subunit of the rod cGMP phosphodiesterase 6. Pathologic changes in rods occur already 8 days after birth. At 4 weeks after birth, photoreceptor degeneration is clearly visible in cross-sectional images of the OCT and accordingly, retinal thickness is reduced. Funduscopically, vessel attenuation and formation of pigment patches can be distinguished (Fig. 18). The ERG response disappears after 20–28 days (19, 40).

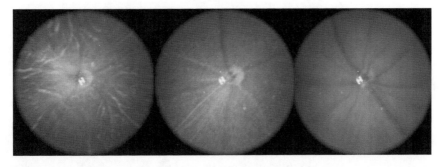

Fig. 18. Fundus image of retinal degeneration mouse models. Rd1 (*left*) with degenerative changes at 3 months of age, rd3 (middle) with milder fundus changes at 7 months of age, and cpfl1 (*right*) with a normal fundus at 3 months of age (images were kindly supplied by Bo Chang, The Jackson Laboratory, Bar Harbor, ME, USA).

Rd3 mutation leads to an early-onset retinal degeneration. Normally, both alleles have to be mutated for a full development of retinal degenerative changes. In *rd3/rd3* homozygous mice, degeneration becomes visible already at the age of 2 weeks. Photoreceptors begin to degenerate. After 8 weeks, all photoreceptors are gone. The *rd3* mutation could be assigned to Chromosome 1 in mice, in a region that is homologous to the region of the human Chromosome 1q. Usher syndrome type IIA has been linked to this chromosome mutation. Figure 20 shows an *rd3* mutation with a milder fundus degeneration at 7 months of age (19).

Slower rod degeneration is found in the *rds* mouse (retinal degeneration slow), where the gene defect is located on chromosome 17 (allele *Prph2^{Rd2}*). In this model, both photoreceptor outer segments are affected. Degeneration proceeds over a time frame of 9–12 months with a corresponding slow fundus alteration (19, 41).

Cone photoreceptor function loss 1 (*cpfl1*) mutation on chromosome 19 does not affect the retinal fundus phenotype (Fig. 18). A pathologic ERG appears from 3 weeks of age. With aging, the number of viable cone photoreceptors diminishes. Rods are unaffected. *Achromatopsia*, a congenital color vision disorder with reduced visual acuity, is determined by cone photoreceptor degeneration (19).

RPE65-deficiency in mice (*RPE65^{-/-}*) leads to a blockage in the visual cycle with accumulation of all-trans-retinyl esters and absence of 11-*cis*-retinal and rhodopsin. Rod photoreceptor degeneration develops. *RPE65* mutations account for 10% of Leber congenital amourosis (42). Accumulated retinyl esters form large lipid droplets with a strong autofluorescence and are visible in the autofluorescence mode in the cSLO (43).

The progression of photoreceptor degeneration can in general be monitored by OCT in vivo.

A further development is the combination of the presented mouse models. Combination of genetically modified mouse models with manually induced pathologies, for example laser application for induction of CNV in CX3CR1 knock-in mice, enables the investigation of the role of these immune cells in a CNV model. Immune cell behavior in the pathologic model of CNV can be studied (20). Same can be done in an ROP mouse model.

4. Notes

1. Variation of the CNV size in the models of laser-induced neovascularization

   The optical properties of a mouse eye and of all other rodents are different from those of a human eye. Due to the relatively short axial bulb length (anterior–posterior mouse bulb length about 3.02 mm; anterior–posterior human bulb length about 24.00 mm) (44), mice need a highly refractive lens, and they have a spherical lens that fills almost the whole eyecup. The vitreous constitutes only a thin layer with a volume of approximately 10 μl. Consequently, mice (and other small rodents) are very hyperopic. The imaging device has to be adjusted to this optical peculiarity. Therefore, a contact lens (+35 spherical diopters) can be put on the mouse cornea. Alternatively, when using the SPECTRALIS® high-resolution angiography and SD-OCT (HRA+OCT), an additional add-on lens (+25 spherical diopters) on top of the objective can be purchased. Difficulties may appear with an equal acuity of the whole image, as the steep concavity of the small posterior pole leads to unequal light reflectance from the retina back into the OCT device. Consequently, the outer lane of one OCT slice might be not as clear as the center of the image. Therefore, it is sometimes beneficial, particularly with the OCT, to choose a smaller window image and though avoid distinct light scattering

It is not possible to simultaneously display infrared images and OCT sections in the mouse with the SPECTRALIS® HRA+OCT in its basic configuration. The challenge is to match the length of the reference arm to the length of the sample arm within the mouse eye. In the OCT debug window, which can be opened by pressing the keys *Ctrl Alt Shift O* at the same time, you can adjust the reference arm for a focussed OCT image parallel to a focussed infrared image (Fig. 19).

During the whole imaging procedure, the cornea should regularly be moistened with artificial tears.

2. Evaluation of neovascularization size
   The variation of parameters of the laser beam leads to a variation of induced CNV area size (21). The variation of the focus plane of the laser beam on the retina leads to different spot sizes and can therefore be responsible for different morphological and functional changes. Due to the anatomic structure of the eye, the laser beam does not reach the fundus in an exact vertical angle, but might impinge slightly tilted on the retinal fundus. Thereby, the energy is not equally distributed in the area of the laser and the laser spot becomes distorted.

3. ICG angiography in mice
   The differences in the extent of CNV between different animals and/or different therapeutic approaches can be evaluated either in vivo with the fluorescence angiography or ex vivo in choroidal and/or retinal flatmounts. Marneros et al. developed a grading system of four gradations for fluorescein angiography (45):

   Grade 0: Lesions without hyperfluorescence.

   Grade 1: Lesions exhibit hyperfluorescence without leakage.

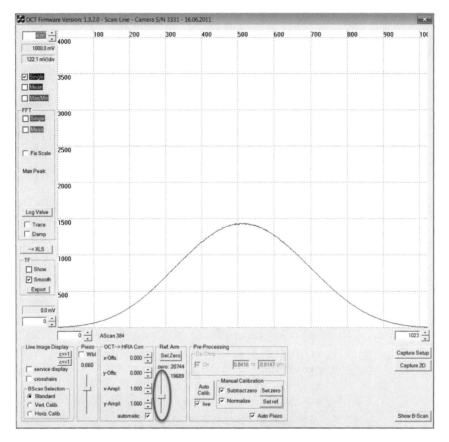

Fig. 19. OCT debug window opened by simultaneously pressing the key combination "Ctrl Alt Shift 0".

Grade 2A: Lesions exhibit hyperfluorescence in the early or midtransit images and late leakage.

Grade 2B: Lesions show bright hyperfluorescence in the transit images and late leakage beyond treated areas (grade 2B lesions are defined as clinically significant).

The relative distribution of fluorescein angiographic grades for CNV lesions was determined within each experimental group of mice. In the case of confluent CNV lesions, the same fluorescein angiographic grade should be assigned for all lesions within the confluent hyperfluorescent area (45, 46).

4. Imaging of rodents

Fundus color imaging in small rodents, especially in mice, is a challenge to the present imaging tools. The difficulty in the proper conduction of color fundus images with cameras constructed for the human eye is the large area of illumination. This illumination area has to be reduced on a size equal or smaller to the dilated mouse pupil (around 3–4 mm). Otherwise,

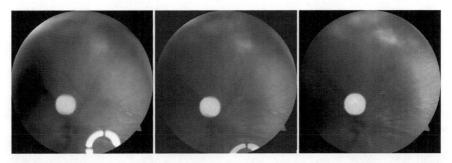

Fig. 20. Mouse fundus of a C57Bl/6 mouse. Light reflections are visible on the fundus image. By variation of the position of the Volk 20D lens, reflections can be reduced (images were taken by Constantin E. Uhlig, University Hospital Muenster, Department of Ophthalmology, Muenster, Germany).

the reflected light cannot emerge from the eye. A non-mydriatic fundus camera has the advantage that it uses a focussed light beam. It is possible to extend into the eye also through small pupils. Anyway, light reflections by other tissues, especially by the cornea, occur. These are hard to avoid. It is important to choose the optimal angle to take the pictures so that the reflection circle shifts into the periphery of the image. Also, the Volk 20D lens, which is held in front of the objective, should be varied slightly in its position to reduce light reflections (Fig. 20). Afterwards, improvements can be made with image software (e.g., Photoshop®).

5. Fundus color imaging

   With the ICG dye, at all less leakage occurs compared to fluorescein angiography because of its very high affinity to plasma protein binding (98%) (43). Choroidal vessels are pictured more detailed but the resolution of retinal vessel morphology declines. In our experience, the amount of injected dye volume is similar to fluorescein. Both dyes are metabolized and excreted by the kidney.

References

1. van Leeuwen R et al (2003) Epidemiology of age-related maculopathy: a review. Eur J Epidemiol 18:845–854

2. Grossniklaus HE et al (2010) Animal models of choroidal and retinal neovascularization. Prog Retin Eye Res 29:500–519

3. Barber AJ (2003) A new view of diabetic retinopathy: a neurodegenerative disease of the eye. Prog Neuropsychopharmacol Biol Psychiatry 27:283–290

4. Joussen AM et al (2003) Molecular mechanisms of vasculogenesis and angiogenesis. What regulates vascular growth? Ophthalmologe 100: 284–291

5. Sharp PF, Manivannan A (1997) The scanning laser ophthalmoscope. Phys Med Biol 42: 951–966

6. Paques M et al (2007) Panretinal, high-resolution color photography of the mouse fundus. Invest Ophthalmol Vis Sci 48:2769–2774

7. Bermudez MA et al (2011) Time course of cold cataract development in anesthetized mice. Curr Eye Res 36:278–284

8. Terman A (2006) Catabolic insufficiency and aging. Ann N Y Acad Sci 1067:27–36

9. Brunk UT, Terman A (2002) Lipofuscin: mechanisms of age-related accumulation and influence on cell function. Free Radic Biol Med 33:611–619

10. Seehafer SS, Pearce DA (2006) You say lipofuscin, we say ceroid: defining autofluorescent storage material. Neurobiol Aging 27: 576–588

11. Eldred GE et al (1982) Lipofuscin: resolution of discrepant fluorescence data. Science 216: 757–759

12. Marmorstein AD et al (2002) Spectral profiling of autofluorescence associated with lipofuscin, Bruch's Membrane, and sub-RPE deposits in normal and AMD eyes. Invest Ophthalmol Vis Sci 43:2435–2441

13. Eldred GE, Lasky MR (1993) Retinal age pigments generated by self-assembling lysosomotropic detergents. Nature 361:724–726

14. Sparrow JR et al (1999) A2E, a lipofuscin fluorophore, in human retinal pigmented epithelial cells in culture. Invest Ophthalmol Vis Sci 40:2988–2995

15. Schmitz-Valckenberg S et al (2008) Fundus autofluorescence imaging: review and perspectives. Retina 28:385–409

16. Bridges CD (1977) Rhodopsin regeneration in rod outer segments: utilization of 11-cis retinal and retinol. Exp Eye Res 24:571–580

17. Jaffe GJ, Caprioli J (2004) Optical coherence tomography to detect and manage retinal disease and glaucoma. Am J Ophthalmol 137:156–169

18. Hawes NL et al (1999) Mouse fundus photography and angiography: a catalogue of normal and mutant phenotypes. Mol Vis 5:22

19. Chang B et al (2002) Retinal degeneration mutants in the mouse. Vision Res 42:517–525

20. Eter N et al (2008) In vivo visualization of dendritic cells, macrophages, and microglial cells responding to laser-induced damage in the fundus of the eye. Invest Ophthalmol Vis Sci 49:3649–3658

21. Tobe T et al (1998) Evolution of neovascularization in mice with overexpression of vascular endothelial growth factor in photoreceptors. Invest Ophthalmol Vis Sci 39:180–188

22. Smith LE et al (1994) Oxygen-induced retinopathy in the mouse. Invest Ophthalmol Vis Sci 35:101–111

23. Spilsbury K et al (2000) Overexpression of vascular endothelial growth factor (VEGF) in the retinal pigment epithelium leads to the development of choroidal neovascularization. Am J Pathol 157:135–144

24. Schmack I et al (2009) Modulation of choroidal neovascularization by subretinal injection of retinal pigment epithelium and polystyrene microbeads. Mol Vis 15:146–161

25. Shen D et al (2006) Exacerbation of retinal degeneration and choroidal neovascularization induced by subretinal injection of matrigel in CCL2/MCP-1-deficient mice. Ophthalmic Res 38:71–73

26. Giove TJ et al (2009) Increased neuronal nitric oxide synthase activity in retinal neurons in early diabetic retinopathy. Mol Vis 15:2249–2258

27. Zhu SS et al (2011) Wld (S) protects against peripheral neuropathy and retinopathy in an experimental model of diabetes in mice. Diabetologia 54(9):2440–2450

28. Kern TS et al (2010) Validation of structural and functional lesions of diabetic retinopathy in mice. Mol Vis 16:2121–2131

29. Larina IV et al (2009) A membrane associated mCherry fluorescent reporter line for studying vascular remodeling and cardiac function during murine embryonic development. Anat Rec (Hoboken) 292:333–341

30. Poche RA et al (2009) The Flk1-myr::mCherry mouse as a useful reporter to characterize multiple aspects of ocular blood vessel development and disease. Dev Dyn 238:2318–2326

31. Jung S et al (2000) Analysis of fractalkine receptor CX(3)CR1 function by targeted deletion and green fluorescent protein reporter gene insertion. Mol Cell Biol 20:4106–4114

32. Kuziel WA et al (1997) Severe reduction in leukocyte adhesion and monocyte extravasation in mice deficient in CC chemokine receptor 2. Proc Natl Acad Sci USA 94:12053–12058

33. Ambati J et al (2003) An animal model of age-related macular degeneration in senescent Ccl-2- or Ccr-2-deficient mice. Nat Med 9:1390–1397

34. Tuo J et al (2007) Murine ccl2/cx3cr1 deficiency results in retinal lesions mimicking human age-related macular degeneration. Invest Ophthalmol Vis Sci 48:3827–3836

35. Takeda A et al (2009) CCR3 is a target for age-related macular degeneration diagnosis and therapy. Nature 460:225–230

36. Malek G et al (2005) Apolipoprotein E allele-dependent pathogenesis: a model for age-related retinal degeneration. Proc Natl Acad Sci USA 102:11900–11905

37. Okamoto N et al (1997) Transgenic mice with increased expression of vascular endothelial growth factor in the retina: a new model of intraretinal and subretinal neovascularization. Am J Pathol 151:281–291

38. Heckenlively JR et al (2003) Mouse model of subretinal neovascularization with choroidal anastomosis. Retina 23:518–522

39. Won J et al (2011) Mouse model resources for vision research. J Ophthalmol 2011:391384

40. Huber G et al (2009) Spectral domain optical coherence tomography in mouse models of retinal degeneration. Invest Ophthalmol Vis Sci 50:5888–5895

41. Kohler K et al (1997) Animal models for retinitis pigmentosa research. Klin Monbl Augenheilkd 211:84–93

42. Van Hooser JP et al (2000) Rapid restoration of visual pigment and function with oral retinoid in a mouse model of childhood blindness. Proc Natl Acad Sci USA 97:8623–8628

43. Seeliger MW et al (2005) In vivo confocal imaging of the retina in animal models using scanning laser ophthalmoscopy. Vision Res 45:3512–3519

44. de la Cera EG et al (2006) Optical aberrations in the mouse eye. Vision Res 46:2546–2553

45. Marneros AG et al (2007) Endogenous endostatin inhibits choroidal neovascularization. FASEB J 21:3809–3818

46. Sheets KG et al (2010) Neuroprotectin D1 attenuates laser-induced choroidal neovascularization in mouse. Mol Vis 16:320–329

Chapter 4

Functional Phenotyping of Mouse Models with ERG

Naoyuki Tanimoto, Vithiyanjali Sothilingam, and Mathias W. Seeliger

Abstract

In many situations it is important to be able to assess the degree of retinal function, e.g., for the characterization of mouse models with unknown retinal involvement, when studying degenerative processes, for the
analysis of visual signal processing, and during the follow-up of therapeutic interventions. Full-field
electroretinography (ERG), yielding a sum response of event-related transient electrical activity of the
entire retina to light stimulation, is widely applied in human as well as experimental functional diagnostics.
ERG examinations normally include initial dark-adapted (scotopic) measurements that enable rod-driven
activity to be studied, followed by light-adapted (photopic) recordings to obtain information about cone
system contributions. The results allow the correlation of acute or long-term disease-related changes or
their alleviation by therapy with morphological data, in order to obtain a comprehensive understanding of
the underlying processes and mechanisms.

Key words: Electroretinography, Rod, Cone, Single flash, Flicker, Mouse

1. Introduction

Due to recent advances in molecular biology, a variety of animal
models have been established for use in basic research, and today,
major advances in the understanding of human retinal disorders
are based on such animal models carrying identical genetic defects.
Subsequent to the generation of an animal model, a thorough
characterization is the first indispensable step to confirm that it has
a phenotype comparable to the corresponding human disease (1, 2).
Once established, therapeutic interventions may be designed and
their effects evaluated (3–5) after or in parallel with the investigation of pathophysiological mechanisms of the disease. The use of
corresponding test methods allows a direct comparison of the phenotypes of animal models and human diseases. Electroretinography
(ERG) is an established and standardized functional diagnostic
method in humans (6) which provides objective information about

Bernhard H.F. Weber and Thomas Langmann (eds.), *Retinal Degeneration: Methods and Protocols*, Methods in Molecular Biology,
vol. 935, DOI 10.1007/978-1-62703-080-9_4, © Springer Science+Business Media, LLC 2013

retinal activity following a flash of light, and which can also be applied to mice noninvasively under anesthesia. ERG data in mice are generally well comparable to those in humans, providing a strong link between basic research and clinical findings in many retinal disorders. In our laboratory, many genetically engineered mouse models have been examined with ERG using white full-field (Ganzfeld) stimulation. According to our experience, several important aspects should be considered when recording mouse full-field ERG in order to assess retinal functional phenotype properly. Such aspects, as well as details of the experimental procedure in our laboratory, are described in this chapter.

2. Materials

2.1. Equipment

1. Ganzfeld ERG system, composed of a light source for stimulation, a Ganzfeld bowl, a signal amplification system, a PC-based control and recording unit, and a monitor screen (see Notes 1 and 2).

2. Two active electrodes (e.g., Ring electrode made of gold wire) (see Note 3).

3. Two short needle electrodes: For a reference and a ground electrode.

4. Heating pad: For control of body temperature of the anesthetized mouse during ERG measurements.

5. Small box on which the anesthetized mouse lies and the subsequent preparations, such as positioning of electrodes, are made: A heating pad is fixed on top of the box. It is ideal if a transparent plastic plate protrudes from the front edge of the box on which the mouse head is placed, in order to allow equal amounts of stimulus light to reach the eyes from all directions.

6. Two arms, each of which is composed of multiple segments and joints: They are attached to the small box described above, and each arm features an active electrode at the free end. Active electrodes can be controlled in all three dimensions of space precisely through the joints of each arm.

7. A long plastic plate, on which the small box slides: This plate has to be fixed horizontally, because it guides the small box into the center of the Ganzfeld bowl.

2.2. Other Materials

1. Mydriatic (e.g., tropicamide eye drops) (see Note 4).

2. Methylcellulose: For corneal surface protection.

3. Anesthetics (e.g., ketamine and xylazine).

4. Normal saline (0.9% NaCl).

5. Large syringe (e.g., 10 ml syringe): For mixture of anesthetics and saline.

6. Small syringe and narrow needle (e.g., 1 ml syringe and 27 gauge needle): For subcutaneous injection of mixed anesthetic solution.

7. Balance scale, which can measure to the first decimal place in gram.

8. Mouse cage and cage lid.

9. Large container with lid, in which mouse cages are put, and a dark-colored thick cloth/curtain that can cover the container: For maintenance of dark adaptation of mice independent of surrounding light conditions.

2.3. Mice

1. Since several potentially influential parameters may change over time, control animals should be included in every set of measurements. The best controls are littermates from heterozygote breeding pairs so that the genetic background and the raising conditions are the same. Only the gene of interest is different (see Note 5).

2. Examination time point (mouse age) is chosen depending on the question to be answered. For the analysis of a primary change due to a genetic defect/modification, 4-week-old mice are ideal, because retinal development is usually complete up to that age but no secondary change, i.e., degeneration, has yet taken place in most cases, even when rod outer segments are completely abolished by rod opsin knockout (7) (see Note 6). The examination of older mice is predominantly valuable for the detection and analysis of an ongoing retinal degeneration (8–11).

3. Methods

3.1. One Day Before Examination

1. Check information of the mouse list and compare it with actual mouse marks/numbers, e.g., ear clip, ear mark, finger mark, and finger tattoo. It is much more difficult to identify a particular mouse before anesthesia in the dark under a dim red light. Therefore, if necessary, mark the tail with a black marker additionally so that you can identify each mouse without any difficulty in the dark.

2. Make the room completely dark for an overnight dark adaptation (longer than 6 h), which usually allows the examination of the maximal performance of the rod system. "Completely dark" means that after ca. 20 min in the room you still consider it dark yourself. Make sure that you can enter/leave the room without light entering it, to avoid interfering with the dark adaptation process.

3.2. Preparation for ERG Recordings

1. Put all mouse cages into a large container under a dim red light, put a lid on the container, and cover the whole container with a dark-colored thick cloth/curtain. Dark adaptation of all mice is thus maintained independent of surrounding light conditions.

2. Turn on the room light. Switch on the equipment and the heating pad. Prepare anesthetic solution. In our laboratory, ketamine and xylazine are diluted with normal saline in a 10 ml syringe which are given subcutaneously at 66.7 mg/kg body weight and 11.7 mg/kg body weight, respectively (see Note 7).

3. Turn off the room light. All procedures until the end of preparation have to be done under a dim red light, in order to preserve dark adaptation.

4. Open the container, and select a mouse to examine (see Note 8).

5. Measure the body weight of the mouse, and calculate the amount of anesthetic solution to be given to the mouse.

6. Inject the anesthetic solution into the mouse subcutaneously.

7. Put the mouse into a cage, and cover it with a cage lid (see Note 9). Wait until the mouse is unconscious.

8. Apply mydriatic eye drops to both eyes, and wait until the pupils are dilated. The duration depends on the type of mydriatic. We use tropicamide eye drops (Mydriaticum Stulln, Pharma Stulln, Stulln, Germany), and wait for 3 min until the next step.

9. Place the anesthetized mouse on the small box. The mouse body should be placed on the heating pad to stabilize the body temperature, whereas the mouse head should be positioned on a transparent plate so that the eyes are stimulated uniformly from all directions (see Note 10).

10. Apply two needle electrodes (Fig. 1b, center) subcutaneously at the middle of the forehead region and the back near the tail as a reference and a ground electrode, respectively. Check each impedance.

11. Moisten active electrodes (Fig. 1b, right) with methylcellulose, and position them on the surface of both corneae (see Notes 11 and 12).

12. Slide the small box carefully into the Ganzfeld bowl (Fig. 1a) so that the mouse eyes are placed well into the center of it.

13. Wait for 1 min in the dark. During this period, all impedances as well as fluctuation of the signal baseline should be checked to confirm that the preparations have been made properly.

14. Start ERG recordings.

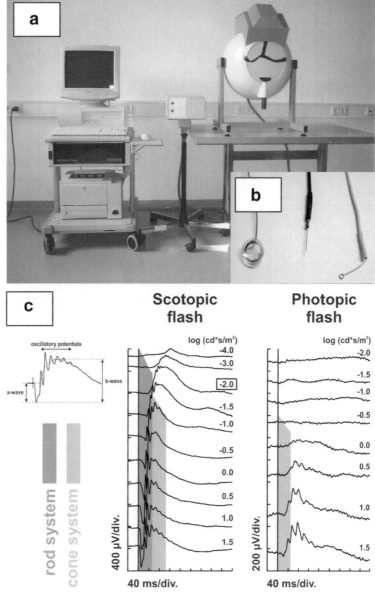

Fig. 1. (**a**) Ganzfeld ERG recording unit (here: Jaeger/Toennies Multiliner Vision). The Ganzfeld (full-field) bowl on the right comes with a chin rest that may be replaced with a table for mouse positioning. *In the center*, the preamplifier is visible (2 channels: one for the *left* and one for the *right eye*). The main unit used for the control of sequences and settings, recording and storing of data, and evaluation of results is shown on the *left*. (**b**) Typical electrode types used in animal recordings. *From the left*: Jet electrode (plastic contact lens with inside ring of gold coating) usually used in larger animals, atraumatic needle electrode used for reference and ground, and gold ring electrode for mice. (**c**) Basic murine ERG recording. *Left*: Sketch of ERG waveform and reference lines for evaluation. *Center*: Scotopic (*dark adapted*) recording series in a normal C57BL/6 mouse. *Right*: Photopic (*light adapted*) recording series in the same mouse. *The dark* and *light gray areas* indicate contributions of the rod and cone system, respectively. (Important note: This may be altered in disease models.) The square around −2.0 log cd × s/m² indicates that up to this intensity only the rod system contributes to the waveform.

3.3. ERG Recording Protocols

In this section, we describe four recording protocols, which we routinely use in the first examinations of retinal activity, i.e., with mice of unknown retinal phenotype. Single flash protocols (Fig. 1c) are considered a minimum requirement. It takes about 1 h to measure one mouse with all four protocols.

1. Dark-adapted (scotopic) single flash intensity series (Fig. 1c, left): Stimulus intensities for this series are -4.0, -3.0, -2.0, -1.5, -1.0, -0.5, -0.0, 0.5, 1.0, and 1.5 log cd$\times$s/m^2. Ten responses are averaged with interstimulus intervals of 5 or 17 s (for $0-1.5$ log cd$\times$s/m^2), in order to minimize fluctuations of the baseline and increase the signal-to-noise ratio. Band-pass filter cutoff frequencies are 0.3 and 300 Hz, as described as the least range for the human standard ERGs (6).

2. Scotopic flicker frequency series at the International Society for Clinical Electrophysiology of Vision (ISCEV) standard flash (SF) intensity (0.5 log cd$\times$s/m^2) (6): Stimulus frequencies for this series are 0.5, 1, 2, 3, 5, 7, 10, 12, 15, 18, 20, and 30 Hz. Flicker responses are averaged either 20 times (for 0.5–3 Hz) or 30 times (for 5 Hz and above).

3. Light adaptation: A 10-min exposure of a static background light of 30 cd/m^2.

4. Light-adapted (photopic; on a 30 cd/m^2 background light) single flash intensity series (Fig. 1c, right): The lowest intensity in this protocol is -2.0 log cd$\times$s/m^2. Other parameters are the same as those in the scotopic single flash intensity series.

5. Photopic flicker frequency series at the ISCEV SF intensity: Parameters except for the background light are the same as those in the scotopic SF flicker frequency series (see Note 13).

3.4. ERG Response Analysis

An ERG response (see Fig. 1c for a sketch) typically begins with a photoreceptor-initiated negative deflection, termed the a-wave. The following positive deflection, the b-wave, reflects the activity of depolarizing (ON-) bipolar cells (for further details about origins of ERG components, see (12)). Rod and cone system contributions to the single flash and the SF flicker ERG responses have also been described for mice with regular rod sensitivity to light (13). The contributions are altered in mice with strongly desensitized rods. In such a case, a proper functional diagnosis with ERG may be achieved by cross-breeding with functionally specific models (14, 15).

1. Measure amplitude and latency of single flash ERG responses: b-wave analysis is generally a good starting point to check overall retinal functionality, because ON-bipolar cell responses are dependent on photoreceptor activities (see Note 14).

2. Measure amplitude of flicker ERG responses (see Note 15).

3. Plot the amplitude and the latency data on a graph: Data should not be presented with mean and standard deviation, if it cannot be assumed that they are normally distributed. In our experience, the 5, 25, 50 (median), 75, and 95% quantiles, presented by box-and-whisker plot, provide a good overview of the data distribution.

4. Choose a representative response series from each group, and make an overlay of the responses: In this overlay analysis, response configurations can be compared, i.e., it is a qualitative analysis. This analysis is indispensable, because the time course of the voltage change cannot be fully analyzed and described only by the statistical analysis of the response peaks (1, 13, 16, 17).

4. Notes

1. ERG systems produced commercially for clinical application can be used for mouse ERG. They should however comply with the current industrial standard issued by the ISCEV.

2. Additional light sources and control systems may be combined with the basic ERG system for an in-depth analysis. We added a strobe flash lamp (Mecablitz 60CT4 flash gun, Metz, Germany) for bright flash experiments and paired-flash ERG, as well as an ON–OFF light pulse unit.

3. ERG recording from both eyes is valuable especially for evaluation of therapeutic effects, because the contralateral eye may be used as an internal control if not treated (3–5).

4. Phenylephrine and/or atropine eye drops can also be used.

5. We use a minimum of four mutants and four controls in the first experiment. This allows us to examine all mice in one day and to see a tendency of alteration of retinal functionality in mutants.

6. There are a few exceptions, e.g., the *rd1* mouse, in which retinal degeneration starts at around postnatal day 11 and the outer retina is usually completely destroyed at the age of 4–5 weeks (18, 19). The same deleterious mutation is also present in the C3H strain.

7. Mixtures of ketamine and xylazine are not stable; therefore, once mixed, they should be used within a day.

8. Since several parameters are changing even within a day, control and mutant mice should be analyzed alternately, not in a blind fashion. Usually, a control mouse is used for the first measurement of the day in order to detect any unexpected problems regarding animal conditions, equipment conditions, or effectiveness of mydriatic and anesthetic.

9. As mice sometimes jump heavily during the excitement stage of anesthesia in the vertical direction higher than the cage, it should be covered with a cage lid. Similarly, mice topple many times before they go to sleep and during the wake-up period; therefore, do not cover the bottom of the cage with any bedding to avoid corneal injury. In our laboratory, we cover the bottom of the cage with a disposable soft paper towel.

10. Try to control everything symmetrically from this step, which is important for equal stimulation of both retinae.

11. The spatial relationship between active electrode and cornea is quite important, because it influences the noise level as well as the fluctuation of the signal baseline. Check the impedance during the positioning of the active electrodes. Large impedances usually mean an inadequate contact between active electrode and cornea, whereas too small impedances suggest that the electrode might press the corneal surface too strongly, which may cause insufficient ocular circulation.

12. The position of the active electrode does not have to be final immediately. It is even better to repeat the procedure from the right and the left side alternately, which results in an optimized symmetrical balance between the right and the left side.

13. We sometimes perform photopic bright flash experiments directly after this photopic flicker frequency series to answer a specific question (8, 15, 17).

14. The maximal positive excursion immediately following the a-wave may not resemble the peak of b-wave. In our laboratory, an imaginary curve (see Fig. 1c, left) is fitted to approximately run through the midpoints between adjacent minimum and maximum of oscillations to account for the contribution of oscillations to the b-wave (13).

15. In the scotopic SF flicker frequency series, a- and b-wave analogues and oscillations of the b-wave analogue merge at very low frequencies with increasing flicker frequency. Therefore, unlike in the single flash ERG response analysis, the size of flicker responses is measured from the trough to the peak of each response so that all responses of the frequency series are analyzed using the same definition.

Acknowledgements

We thank Anne Kurtenbach for critical reading of the manuscript. This work was supported by the Deutsche Forschungsgemeinschaft (DFG, grants KFO134-Se837/5-2 and Se837/6-1) to M.W.S., and the Kerstan Foundation to N.T.

References

1. Biel M, Seeliger M, Pfeifer A, Kohler K, Gerstner A, Ludwig A, Jaissle G, Fauser S, Zrenner E, Hofmann F (1999) Selective loss of cone function in mice lacking the cyclic nucleotide-gated channel CNG3. Proc Natl Acad Sci U S A 96:7553–7557

2. Weber BH, Schrewe H, Molday LL, Gehrig A, White KL, Seeliger MW, Jaissle GB, Friedburg C, Tamm E, Molday RS (2002) Inactivation of the murine X-linked juvenile retinoschisis gene, Rs1h, suggests a role of retinoschisin in retinal cell layer organization and synaptic structure. Proc Natl Acad Sci U S A 99: 6222–6227

3. Min SH, Molday LL, Seeliger MW, Dinculescu A, Timmers AM, Janssen A, Tonagel F, Tanimoto N, Weber BH, Molday RS, Hauswirth WW (2005) Prolonged recovery of retinal structure/function after gene therapy in an Rs1h-deficient mouse model of x-linked juvenile retinoschisis. Mol Ther 12:644–651

4. Janssen A, Min SH, Molday LL, Tanimoto N, Seeliger MW, Hauswirth WW, Molday RS, Weber BH (2008) Effect of late-stage therapy on disease progression in AAV-mediated rescue of photoreceptor cells in the retinoschisin-deficient mouse. Mol Ther 16:1010–1017

5. Michalakis S, Mühlfriedel R, Tanimoto N, Krishnamoorthy V, Koch S, Fischer MD, Becirovic E, Bai L, Huber G, Beck SC, Fahl E, Büning H, Paquet-Durand F, Zong X, Gollisch T, Biel M, Seeliger MW (2010) Restoration of cone vision in the CNGA3-/- mouse model of congenital complete lack of cone photoreceptor function. Mol Ther 18:2057–2063

6. Marmor MF, Holder GE, Seeliger MW, Yamamoto S (2004) Standard for clinical electroretinography (2004 update). Doc Ophthalmol 108:107–114

7. Jaissle GB, May CA, Reinhard J, Kohler K, Fauser S, Lütjen-Drecoll E, Zrenner E, Seeliger MW (2001) Evaluation of the rhodopsin knockout mouse as a model of pure cone function. Invest Ophthalmol Vis Sci 42:506–513

8. Wenzel A, von Lintig J, Oberhauser V, Tanimoto N, Grimm C, Seeliger MW (2007) RPE65 is essential for the function of cone photoreceptors in NRL-deficient mice. Invest Ophthalmol Vis Sci 48:534–542

9. Samardzija M, von Lintig J, Tanimoto N, Oberhauser V, Thiersch M, Remé CE, Seeliger M, Grimm C, Wenzel A (2008) R91W mutation in Rpe65 leads to milder early-onset retinal dystrophy due to the generation of low levels of 11-cis-retinal. Hum Mol Genet 17:281–292

10. Beck SC, Schaeferhoff K, Michalakis S, Fischer MD, Huber G, Rieger N, Riess O, Wissinger B, Biel M, Bonin M, Seeliger MW, Tanimoto N (2010) In vivo analysis of cone survival in mice. Invest Ophthalmol Vis Sci 51:493–497

11. Lange C, Heynen SR, Tanimoto N, Thiersch M, Le YZ, Meneau I, Seeliger MW, Samardzija M, Caprara C, Grimm C (2011) Normoxic activation of hypoxia inducible factors in photoreceptors provides transient protection against light-induced retinal degeneration. Invest Ophthalmol Vis Sci 52:5872–5880

12. Frishman LJ (2006) Origins of the electroretinogram. In: Heckenlively JR, Arden GB (eds) Principles and practice of clinical electrophysiology of vision, 2nd edn. The MIT press, Massachusets, pp 139–183

13. Tanimoto N, Muehlfriedel RL, Fischer MD, Fahl E, Humphries P, Biel M, Seeliger MW (2009) Vision tests in the mouse: functional phenotyping with electroretinography. Front Biosci 14:2730–2737

14. Seeliger MW, Grimm C, Ståhlberg F, Friedburg C, Jaissle G, Zrenner E, Guo H, Remé CE, Humphries P, Hofmann F, Biel M, Fariss RN, Redmond TM, Wenzel A (2001) New views on RPE65 deficiency: the rod system is the source of vision in a mouse model of Leber congenital amaurosis. Nat Genet 29:70–74

15. Samardzija M, Tanimoto N, Kostic C, Beck S, Oberhauser V, Joly S, Thiersch M, Fahl E, Arsenijevic Y, von Lintig J, Wenzel A, Seeliger MW, Grimm C (2009) In conditions of limited chromophore supply rods entrap 11-cis-retinal leading to loss of cone function and cell death. Hum Mol Genet 18:1266–1275

16. Knop GC, Seeliger MW, Thiel F, Mataruga A, Kaupp UB, Friedburg C, Tanimoto N, Müller F (2008) Light responses in the mouse retina are prolonged upon targeted deletion of the HCN1 channel gene. Eur J Neurosci 28:2221–2230

17. Schaeferhoff K, Michalakis S, Tanimoto N, Fischer MD, Becirovic E, Beck SC, Huber G, Rieger N, Riess O, Wissinger B, Biel M, Seeliger MW, Bonin M (2010) Induction of STAT3-related genes in fast degenerating cone photoreceptors of cpfl1 mice. Cell Mol Life Sci 67:3173–3186

18. Sahaboglu A, Tanimoto N, Kaur J, Sancho-Pelluz J, Huber G, Fahl E, Arango-Gonzalez B, Zrenner E, Ekström P, Löwenheim H,

Seeliger M, Paquet-Durand F (2010) PARP1 gene knock-out increases resistance to retinal degeneration without affecting retinal function. PLoS One 5:e15495

19. Paquet-Durand F, Beck S, Michalakis S, Goldmann T, Huber G, Mühlfriedel R, Trifunović D, Fischer MD, Fahl E, Duetsch G, Becirovic E, Wolfrum U, van Veen T, Biel M, Tanimoto N, Seeliger MW (2011) A key role for cyclic nucleotide gated (CNG) channels in cGMP-related retinitis pigmentosa. Hum Mol Genet 20:941–947

Chapter 5

Phenotyping of Mouse Models with OCT

M. Dominik Fischer, Ahmad Zhour, and Christoph J. Kernstock

Abstract

Optical coherence tomography (OCT) is an invaluable technique to perform noninvasive retinal imaging in small animal models such as mice. It provides virtual cross sections that correlate well with histomorphometric data with the advantage that multiple iterative measurements can be acquired in time line analyses to detect dynamic changes and reduce the amount of animals needed per study.

Key words: Optical coherence tomography, Confocal scanning laser ophthalmoscopy, Retina, Animal models, Morphology

1. Introduction

Optical coherence tomography (OCT) has evolved over the past two decades to become an important diagnostic tool in clinical and experimental ophthalmology (1, 2). Advances in OCT technology provided the required resolution needed for small animal imaging and proved to be ideally suited for, e.g., studying changes of retinal integrity in mouse models of retinal disorders (3).

Morphometric assessment was traditionally performed ex vivo using light and electron microscopy providing (ultra-)high structural resolution. However, fixation and handling protocols are potential sources for variance in terms of tissue integrity and dimensions. In vivo analyses provide significant benefits as delicate, but functionally important changes such as edema formation or focal detachments can readily be detected while potentially being misinterpreted or masked by handling procedures in histologic analysis (4). First digital in vivo imaging techniques in small laboratory animals were based on confocal scanning laser ophthalmoscopy (cSLO) providing en face images with limited depth resolution (5). Benefits of cSLO imaging stem from the use of different light sources and barrier filters to specifically investigate autofluorescence patterns, perform

Bernhard H.F. Weber and Thomas Langmann (eds.), *Retinal Degeneration: Methods and Protocols*, Methods in Molecular Biology, vol. 935, DOI 10.1007/978-1-62703-080-9_5, © Springer Science+Business Media, LLC 2013

angiography, or analyze retinal nerve fibers. Combination of these en face modalities with OCT imaging now allows for a noninvasive, detailed phenotypic analysis of small animal models such as mice. Because individual animals may be investigated at multiple time points, OCT imaging can also help to reduce the number of animals needed for each study.

2. Materials

2.1. OCT Device

There are currently multiple devices commercially available featuring spectral domain OCT technology for diagnostic purposes. Among them are Spectralis® HRA + OCT (Heidelberg Engineering), Cirrus™ HD-OCT (Carl Zeiss Meditec, Inc.), Spectral OCT/SLO (Opko/OTI, Inc.), SOCT Copernicus HR (OPTOPOL Technologies S. A.), RTVue-100 (Optovue Corporation), and Envisu R4300 (Bioptigen Inc.). Currently, only the Spectralis™ platform allows simultaneous cSLO recordings with precise realignment of the retina during and in between OCT recordings (automatic real-time and follow-up modes, respectively). In the following, the protocol specifically describes the use of the Spectralis™ platform. Please contact the provider of other devices on how to adapt for the differences where appropriate.

2.2. Equipment to Adapt the OCT for Animal Use

1. Commercially available chinrest replacement for use in laboratory animals. If such a chinrest is not available, use a separate table or manufacture a custom chinrest replacement mounting plate (for this drill two holes of 13 mm diameter into a plate, with centers 28.8 cm apart; these dimensions may be subject to change in future models).

2. XYZ-table (mountable on the chinrest replacement).

3. Optional: Heat mat to maintain body temperature during anesthesia.

4. 78 dpt standard ophthalmologic non-contact slit lamp lens, e.g., Volk 78D (Volk Optical Inc., Ohio, USA).

5. Aspherical collimator lens: 100 dpt, 6.28 mm diameter, e.g., Philips CAX100 (IMM Photonics Ltd, Unterschleissheim, Germany).

2.3. Drugs

1. Anesthesia: Subcutaneous injection of ketamine (Bayer AG, Leverkusen, Germany) and xylazine (Bela-Pharm, Vechta, Germany).

2. Mydriasis: Tropicamide eye drops 5 mg/ml (Mydriaticum Stulln, Pharma Stulln, Stulln, Germany).

3. Hydroxypropylmethylcellulose (Methocel®) 2 % to negate the refractive power of the air corneal interface and reduce the risk of corneal dehydration.

3. Methods

3.1. Device Modifications

Prior to acquisition, some modifications are necessary to adapt the device from human use to mouse use (Fig. 1).

1. Remove the regular headrest and the chinrest if already installed. Install the chinrest replacement.

2. Mount the XYZ-table to the special chinrest replacement. If not available, the XYZ-table can be fixed to a separate table. Place the entire construction in front of the OCT-System so that the XYZ-table is positioned approximately at the same height with the camera lens.

3. Fixate the 78 dpt lens to the front element of the camera head (i.e., directly to the outlet of the device, see Notes 1–2).

4. Disconnect the cable for left/right eye detection. Manually choose left or right eye when starting the software.

3.2. Preparing the Animal

To achieve best results it is important to fully dilate the pupils of the animal and to ensure deep anesthesia with as little body movement due to heart beat and respiratory excursions as possible.

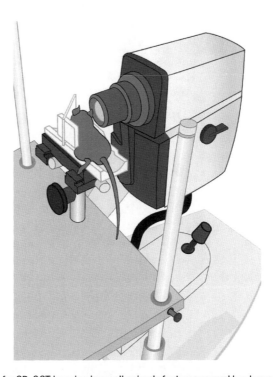

Fig. 1. Setup for SD-OCT imaging in small animals features several hardware adaptations. Mounted to the outlet of the camera head is a 78 dpt Volk lens for routine clinical biomicroscopy. The headrest for patients has been removed and a XYZ table with custom placement of mice fixed to the vertical columns attached to the instrument table.

Once the animal is anesthetized, care has to be taken to prevent cornea exposure/edema.

1. Anesthetize the mouse with ketamine (66.7 mg/kg body weight) and xylazine (11.7 mg/kg body weight) subcutaneous injection.

2. Apply the mydriatic eye drops to dilate the pupil. Complete mydriasis is achieved after 10 min.

3. Carefully wipe the eyelids with outward movements to remove eyelashes from the corneal surface.

4. Place one drop of Methocel onto the flat surface of the contact lens (see Note 3).

5. Gently press the contact lens centrally onto the eye with the Methocel between cornea and lens while holding the eyelids apart (see Note 4).

6. Drop some Methocel on the other eye to prevent corneal exposure (see Notes 5–6).

7. Place the mouse onto the XYZ-table, and adjust the head to align the longitudinal axis of the eye ("viewing direction") in line with the device's optic path (laser beam direction, see Note 7). Use a soft underlayment to minimize transmission of breathing movements to the head.

8. Optionally, use the heat mat to maintain body temperature.

3.3. Software and Device Settings

Please follow the hardware operating instructions of the manufacturer of the OCT system in use. If using the Spectralis® HRA + OCT the following steps and settings are advised:

1. Switch on the power supply and the laser box. The laser source will warm up (takes approx. 15 min) to provide a constant laser quality during the measurement.

2. Start the Heidelberg Eye Explorer Software (HEYEX™).

3. Create or open a "Patient File" for the animal. After entering the "Patient Data" an Eye Data Dialogue Box appears. It is important to enter the right value for cornea curvature ("C-Curve"). When using a contact lens that defines the air/subject interface, the value of the lens curvature should be entered (curvature of the recommended lens is 5.8 mm).

4. Start the laser with the Laser on/off button on the control panel. Switch to IR mode (Infrared Reflectance Imaging). A frame with a live image appears on the monitor.

5. Adjust the camera head, first start to center and focus the whole eye from a distance of about 5 cm. Slowly move the camera closer towards the eye; parts of the retina will appear on the screen. Continuously realign the XY position of the camera

head and readjust the focus until the distance to the contact lens is reduced to about 5 mm.

6. Pan and tilt the camera head until the optic nerve is centered in the frame.

7. Fine-tune the focus.

3.4. Image Acquisition Settings

For detailed instructions please read instructions provided by the manufacturer (see Note 8). When using the Spectralis® HRA + OCT system the following settings are advised for basic phenotypic analysis. However, a major strength of the noninvasive in vivo imaging is its versatility for screening and the option to adapt the analysis according to the phenotype (e.g., use of different imaging modalities and scan protocols).

1. IR mode.

2. Scan angle of 30°.

3. Manually adjustable image brightness control.

4. Reflection mode (turn the filter lever on the camera head to "R").

5. For Single IR fundus image acquisition press "Acquire."

6. To achieve averaged recordings with improved signal-to-noise ratio use the Automatic Real-Time (ART) mode. It averages an individually defined number of fundus images. An averaging of 16 frames reduces speckle noise by a factor of four.

7. When switching to Red Free mode, readjust the focus and the detector sensitivity.

8. When switching to autofluorescence mode, turn the filter lever on the camera head to "A."

The following settings are useful for initial OCT screening:

1. IR + OCT mode.

2. HR (high resolution) or HS (high speed) mode.

3. Line scan or volume scan.

4. Scan orientation (horizontal, vertical, or circular).

5. ART mode with defined no. of averaged frames.

Once the settings are defined follow the steps:

1. Start the ART mode by pressing the black dial on the touchscreen unit.

2. Wait until the grey bar in the ART setting has reached the chosen no. of averaged frames.

3. Press "acquire" on the touchscreen unit.

4. Leave the ART mode by pressing the black dial on the touchscreen unit and continue with 1. for additional scans.

5. Click "Exit" to exit and save the acquired scans to the database.

3.5. Data Analysis   Detailed analysis may be limited when using the proprietary software provided by the manufacturer (see Note 9). However, a number of third-party software programs are available for post hoc analysis.

1. The Heidelberg Eye Explorer Software (HEYEX) provides the option to determine retinal thickness based on segmentation lines. The software features an algorithm to automatically detect inner and outer retinal borders. Segmentation lines can be modified so that separate thickness measurements of the different retinal layers can be performed. However, there is no option to export the data for, e.g., statistical analysis.

2. Raw data export can be enabled in case of the Heidelberg Eye Explorer Software according to the manufacturer's instructions (please contact your local representative of the manufacturer for further information). These raw data can be further analyzed using the following ImageJ plugin (6): http://rsb.info. nih.gov/ij/plugins/heyex/index.html.

3. Raw data can also be imported into custom-designed Multi-Modal Mapping Software (7, 8). Multiple segmentation lines can be defined for detailed structural analysis and data exported for use in spreadsheet software.

4. Notes

1. Device modification: The Volk 78 dpt ophthalmic slit lamp lens has the same outer diameter as the lens barrel of the camera head. The 78 dpt lens can be mounted using a custom-made adaptor that holds the lens directly at the outlet. Alternatively, fixate the lens with tape for quick removal taking care to precisely align and center the optical pathways of the lens systems.

2. Care should be taken to regularly clean the camera objective lens, the 78 dpt, and the contact lens. Even small specks can produce significant alterations of high-resolution imaging data.

3. Stability of the contact lens is determined by the use of the right amount of Methocel. Too much Methocel on the contact lens makes it slide off and may spread to the front side of the lens. Too little Methocel may lead to air pockets between cornea and lens, thus disturbing the optical pathway and adhesion between lens and eye.

4. Take care to place the lens centrally on the mouse eye as precisely as possible. Otherwise the oblique optical pathway will cause distortion of the fundus image and lead to poor quality with a decentralized optic nerve head.

5. One may put contact lenses on both eyes at the same time when iterative examination of both eyes is necessary. This provides optimal protection of the cornea.

6. Contact lenses may be cleaned with 70 % (v/v) Ethanol for reuse.

7. As the animal has to be manipulated occasionally during image acquisition, the orientation of the camera base is preferably mounted in reverse orientation (i.e., "patient" and investigator on the same side).

8. The acquisition time per eye is limited by default settings. This can be canceled by changes in the heyex.ini file according to the manufacturer's instructions.

9. Note that raw data export is disabled in the latest HEYEX Software Version 5.3. Please contact the local representative of the manufacturer for further assistance.

Acknowledgements

The authors wish to acknowledge the continued support and mentoring by Drs. Zrenner, Bartz-Schmidt, Ueffing, and MacLaren.

References

1. Huang D, Swanson EA, Lin CP, Schuman JS, Stinson WG et al (1991) Optical coherence tomography. Science 254:1178–1181

2. Drexler W, Fujimoto JG (2008) State-of-the-art retinal optical coherence tomography. Prog Retin Eye Res 27:45–88

3. Huber G, Beck SC, Grimm C, Sahaboglu-Tekgoz A, Paquet-Durand F et al (2009) Spectral domain optical coherence tomography in mouse models of retinal degeneration. Invest Ophthalmol Vis Sci 50:5888–5895

4. Fischer MD, Huber G, Beck SC, Tanimoto N, Muehlfriedel R et al (2009) Noninvasive, in vivo assessment of mouse retinal structure using optical coherence tomography. PLoS One 4:e7507

5. Seeliger MW, Beck SC, Pereyra-Munoz N, Dangel S, Tsai JY et al (2005) In vivo confocal imaging of the retina in animal models using scanning laser ophthalmoscopy. Vision Res 45:3512–3519

6. Knott EJ, Sheets KG, Zhou Y, Gordon WC, Bazan NG (2011) Spatial correlation of mouse photoreceptor-RPE thickness between SD-OCT and histology. Exp Eye Res 92:155–160

7. Troeger E, Sliesoraityte I, Charbel Issa P, Scholl HN, Zrenner E et al (2010) An integrated software solution for multi-modal mapping of morphological and functional ocular data. Conf Proc IEEE Eng Med Biol Soc 2010:6280–6283

8. Charbel Issa P, Troeger E, Finger R, Holz FG, Wilke R et al (2010) Structure-function correlation of the human central retina. PLoS One 5:e12864

Chapter 6

Light Damage as a Model of Retinal Degeneration

Christian Grimm and Charlotte E. Remé

Abstract

The induction of retinal degeneration by light exposure is widely used to study mechanisms of cell death. The advantage of such light-induced lesions over genetically determined degenerations is that light exposures can be manipulated according to the needs of the experimenter. Bright white light exposure can induce a synchronized burst of apoptosis in photoreceptors in a large retinal area which permits to study cellular and molecular events in a controlled fashion. Blue light of high energy induces a hot spot of high retinal irradiance within very short exposure durations (seconds to minutes) and may help to unravel the initial events after light absorption which may be similar for all damage regimens. These initial events may then induce various molecular signaling pathways and secondary effects such as lipid and protein oxidation, which may be varying in different light damage setups and different strains or species, respectively. Blue light lesions also allow to study cellular responses in a circumscribed retinal area (hot spot) in comparison with the surrounding tissue.

Here we describe the methods for short-term exposures (within the hours range) to bright full-spectrum white light and for short exposures (seconds to minutes) to high-energy monochromatic blue or green light.

Key words: Light damage, White light setup, Blue light setup, Retinal degeneration, Apoptosis, Mouse, Rat, Visual pigment, Anesthesia, Monochromatic light

1. Introduction

Many animal models of inherited retinal degeneration exist (1) and can be used to analyze cellular, molecular, and biochemical mechanisms during photoreceptor cell death. However, degeneration in most of these models proceeds rather slowly and it takes several weeks to months until degeneration is complete. Therefore, only few cells are in the same stage of the dying process at any given time during the course of the degeneration. This makes it difficult to investigate the molecular processes in detail and it may be especially difficult to detect subtle changes in levels, localization, modifications, and/or activity of molecules involved in the regulation of the degeneration.

Bernhard H.F. Weber and Thomas Langmann (eds.), *Retinal Degeneration: Methods and Protocols*, Methods in Molecular Biology, vol. 935, DOI 10.1007/978-1-62703-080-9_6, © Springer Science+Business Media, LLC 2013

Visible light is discussed as a contributing factor in human retinal degenerations such as retinitis pigmentosa (RP) and age-related macular degeneration (AMD). In fact, light exposure can induce photoreceptor death in wild-type mice, rats, and several other species, and progression of photoreceptor degeneration in many of the inherited animal models is accelerated by normal environmental light. Thus, light is not only a factor which needs to be considered when studying retinal degeneration but light can also be used in experimental settings to control induction, timing, and extent of photoreceptor degeneration. Exposure to bright visible light simultaneously induces cell death in a large number of photoreceptor cells synchronizing the molecular mechanisms which greatly facilitates their detection and analysis. Four general light exposure protocols have to be distinguished: short-term exposure to high levels of white light, long-term exposure to low levels of white light, broadband blue–green–yellow light (490–580 nm), and exposure to monochromatic light of a specific wavelength. All of these protocols may share common mechanisms but are also characterized by the activation of distinct pathways. Short-term exposure to bright light, for example, depends on the transcription factor AP-1 and is independent of phototransduction whereas long-term exposure to low levels of white light is independent of AP-1 but requires active phototransduction (2). Thus, to find and define possible common mechanisms for all (or at least most) forms of retinal degeneration, it seems important to test findings made with a particular protocol in additional animal models of induced and inherited retinal degeneration.

To date, none of the "classical" factors seem to be involved in the regulation of blue light damage. However, since practically all experimental data appear to suggest that light damage follows the action spectrum of blue light (3), it is conceivable that all light exposure regimens will show that absorption of light by the same initial chromophore precedes the subsequent diversity of regulatory mechanisms (see Note 1). Since the initial chromophore inducing light damage remains elusive to date it is relevant to study the initial events after light absorption leading to retinal lesions. As all light damage models depend on the presence of visual pigments (rhodopsin or cone pigments) but do not follow their action spectrum (3), more studies are needed to clarify this basic issue.

Here we describe the protocols for short-term exposure to high levels of white light and to high-intensity monochromatic green or blue light. For the sake of simplicity we will call the latter type of exposure "blue light" even though this light includes the violet as well as the short-wavelength blue part of the spectrum (410 ± 10 nm). Since the exposure to green (550 ± 10 nm) light follows the same protocol, it will not be described separately.

2. Materials

2.1. Short-Term Exposure to High Levels of White Light

1. Room/box for dark adaptation: Any lighttight room, box, or cupboard large enough to host at least one normal animal cage with sufficient ventilation will do. Pay attention that normal oxygen levels are maintained during dark adaptation since hypoxia may strongly influence light damage susceptibility (4).

2. 1% cyclogyl (Alcon, Cham, Switzerland), 5% phenylephrine (Ciba Vision, Niederwangen, Switzerland).

3. Light exposure device (Fig. 1): Our light exposure device is custom-made but any device holding the respective light bulbs might work if sufficiently high levels of light can be reached. The light exposure device consists of a holder for eight light bulbs placed above the animal cages. A diffusion screen is positioned between exposure cages and light bulbs to filter UV light below a wavelength of 400 nm. The screen also prevents an increase of the temperature within the animal cages. The distance between the light-bulb holder and the cages is adjustable to reduce or increase light intensity at cage level, respectively.

4. Light bulbs (Master TL-D 90 De Luxe 36W/965 1SL, Philips, Hamburg, Germany) (see Note 2).

5. Luxmeter (Luminance meter T-10, Konica Minolta Sensing, Inc., Osaka, Japan) (see Note 3).

6. Cages with reflective interior (Fig. 2): We use normal housing cages (type T2) without lid or grid. Cages are lined with aluminum foil to reflect light from the walls and the bottom of the cage.

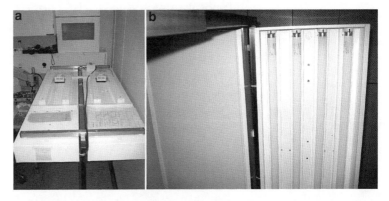

Fig. 1. Light exposure device. (**a**) View from top. (**b**) View from below showing the mounting of the light bulbs. The bulbs on the left side are shielded by the diffusion screen. On the right side of the device, the screen has been removed to reveal the arrangement of the light bulbs.

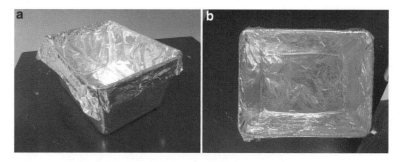

Fig. 2. Exposure cage lined with aluminum foil. (**a**) Side view. (**b**) Top view.

2.2. Short-Term Exposure to High-Intensity Blue or Green Light

1. Room/box for dark adaptation: Any lighttight room, box, or cupboard large enough to host at least one normal animal cage with sufficient ventilation will do.

2. Pupil dilation: 1% cyclogyl (Alcon, Cham, Switzerland), 5% phenylephrine (Ciba Vision, Niederwangen, Switzerland), Methocel drops (isotonic hydroxypropyl methylcellulose 2% with the same refractive index as air; Omnivision AG, Neuhausen, Switzerland) for corneal moistening.

3. Anesthesia: Ketamine (75 mg/kg; Parke Davis, Zug, Switzerland), Xylazine 2% (23 mg/kg; Bayer AG, Leverkusen, Germany), sodium chloride. Make a mixture of 0.84 ml Ketamine, 0.51 ml Xylazine, 0.35 ml NaCl or a multiple of that mixture. Mixture can be stored in the refrigerator for several weeks. Take 0.03–0.06 ml for 20–30 g mouse, depending on the duration of light exposure and mouse strain. Albino mice generally need a higher dose of anesthetics than pigmented strains.

4. Light exposure device (Fig. 3): The aim is to achieve a high and quantifiable light output, to generate a homogeneous light spot with reproducible size on the cornea and the retina, and to provide a choice of two monochromatic light types (blue and green).

   The light source is a modified xenon arc lamp (Xenon 100W reflector bulb) for photodynamic tumor therapy for dermatological use (Intralux MDR 100, purchased at VOLPI AG, Schlieren, Switzerland) with a liquid fiber-optic light guide. Color temperature is 5,600 °K, spectrum is 400–780 nm (see Note 4).

   For our experiments the following additions to the system were made:

   (a) An aluminum holder with two lenses and an infrared filter is positioned at the outlet of the fiber-optic light guide. The first lens spreads the light beam parallel; the second lens focuses the light to a beam of 5 mm diameter. In front

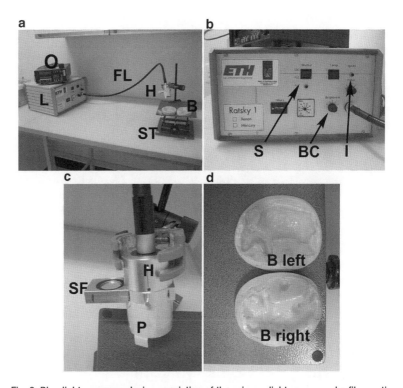

Fig. 3. Blue light-exposure device consisting of the primary light source and a fiber-optic light guide. An aluminum holder at the end of the light guide contains two lenses, the filter slider for blue and green filter and an infrared heat filter. The mouse is placed on a mouse bed on a stage with adjustable height. The distance from the light outlet to the mouse cornea is 1 cm, marked by a paper bar. (**a**) Overview over the complete system. (**b**) Detail-view of the control panel of the light source. (**c**) Detail-view of the aluminum holder. (**d**) Detail-view of the mouse beds. *L* light source, *O* optical power meter, *FL* fiber-optic light guide, *H* aluminum holder for the lens system and filter slider, *B* mouse bed, *ST* adjustable stage to hold the mouse bed, *S* shutter switch for the light outlet within the body of the light source, *BC* brightness controller, *I* button to ignite the light bulb, *SF* slider with filter, *P* paper clip as 1 cm-ruler, *B left* mouse bed for exposure of the left eye, *B right* mouse bed for exposure of the right eye.

of the lenses before the light exits the system is an infrared heat filter. The distance of the holder from the mouse cornea should be 1 cm. Hold a sheet of white paper under the light beam and see at which distance the edges of the light spot are sharpest and the illumination within the spot is homogeneous. This is the 1 cm distance. The procedure is similar to "Koehlern" with the Kondensor lens and Kondensor diaphragm in a light microscope.

(b) A slider containing two holes for changeable filters is placed between the lens system and the infrared filter. We use a blue filter (410 ± 10 nm bandwidth) and a green filter (550 ± 10 nm bandwidth). The slider allows the quick change between blue and green filters, if required (see Note 5).

5. Mouse "bed" with caved contours of a mouse lying on its side for reproducible positioning of head and eye, one for left eye, one for right eye (Fig. 3).

6. Stage with adjustable height to place the mouse bed.

7. Optical Power Meter (Model 835, Newport Corporation, Fountain Valley, CA, USA) to measure irradiance levels for different wavelengths.

8. Timer for short light exposures.

9. Laboratory paper towels to wrap mouse for warming.

3. Methods

3.1. Short-Term Exposure to High Levels of White Light

1. House mice in normal cages with food and water ad libitum and a 12:12-h light–dark cycle with less than 60 lx at cage level.

2. Dark adapt mice (see Notes 6–8) for 16 h overnight. Start at 6 pm.

3. Switch light bulbs in the light exposure device on at 9 am (see Notes 9 and 10).

4. Dilate pupils at 9:30 in dim red light (see Note 11).

5. Adjust light levels at 9:45 am (see Note 12).

6. Place mice in aluminum foil-lined cages and expose mice to light from 10 to 12 am (see Note 13).

7. After exposure, return mice to their housing cage with food and water ad libitum and place cages in darkness until next morning.

8. Return animals to the normal light–dark cycle the next day until mice are sacrificed for analysis.

3.2. Exposure to Blue or Green Light

1. Keep mice (see Note 14) in normal cages in a 12:12-h light–dark cycle with food and water ad libitum and an illuminance of 60 lx at cage level.

2. Dark adapt mice for 12–16 h.

3. Turn on the light of lamp ("ignite" button), switch open the light shutter, and adjust desired irradiance with the optical power meter for wavelength of blue or green. We use 30 mW/cm^2 at the corneal level. Close shutter by switch but keep lamp turned on.

4. Dilate pupils in dim red light and keep mice dark adapted for additional 20–30 min.

5. Control irradiance level (see Note 15).

6. Anesthetize mice with ketamine–xylazine (see Note 16), two to three mice at a time, depending on the following exposure duration.

7. Place mouse on mouse bed with shutter of lamp closed. Choose the filter (blue or green) by using the slider. Apply a drop of methocel to the cornea, adjust mouse head and eye, and place mouse under light source. Adjust the distance of the mouse eye to the lens holder to 1 cm (we have a small paper clip of 1 cm length fixed at the margin of the lens holder). Cover mouse with a paper towel (see Note 17).

8. Switch open the shutter and very quickly fine adjust the mouse eye to the light beam (see Note 18). Use timer for short exposures.

9. Place exposed and still anesthetized mouse in extra cage and wrap in paper towel.

10. When all mice of a group/cage are exposed, put them together again in their original cage, still wrapped in paper towels. Control their awakening during the rest of the day and keep them in darkness until next morning.

11. Return animals to the normal light–dark cycle the next day until mice are sacrificed for analysis.

4. Notes

1. The majority of light damage studies indicate that light damage follows the action spectrum of short-wavelength light (violet–blue) (3). Therefore it seems essential to study mechanisms of "pure" (monochromatic) blue light damage in order to try to understand white light and broadband green light (5) lesions. Monochromatic blue light damage is independent of most of the known "classical" factors like AP1, phototransduction, rhodopsin regeneration rate, time of day, and others. The only known common mechanism is the dependence on the rhodopsin molecule but not the rhodopsin action spectrum. Thus it may be that to date only partially known products of rhodopsin bleaching are the primary absorbing chromophores leading to the damaging molecular and cellular events, which may be different in various damage regimens and diverse strains and species. Those secondary events can comprise a multitude of factors which include DNA-damage, transcription factor expression, lipid and protein oxidation, release of lipid mediators, a spectrum of inflammatory responses including chemokine and cytokine expression, activation of macrophages and microglia, and induction of apoptosis and necrosis (6).

Thus we may tentatively conclude that the initial chromophore for most light damage regimens may be visual pigment bleaching products whereas a host of secondary events are then distinguished in the different light damage studies.

2. Before using new light bulbs in an experiment, keep the bulbs turned on for at least 48 continuous hours. This will stabilize the light.

3. Always use the same luxmeter for measuring light intensity. Numbers may vary considerably depending on the form of the light-sensitive head of the luxmeter.

4. We use a dermatological lamp with high irradiance output because the monochromatic light needs high energy to be able to induce damage. Light levels of blue LEDs were insufficient for this type of light damage experiments when we checked this in 2008. Perhaps new ones are on the market since that time.

   At 30 mW/cm^2 irradiance at the mouse cornea, the irradiance in our hot spot area on the retina is about 62 mW/cm^2 (calculation by François Delori). Photon flux calculated is 6.2×10^9 photons μm^{-2} s^{-1} at 410 nm and rate of rhodopsin isomerization is 1.45×10^9 s^{-1} at 410 nm, calculations by Ed Pugh jr. (7). The size of the hot spot is 5 mm^2 on the cornea and about 2 mm^2 on the retina.

   A practical advice: The fiber-optic light guide should not be bent strongly, because fibers may break.

   One could use laser light for this type of experiment. However, the resulting hot spot may be much smaller unless the light beam is spread by a lens system. For morphological and biochemical studies it is recommended to have a large hot spot.

5. We used the combination of green followed by blue exposure to study photoreversal of rhodopsin bleaching (8) and mechanisms of blue light-damage (9).

   Furthermore, exposure to green of 550 nm does not induce any lesions due to a rapid and strong bleach of rhodopsin, indicating that rhodopsin bleaching per se is not damaging provided that the bleaching products are quickly transported into the pigment epithelium and further that the bleaching products are not exposed to blue light (8, 9).

6. Photoreceptors of young mice (freshly weaned) are less susceptible to light damage than photoreceptors of adult mice. Therefore, mice should be at least 6 weeks of age for consistent results.

7. The genetic background of the mice is important and influences light damage susceptibility. Bl6 mice are generally not susceptible to light damage by the protocol presented here. An important genetic factor to be considered is the sequence variation in the *Rpe65* gene. The *Rpe65$_{450Met}$* variant renders

the retina less susceptible to damage than the $Rpe65_{450Leu}$ variant (10). Most wild-type strains, with the exception of C57Bl6, express the $Rpe65_{450Leu}$ variant. Many transgenic animals are on a mixed background and may express the $Rpe65_{450Met}$ variant. Always test transgenic mice for their $Rpe65$ variant to decide on the exposure protocol. Photoreceptor damage in mice with the $Rpe65_{450Met}$ variant may need longer exposure durations and/or higher light intensities. Good wild-type strains to be used with this protocol are albino mice like Balb/c and pigmented mice like 129S6/SvEvTac (Taconics, Eiby, Denmark).

8. It is important that mice are stressed as little as possible before and during light exposure. Stress induces expression of glucocorticoids which may modulate AP-1 activity. Stressed mice are resistant to damage induced by exposure to short-term high-level white light (11). It is best if animals can be housed and dark adapted in—or very close to—the room with the light exposure device in order to minimize transport before the experiment. Also, do not mix animals for dark adaptation. This may cause stress, especially among males.

9. For highest reproducibility, expose mice during the same period of the day. Circadian variations in light damage susceptibility have been reported (5).

10. Do not dim the light bulbs to reduce light intensity. Dimming may change the spectrum of the emitted light. Instead, vary the distance between exposure cages and light bulbs.

11. Dilation of pupils is essential for pigmented animals and should be done under dim red light (above 600 nm). Avoid stressing the animals as much as possible. First, use one drop of cyclogyl per eye. Release the animal until all eyes of the animals in the respective exposure series are treated. Then start over with the first animal using one drop of 5% phenylephrine per eye. Cyclogyl (cyclopentolate hydrochloride, 10 mg/ml) blocks the response of the sphincter muscle of the iris (and of the accommodative muscle of the ciliary body) to cholinergic stimulation. This produces pupillary dilation (mydriasis). Phenylephrine (phenylephrine hydrochloride) is an α-adrenergic receptor agonist, which causes vasoconstriction and mydriasis through stimulation of the dilator muscle of the pupil. After application of both drops, return the animals to their cages and continue dark adaptation for an additional 30 min.

12. Adjust light levels by placing the light-sensitive head of the luxmeter face-up into the middle of one exposure cage lined with aluminum foil. Change the distance between cage and light source until the required light level is reached. Measure light levels in all cages which will hold mice during exposure.

Do not dim the light bulbs. Adjust light levels by varying the distance between exposure cage and light bulbs. Use an exposure time according to your experimental needs. A 10-min exposure to 5,000 lx of white light is borderline to damage photoreceptors in Balb/c mice. One hour of illumination to 5,000 lx induces severe photoreceptor degeneration in Balb/c. To reach a similarly severe damage in 129S6 pigmented animals, a 2-h exposure to 13,000 lx may be required.

13. Place the animals as quickly as possible into the aluminum foil-lined exposure cages under the light bulbs. Cages do not contain food or water and are not covered by a grid or a lid. One animal per cage is optimal. If more than one animal is placed into one cage, animals tend to stick together to shield their eyes. Monitor the mice frequently (at least every 10 min). Some mice make holes into the aluminum foil and hide between foil and cage wall. If this happens, replace cage with a new cage lined freshly with aluminum foil.

14. In contrast to white light exposures, the genetic background of mice appears to be less important for blue light-mediated damage. For example, the $Rpe65$ variants $Rpe65_{450Leu}$ and $Rpe65_{450Met}$ are not distinctly different in their blue light-damage susceptibility (Wenzel A., Grimm C., Remé C.E., unpublished observations), supporting the finding that metabolic rhodopsin regeneration does not determine blue light-damage in mice (12). Furthermore, blue light-damage is independent of the transcription factor AP1 and of phototransduction (Wenzel A., Grimm C., Remé C.E., unpublished observations).

15. It is important to control the light output of the lamp at least 15 min after the lamp was switched on, since the output of a cold lamp can be higher.

16. We apply anesthesia intramuscularly (i.m.) into the gluteus muscle, by holding the hind leg while the mouse can grasp the metal bars of the cage cover. We found that the procedure of i.m. injection is faster than the intraperitoneal injection and for that reason i.m. anesthesia is less stressful for the animal.

17. We use paper towels and wrap them around the mouse to keep it warm for safety reasons, since a heating pad with insufficient thermostat can easily increase in temperature. Overheating the animal might accelerate damage.

18. In order to center the light beam on the mouse eye, an autofluorescence of the mouse lens is helpful for orientation. This can be nicely seen through the maximally dilated pupil.

Acknowledgement

We thank the late Theodore P. Williams for numerous stimulating discussions, help with setting up the light damage systems, analyzing data, and providing crucial insights into the function and metabolism of rhodopsin.

We also cordially thank François Delori and Ed Pugh jr. for contributing to the blue light damage setup by calculating retinal irradiance, photon flux, and rate of rhodopsin isomerizations.

The late Pascal Rol helped to build the first blue light setup, which was later refined by Michael Mrochen and Thomas Menzi.

Discussions with and ideas from all past and present members of the Lab for Retinal Cell Biology helped to improve the light exposure systems. Without their input and experiments, many of the potential pitfalls would not have been recognized and eliminated.

References

1. Samardzija M, Neuhauss SCF, Joly S, Kurz-Levin M, Grimm C (2010) Animal models for retinal degeneration. In: Pang I-H, Clark AF (eds) Advances in experimental medicine and biology, Retinal degenerative diseases. Humana, New York, pp 52–80

2. Hao W, Wenzel A, Obin MS, Chen CK, Brill E, Krasnoperova NV, Eversole-Cire P, Kleyner Y, Taylor A, Simon MI, Grimm C, Reme CE, Lem J (2002) Evidence for two apoptotic pathways in light-induced retinal degeneration. Nat Genet 32:254–260

3. van Norren D, Gorgels TG (2011) The action spectrum of photochemical damage to the retina: a review of monochromatic threshold data. Photochem Photobiol 87:747–753

4. Grimm C, Wenzel A, Groszer M, Mayser H, Seeliger M, Samardzija M, Bauer C, Gassmann M, Reme CE (2002) HIF-1-induced erythropoietin in the hypoxic retina protects against light-induced retinal degeneration. Nat Med 8:718–724

5. Organisciak DT, Darrow RM, Barsalou L, Kutty RK, Wiggert B (2000) Circadian-dependent retinal light damage in rats. Invest Ophthalmol Vis Sci 41:3694–3701

6. Joly S, Francke M, Ulbricht E, Beck S, Seeliger M, Hirrlinger P, Hirrlinger J, Lang KS, Zinkernagel M, Odermatt B, Samardzija M, Reichenbach A, Grimm C, Remé CE (2009) Cooperative phagocytes. Resident microglia and bone marrow immigrants remove dead photoreceptors in retinal lesions. Am J Pathol 174:2310–2322

7. Breton ME, Schueller AW, Lamb TD, jr Pugh EN (1994) Analysis of ERG a-wave amplification and kinetics in terms of the G-protein cascade of phototransduction. Invest Ophthalmol Vis Sci 35:295–309

8. Grimm C, Remé CE, Rol PO, Williams TP (2000) Blue light's effects on rhodopsin: photoreversal of bleaching in living rat eyes. Invest Ophthalmol Vis Sci 41:3983–3990

9. Grimm C, Wenzel A, Williams TP, Rol PO, Hafezi F, Remé CE (2001) Rhodopsin-mediated blue-light damage to the rat retina: effect of photoreversal of bleaching. Invest Ophthalmol Vis Sci 42:497–505

10. Wenzel A, Grimm C, Samardzija M, Reme CE (2003) The genetic modifier Rpe65Leu(450): effect on light damage susceptibility in c-Fos-deficient mice. Invest Ophthalmol Vis Sci 44:2798–2802

11. Wenzel A, Grimm C, Seeliger MW, Jaissle G, Hafezi F, Kretschmer R, Zrenner E, Reme CE (2001) Prevention of photoreceptor apoptosis by activation of the glucocorticoid receptor. Invest Ophthalmol Vis Sci 42: 1653–1659

12. Keller C, Grimm C, Wenzel A, Hafezi F, Remé CE (2001) Protective effect of halothane anesthesia on retinal light damage: inhibition of metabolic rhodopsin regeneration. Invest Ophthalmol Vis Sci 42:476–480

Chapter 7

N-Methyl-D-Aspartate (NMDA)-Mediated Excitotoxic Damage: A Mouse Model of Acute Retinal Ganglion Cell Damage

Roswitha Seitz and Ernst R. Tamm

Abstract

The animal model of *N*-methyl-D-aspartate (NMDA)-induced excitotoxic damage of retinal ganglion cells (RGC) is widely used to study the molecular mechanisms of RGC apoptosis and/or its prevention by neuroprotective agents. This chapter provides protocols for applying NMDA-induced excitotoxic damage to RGC of mouse eyes and for subsequent measuring of the extent of the resulting damage.

Key words: Retinal ganglion cells, NMDA, Excitotoxicity, Cell death, Glaucoma

1. Introduction

Treatment with the synthetic glutamate analogue *N*-methyl-D-aspartate (NMDA) causes excitotoxicity of neurons by hyperactivation of NMDA-type glutamate receptors, which results in a massive Ca^{2+} influx that subsequently propagates pro-apoptotic signaling cascades (1). In the retina, retinal ganglion cells (RGC) and amacrine cells are particularly sensitive to excitotoxicity, and excess glutamate has been proposed to contribute to RGC apoptosis in common neurodegenerative disorders of the eye, including glaucoma and retinal artery occlusion (2). Since RGC and amacrine cells preferentially express NMDA-type glutamate receptors in the retina, intravitreal injection of NMDA provides a specific model for their acute damage facilitating studies on the molecular mechanisms of RGC apoptosis and/or on neuroprotective signaling pathways preventing their apoptotic death. The goal of this chapter is to provide protocols for NMDA-induced RGC damage in the mouse eye and for methods that can be used for a subsequent readout of the induced cellular and structural changes.

Bernhard H.F. Weber and Thomas Langmann (eds.), *Retinal Degeneration: Methods and Protocols*, Methods in Molecular Biology, vol. 935, DOI 10.1007/978-1-62703-080-9_7, © Springer Science+Business Media, LLC 2013

2. Materials

1. Sterile phosphate-buffered saline (PBS) for control injections.
2. NMDA stock solution: NMDA is dissolved in sterile PBS at a concentration of 100 mM and stored at −20°C (see Note 1).
3. Intravitreal injections are administered with a beveled needle (34 Gauge) which is linked via a tubing (0.4 mm inner diameter) to a 25 μl Hamilton syringe.
4. To perform injections under optimal visual control, intravitreal injections are performed under a binocular microscope. Lack of good visual control can lead to damage of the lens, a scenario that leads to activation of neuroprotective signaling cascades (see Note 2).
5. For anesthesia and antiseptic treatment of the eyes after injection, isoflurane (2–5%), iodine tincture (10%), and antiseptic eye ointment (e.g., containing dexamethasone, neomycin, and polymyxin B) should be available.

3. Methods

In the mouse eye the amount of retinal neurons that are damaged by NMDA-treatment is dose dependent (3). In our hands, an injection of 3 μl of a 10 mM NMDA-solution into the vitreous cavity of 6-week-old C57/BL6-mice will cause substantial (approximately 75%), but not complete, loss of RGC (ref. 4; see Note 3).

3.1. Intravitreal Injections

Before starting intravitreal injections have all working material ready at hand. Make sure that all working solutions are sterile. Preferentially, the injections should be performed by two individuals. It helps considerably if the individual who handles the needle is different from the one who handles the Hamilton syringe.

1. Rinse the Hamilton syringe, the beveled needle, and the tubing three to four times with 70% ethanol and then for additionally three to four times with PBS (see Note 4).
2. Link the beveled needle to the syringe via the tubing (see Note 5).
3. Dilute the 100 mM NMDA-stock-solution with PBS to a 10 mM working solution.
4. Prepare sterile PBS for control injections into the contralateral fellow eye.
5. Prior to injections, mice are deeply anesthetized with isoflurane (about 2% for maintenance, up to 5% for induction) and the ocular surface is disinfected by a 10% iodine tincture.

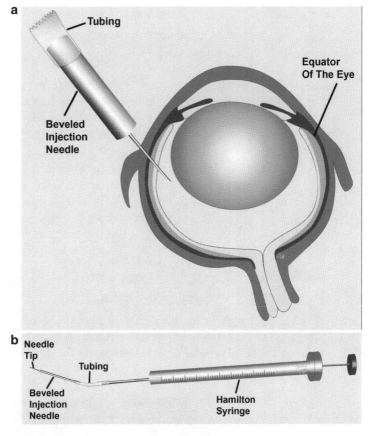

Fig. 1. Schematic drawing of intravitreal injections. (**a**) PBS or NMDA is injected through the equatorial sclera into the vitreous body. (**b**) For injections, a beveled needle is linked to a Hamilton syringe.

6. Insert the needle at the equator of the eye (see Note 6). The tip should point in the direction of the optic nerve to avoid injury of the lens (see Note 2) (Fig. 1).

7. 3 µl of PBS or NMDA are slowly injected into the vitreous body (see Note 7).

8. Leave the needle in the eye for an additional 20 s to allow the eye to adjust to the increase in volume (see Note 8).

9. After removal of the needle, an antiseptic eye ointment should be administered.

10. Rinse syringe and needle thoroughly after each injection.

3.2. Readouts

The full extent of NMDA-induced damage can be analyzed by

1. Quantification of RGC apoptosis.

2. Quantification of the remaining RGC perikarya in the ganglion cell layer (GCL).

3. Quantification of the area of the inner plexiform layer (IPL).

4. Quantification of the total number of axons in the optic nerve (see Note 9).

3.2.1. TUNEL Labeling

A few hours after NMDA-injection, the first apoptotic cells can be observed in the retina. Apoptotic cells can be detected via TdT-mediated dUTP-biotin nick end labeling (TUNEL)-assay. Cleavage of DNA by endonucleases is one of the last events that occur in apoptotic cells. At the ends of the fragmented DNA strands, free OH groups remain. The 3′-OH ends can be marked with conjugated (e.g., fluorescein-conjugated) dNTPs by the use of terminal deoxynucleotidyl transferase (TdT) and labeled apoptotic cells can be then visualized by fluorescence microscopy (5) (Fig. 2).

1. Twenty-four hours after intravitreal injection mice are killed and eyes enucleated (see Note 10).

2. During harvesting of the eyes it is important to avoid squeezing of the eye bulb.

3. For preparation of paraffin sections, eyes are fixed by immersion in 4% paraformaldehyde in 0.1 M phosphate buffer for 4 h. For better fixation, the cornea should be opened.

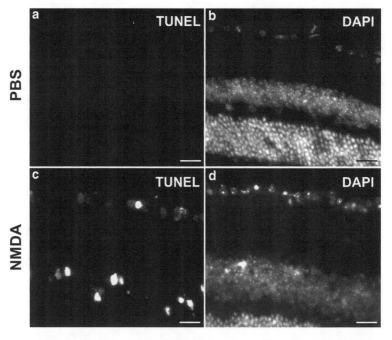

Fig. 2. TUNEL-staining 24 h after intravitreal injection. (**a**, **b**) After injection of PBS no TUNEL-positive cells are observed in the retina. (**c**, **d**) After NMDA-injection about 50% of the cells in the GCL are marked TUNEL positive. Several apoptotic cells are also observed in the inner nuclear layer. These cells represent a subpopulation of amacrine cells which are also expressing NMDA-receptors. Scale bars in **a–d**, 20 μm.

4. Paraffin embedding of the eyes is performed according to standard protocols.

5. For TUNEL-assay, 6 μm sagittal paraffin sections of the eye are cut (see Note 11).

6. For detection of apoptosis in the retina use a commercially available kit for TUNEL-labeling (e.g., Promega). Follow the manufacturer's instructions.

7. For quantification of total cell number in the GCL, a nuclear counterstain should be performed (e.g., DAPI).

8. After labeling of apoptotic cells and nuclear counterstain, the slides are mounted with fluorescent mounting medium.

9. After mounting, the slides can be analyzed by fluorescent microscopy.

10. Take pictures of the entire retina. A microscope with panorama function (e.g., Zeiss Axiovision) is very helpful for this.

11. Quantify the total number of TUNEL-positive cells and the total number of nuclei in the GCL with the help of an image analyzing program (see Notes 12 and 13).

12. Subsequently, the percentage of apoptotic cells per sagittal section is calculated as total number of TUNEL-positive cells per total number of cells in the GCL.

3.2.2. Quantification of Optic Nerve Axons

The protocol below uses light microscopy for axon counting. The total number of axons may be higher if transmission electron microscopy is used, as this method allows including also the smallest axons in the analyses (see Note 14) (Fig. 3).

1. Three weeks after injection of NMDA into the vitreous cavity mice are killed and eyes with optic nerves are harvested (see Note 15).

2. During harvesting of the eyes it is important to avoid squeezing of optic nerves. To make sectioning easier nerves should not bend, but should be fixed as straight as possible.

3. For preparation of semithin sections, eyes with optic nerves attached are fixed by immersion in cacodylate buffer containing 2.5% paraformaldehyde and 2.5% glutaraldehyde for 24 h (6).

4. After fixation, eyes are washed in cacodylate buffer.

5. Epon embedding of the eyes is performed according to standard protocols.

6. Analysis is carried out on 1 μm semithin cross sections of the optic nerve (see Note 16).

7. To facilitate visualization of optic nerve axons, sections are stained with paraphenylenediamine (PPD) to visualize myelin sheaths (7).

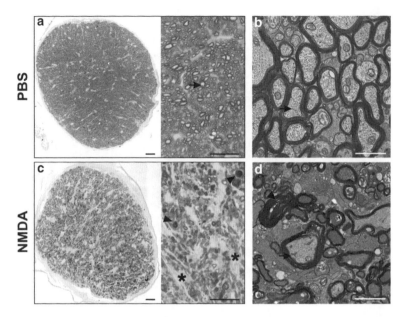

Fig. 3. Light microscopy of semithin (**a**, **c**) or ultrathin cross sections (**c**, **d**) through the optic nerve three weeks after intravitreal injection of PBS or NMDA. (**a**, **c**) Overview and details of optic nerves after intravitreal injection of PBS (**a**) or NMDA (**c**). NMDA leads to a substantial decrease in the number of axons (*arrows*). The area where axons have degenerated are filled by glial scar tissue (*asterisk*). Black axons, mainly seen in NMDA-treated optic nerves, represent degenerating axons (*arrowheads*). The disorganized intensely stained myelin sheath of the axons is clearly visible by electron microscopy (**d**). In contrast, the axons of PBS-treated control eyes appear to be healthy and are still filled with neurofilaments and mitochondria (**b**). Scale bars: (**a**, **c**) 20 μm; (**b**, **d**) 2 μm; paraphenylenediamine (PPD) stain.

8. Prepare the PPD staining solution.

9. Dissolve 500 mg PPD in 50 ml ethanol (100%).

10. Leave the PPD solution 3 days in broad daylight till it turns dark.

11. Cross sections of optic nerves are incubated with PPD solution for 2–3 min. After staining the sections are rinsed with ethanol (100%).

12. When the staining procedure is finished, slides are mounted with DePeX mounting medium for histology.

13. Stained sections can now be analyzed by light microscopy.

14. Take an overview image with high magnification (×100; e.g., by using an Axiovision microscope, Zeiss).

15. Remaining axons are quantified by an image analyzing program (see Notes 12 and 17).

16. Count all axons in the section, but ignore dark black stained axons: here degeneration is still continuing (see Note 18).

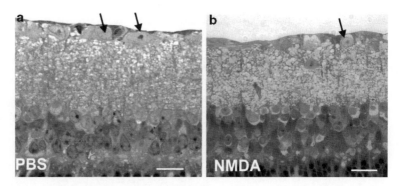

Fig. 4. Sagittal semithin sections through the retinae of mouse eyes 3 weeks after intravitreal injection. After injection of NMDA (**b**), the number of perikarya (*arrows*) in the GCL is markedly decreased when compared to the control retina injected with PBS (**a**). Scale bars: 20 μm, Richardson's stain.

3.2.3. Analyzing RGC Perikarya or IPL Thickness on Semithin Sections

In addition to the number of remaining perikarya in the GCL after NMDA-induced apoptosis, the area of the IPL, where the synapses of RGC and bipolar cells are located, can be measured (Fig. 4). After degeneration of RGC and their dendrites, the area of the IPL is substantially reduced.

1. Three weeks after injection of NMDA into the vitreous cavity mice are killed and eyes are enucleated (see Note 19).

2. During enucleation of the eyes, it is important to avoid squeezing of the eye bulb.

3. For preparation of semithin sections, eyes are fixed by immersion in cacodylate buffer containing 2.5% paraformaldehyde and 2.5% glutaraldehyde for 24 h (6). For better fixation, the cornea should be opened.

4. After fixation, eyes are washed in cacodylate buffer.

5. Epon embedding of the eyes is performed according to standard protocols.

6. Analysis is carried out on 1 μm sagittal semithin sections through the central eye (see Note 11).

7. For staining, Richardson's stain for plastic sections is recommended (8). Stock and working solutions can be stored at room temperature: Prepare stock solutions: Stock solution A (1% Azur II): Dissolve 5 g Azur II in 500 ml H_2O. Stock solution B (1% methylene blue): Dissolve 5 g methylene blue in 500 ml 1% borax (sodium borate). For staining of semithin sections prepare working solution: Mix 50 ml Solution A with 50 ml Solution B and 100 ml H_2O.

8. Slides are incubated for 15–30 s with the working solution at 60°C.

9. Rinse slides with H_2O.

10. Control the staining intensity by microscopy. If the staining is too weak, repeat steps 8 to 10.

11. After staining, the slides are mounted with DePeX mounting medium for histology.

12. Stained sections can now be analyzed by light microscopy.

13. An overview image with high magnification (×100; e.g., with Axiovision microscope, Zeiss) should be recorded.

14. Remaining perikarya and the area of IPL are quantified by an image analyzing program (see Note 12).

15. The total amount of perikarya in the GCL is plotted against the total length of the retina (see Note 20).

16. For quantification of the IPL, the area of IPL is plotted against the total length of the retina.

4. Notes

1. Aliquot the NMDA stock solution to avoid repeated freeze–thaw cycles.

2. Keep in mind that injury of the lens will have a large influence on the quality of your results, because lens injury induces signaling cascades that are protective for RGC. Upon lens damage, β- and γ-crystallins may be released into the vitreous cavity, a scenario that causes macrophage activation and/or secretion of ciliary neurotrophic factor (CNTF) from astrocytes (9–12). An injured lens will develop cataract and turn white 1 day after injection. This should not be mistaken from an immediate effect after the injection when the whole eye turns opaque due to the transient increase in volume.

3. Be aware that different mouse strains do not only have different numbers of optic nerve axons (13) but may also show a different susceptibility to NMDA-treatment due to their respective genetic background (13–15). Always perform dose–response experiments for your respective mouse model.

4. Make sure that your experimental equipment is as clean as possible and sterile to avoid infections.

5. Check if the tubing is linked to the Hamilton syringe and the needle without any leaks and the liquid is really injected into the eye.

6. If you have problems with the injection, because the eye is evading the needle, you can keep the eye in position with the help of a spatula.

7. Injections should be performed slowly to avoid peaks of very high intraocular pressure, which can lead to mechanical constriction of retinal blood vessels and finally cause retinal ischemia.

8. If the needle is removed too soon, NMDA or PBS may spill out of the eye due to the temporarily increased volume.

9. Quantification of RGC apoptosis, e.g., by TUNEL-labeling 24 h after NMDA-injection (4), is a method to assess the acute effects of excitotoxic RGC damage. Longer term effects are analyzed by counting the number of remaining RGC perikarya in the GCL or by counting the number of their axons in the optic nerve. Counting of RGC perikarya can be done on retinal whole mounts after retrograde labeling of RGC following Fluoro-Gold injection in both superior colliculi (15, 16). A potential and critical pitfall of this method is underestimation of RGC perikarya due to incomplete uptake of the tracer resulting in incomplete labeling. Alternatively, RGC may be labeled on retinal whole mounts by using antibodies against Brn3a, which recognize an epitope that is preferentially expressed on RGC (16, 17). In our opinion, the method of choice to obtain a complete overview on the degree of NMDA-mediated RGC damage is the quantification of the total number of remaining RGC axons in the optic nerve (4). Quantification of the remaining RGC perikarya and measuring of IPL-area after NMDA-treatment on meridional retinal sections are less favorable as RGC are not homogeneously distributed throughout the retina. Such methods should only be used in conjunction with other methods, or if a substantially high number of sections are evaluated per eye.

10. In our hands, a substantial labeling of TUNEL-positive apoptotic RGC is observed 24 h after NMDA-induced damage, when about at least half of the cells in the GCL are TUNEL positive (Fig. 2).

11. For standardization, central meridional sections should be used for analysis. To this end, both the optic nerve head and the open iris should be seen on the section.

12. Counting of cells/axons or measuring of IPL area can be facilitated by microscope-specific software (e.g., Axiovision, Zeiss). In addition to commercially available programs, free image analyzing programs are available, e.g., the *UTHSCSA ImageTool*, which was developed in the Department of Dental Diagnostic Science at the University of Texas Health Science Center (http://ddsdx.uthscsa.edu/Imagetool.asp).

13. Be aware that the apoptotic cells do not only represent RGC, as displaced amacrine cells in the GCL are very likely damaged by NMDA-treatment as well (1, 18). In control retinae, which only received an injection of PBS, only very few apoptotic cells are detectable, predominantly in the outer nuclear layer (ONL), representing spontaneous apoptosis occurring in photoreceptors.

14. Be aware that different mouse strains have different numbers of axons in their optic nerves (5).

15. Degeneration of RGC axons after excitotoxic damage continues for several weeks. Reliable results are already received by quantification of the total amount of axons 3 weeks after NMDA-injection (Fig. 3), although the process of degeneration is still continuing.

16. The degeneration of optic nerve axons starts at the perikarya and extends in direction to the brain. For this reason, 3 weeks after NMDA-injection only those sections should be analyzed which are as close as possible to the optic nerve head.

17. Looking at optic nerves from PBS-treated eyes, numerous healthy axons can be detected which lie close to each other (Fig. 3a, b). There are only small areas of glial tissue. Three weeks after NMDA-injection, the optic nerve shows a substantial loss of axons. Degenerated axons have been replaced by glial scars.

18. Keep in mind that the degeneration of axons is not completed 3 weeks post injection. There are a few dark and intensely stained axons displaying degeneration of their axonal myelin sheath (Fig. 3c, d). Do not count such darkly stained axons, as these are still in the process of degeneration.

19. Three weeks after intravitreal injections, apoptotic processes in the retina have been largely completed and cellular deposits have been removed.

20. Perikarya of RGC can be identified by their size which usually is bigger than that of other cells in the GCL and their less dense chromatin (Fig. 4). Nuclei from endothelial cells which are also present in the GCL are much smaller and their chromatin stains darker because of its density.

Acknowledgments

Antje Zenker provided the schematic drawings.

References

1. Shen Y, Liu XL, Yang XL (2006) N-methyl-D-aspartate receptors in the retina. Mol Neurobiol 34:163–179

2. Seki M, Lipton SA (2008) Targeting excitotoxic/free radical signaling pathways for therapeutic intervention in glaucoma. Prog Brain Res 173:495–510

3. Li Y, Schlamp CL, Nickells RW (1999) Experimental induction of retinal ganglion cell death in adult mice. Invest Ophthalmol Vis Sci 40:1004–1008

4. Seitz R, Hackl S, Seibuchner T, Tamm ER, Ohlmann A (2010) Norrin mediates neuroprotective effects on retinal ganglion cells via activation of the Wnt/beta-catenin signaling pathway and the induction of neuroprotective growth factors in Muller cells. J Neurosci 30:5998–6010

5. Gavrieli Y, Sherman Y, Ben-Sasson SA (1992) Identification of programmed cell death in situ via specific labeling of nuclear DNA fragmentation. J Cell Biol 119:493–501

6. Karnovsky MJ (1965) A formaldehyde-glutaraldehyde fixative of high osmolality for use in electron-microscopy. J Cell Biol 27:137–138

7. Schultze WH (1972) Über das Paraphenylendiamin in der histologischen Färbetechnik und über eine neue Schnellfärbemethode der Nervenmarkscheide am Gefrierschnitt. Zentralbl Pathol 36:639–640

8. Richardson KC, Jarret L, Finke H (1960) Embedding in epoxy resins for ultrathin sectioning in electron microscopy. Stain Technol 35:313–323

9. Fischer D, Pavlidis M, Thanos S (2000) Cataractogenic lens injury prevents traumatic ganglion cell death and promotes axonal regeneration both in vivo and in culture. Invest Ophthalmol Vis Sci 41:3943–3954

10. Fischer D, Hauk TG, Muller A, Thanos S (2008) Crystallins of the beta/gamma-superfamily mimic the effects of lens injury and promote axon regeneration. Mol Cell Neurosci 37:471–479

11. Muller A, Hauk TG, Fischer D (2007) Astrocyte-derived CNTF switches mature RGCs to a regenerative state following inflammatory stimulation. Brain 130:3308–3320

12. Yin Y, Cui Q, Li Y, Irwin N, Fischer D, Harvey AR, Benowitz LI (2003) Macrophage-derived factors stimulate optic nerve regeneration. J Neurosci 23:2284–2293

13. Williams RW, Strom RC, Rice DS, Goldowitz D (1996) Genetic and environmental control of variation in retinal ganglion cell number in mice. J Neurosci 16:7193–7205

14. Dangata YY, Findlater GS, Dhillon B, Kaufman MH (1994) Morphometric study of the optic nerve of adult normal mice and mice heterozygous for the Small eye mutation (Sey/+). J Anat 185(Pt 3):627–635

15. Schori H, Yoles E, Wheeler LA, Raveh T, Kimchi A, Schwartz M (2002) Immune-related mechanisms participating in resistance and susceptibility to glutamate toxicity. Eur J Neurosci 16:557–564

16. London A, Itskovich E, Benhar I, Kalchenko V, Mack M, Jung S, Schwartz M (2011) Neuroprotection and progenitor cell renewal in the injured adult murine retina requires healing monocyte-derived macrophages. J Exp Med 208:23–39

17. Ganesh BS, Chintala SK (2011) Inhibition of reactive gliosis attenuates excitotoxicity-mediated death of retinal ganglion cells. PLoS One 6:e18305

18. Jakobs TC, Ben Y, Masland RH (2007) Expression of mRNA for glutamate receptor subunits distinguishes the major classes of retinal neurons, but is less specific for individual cell types. Mol Vis 13:933–948

Part III

Other Animal Models

Chapter 8

Generation of Transgenic *X. laevis* Models of Retinal Degeneration

Beatrice M. Tam, Christine C.-L. Lai, Zusheng Zong, and Orson L. Moritz

Abstract

Transgenic models are invaluable tools for researching retinal degenerative disease mechanisms. However, they are time-consuming and expensive to generate and maintain. We have developed an alternative to transgenic rodent models of retinal degeneration using transgenic *Xenopus laevis*. We have optimized this system to allow rapid analysis of transgene effects in primary transgenic animals, thereby providing an alternative to establishing transgenic lines, and simultaneously allowing rigorous comparisons between the effects of different transgenes.

Key words: Transgenic *Xenopus laevis*, Retinal degeneration, Dot blot, Confocal microscopy

1. Introduction

We have developed techniques for generating and analyzing transgenic *Xenopus laevis* models of retinal degeneration (RD) based on mutations in the rhodopsin gene responsible for retinitis pigmentosa in humans (1–9); we are also currently applying these techniques to the analysis of other transgenes in our laboratory. In addition, we (and others) have applied these and related techniques to studies of protein localization in photoreceptors (5–19), and to the analysis of promoter activities (20–27). In general, these techniques differ from those typically used for analysis of transgenic rodents in that founder ("F0" or "primary") transgenic animals are analyzed without further breeding to create transgenic lines, and the effects of multiple transgenes can be compared in a single experiment. Transgenic *X. laevis* are generated by injection of transgenic sperm into unfertilized eggs (the REMI/nuclear transplantation method) (28), followed by an antibiotic selection protocol to eliminate

Bernhard H.F. Weber and Thomas Langmann (eds.), *Retinal Degeneration: Methods and Protocols*, Methods in Molecular Biology, vol. 935, DOI 10.1007/978-1-62703-080-9_8, © Springer Science+Business Media, LLC 2013

non-transgenic embryos (29). For antibiotic selection purposes, the DNA construct must contain a second transgene—a neomycin resistance cassette based on the *aphA-2* gene capable of functioning in eukaryotic cells, such as that found in the eGFP-N1 vector (Clontech). The primary transgenic animals generated by these methods are non-chimeric and can therefore be analyzed without further breeding (28). In our experiments, the animals are typically sacrificed and analyzed two weeks after a set of injections, thereby allowing an entire experiment to be completed in under a month.

Using these techniques, two experienced individuals working together can easily generate more than 200 transgenic animals in a single day. A typical experiment would involve at least two transgenes—for example, a comparison of the effects of a wild-type rhodopsin cDNA and a rhodopsin mutant. However, we have often compared multiple transgenes (up to eight) (6). The use of a wild-type rhodopsin cDNA allows us to control for the effects of rhodopsin overexpression, although in contrast to results obtained in mice (30, 31), these effects are typically quite minimal.

In addition, transgenic *X. laevis* containing two transgenes are also readily produced by simultaneously injecting two different transgene constructs (3)—the high success rate is likely due to high transgene copy numbers obtained using this method.

Because each resulting transgenic animal contains unique transgene integration sites and copy numbers, expression levels vary considerably between animals (typically over a range of two orders of magnitude for wild-type rhodopsin), with the highest expression levels approaching or exceeding 50% of total rhodopsin being least common (5–7). Given a sufficient yield of primary transgenic animals, this allows investigators to survey transgene effects at a variety of expression levels, and also to monitor the effects of mutations on protein expression levels (5–8). This requires a relatively high "N," but this is generally easily achieved.

However, this non-normal distribution of expression levels, combined with the likelihood that a threshold expression level is required to achieve a phenotype, requires that special considerations must be made for the analysis of transgene effects and RD—in particular, nonparametric statistical methods (which do not assume normally distributed data) should be employed when analyzing primary transgenic animals (5–8).

One confounding aspect of the system is the presence of position effects that result in transgene silencing in a relatively high proportion of transgenic animals. This silencing can be transient (on and off) or relatively permanent, and can affect a subset or virtually all cells in an animal (15). We have found that position effects can be minimized by two techniques that can be applied in combination: the use of antibiotic selection (29) (presumably because the neomycin resistance cassette is subject to similar silencing and therefore embryos with strong position effects do not survive), and the use of a chicken β-globin "double insulator" sequence in transgene constructs (32, 33).

Although we have attempted to duplicate these procedures in the diploid species *Xenopus tropicalis*, the resulting yield of primary transgenic animals is prohibitively low in our hands. This is likely due to the relatively small size of *X. tropicalis* eggs, which sustain comparatively greater damage on injection. We have also attempted to duplicate these procedures using other published methods for generation of transgenic *X. laevis*, including φC31 integrase (34) and ISce1-mediated transgene integration (35, 36) methods. In our hands, these generate high yields of primary transgenic animals consistent with the original reports. However, the expression levels are insufficient to allow for the development of an RD phenotype in a significant proportion of the animals.

The procedures we have described can also be used to generate transgenic lines with consistent RD phenotypes (2, 37). Our standard approach is to initially conduct experiments with primary transgenic animals while setting aside a population to rear to sexual maturity (requiring 8 months to 1 year).

Here we present protocols for generation of transgenic embryos by nuclear transplantation, antibiotic selection of transgenic embryos, and dot blot analysis of total rod opsin levels to monitor RD. Other valuable resources for *X. laevis* transgenesis procedures are also available (38, 39).

2. Materials

2.1. Generation of Transgenic X. laevis Embryos

1. Special equipment and materials required: Two high-quality dissecting microscopes (e.g., Zeiss Stemi), two micromanipulators (e.g., Narishige MM-3 or similar), a syringe pump (e.g., Harvard pump 11 plus) equipped with two 50 μl syringes, Tygon tubing, microcap pipettes, pipette puller (e.g., Flaming/Brown type pullers manufactured by Sutter Instruments), cold room, adult *X. laevis* females (Fig. 1a shows a typical injection setup).

2. Needles for microinjection—we use microcap pipettes (Drummond, 30 μl) using a single pull to achieve a taper length of approximately 1 cm, which we then break with tweezers to give a hypodermic-like profile, and an opening diameter of 60–80 μm (Fig. 1b, c).

3. Sperm nuclei—prepared according to Murray (40) as modified by Kroll and Amaya (28) and subsequently made up to a final concentration of 30% glycerol and 100 nuclei/nl, then aliquoted, and frozen at –80° for indefinite storage. We will typically do a prep using testes from 1 to 2 animals that will be sufficient for a large number of experiments.

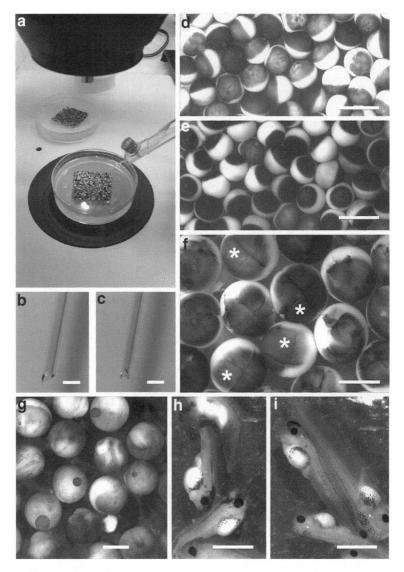

Fig. 1. Generation of transgenic *Xenopus laevis*. (**a**) Eggs ready for injection. (**b**) Needle suitable for injection. (**c**) Unacceptable needle. (**d**) Eggs prior to injection of nuclei. (**e**) Eggs immediately following injection of nuclei—very little noticeable damage, eggs have activated. (**f**) Embryos after two cell divisions—those noted by an *asterisk* will be retained, others show abnormal cell divisions or are nondividing. (**g**) Embryos immediately prior to antibiotic selection (gastrula or neurula stage). Some embryos have an attached bleb consisting of cells that have leaked from the injection site. (**h**) Surviving abnormal (likely non-transgenic) embryos following antibiotic selection. (**i**) Surviving normal (likely transgenic) embryos following G418 selection. ((**b**), (**c**)—bar = 100 μm. (**d**), (**e**), (**h**), (**i**)—bar = 2 mm. (**f**), (**g**)—bar = 1 mm).

4. High-Speed Egg Extract—prepared according to Murray (40) as modified by Kroll and Amaya (28), aliquoted, and frozen at –80°.

5. Human chorionic gonadotropin (Sigma Aldrich)—made up at 1 unit/μl.

6. Linearized transgene DNA—This can be prepared by either linearization of plasmids containing the transgenes with a restriction enzyme followed by gel purification (we use kits available from Qiagen) or amplification of the necessary sequence by long accurate PCR followed by similar gel purification. The final prep should be diluted to 75 ng/μl in dH$_2$O. If the antibiotic selection protocol is to be used, it is critical that a neomycin-resistance cassette is present in the transgene construct, and is not disrupted by the plasmid linearization process. It is also critical to eliminate all circular DNA, and to use DNA at the specified concentration (see Note 1).

7. Mark's modified ringer (MMR): 100 mM NaCl, 2 mM KCl, 1 mM MgCl$_2$, 2 mM CaCl$_2$, 5 mM HEPES pH 7.4 and autoclaved. We prepare 1 and 20× stocks.

8. Tadpole Ringer: 10 mM NaCl, 0.2 mM KCl, 0.1 mM MgCl$_2$, 0.2 mM CaCl$_2$. We prepare as 100× stock.

9. 2% Cysteine solution: 1 g of cysteine hydrochloride added to 50 ml of 1× MMR, pH adjusted to 8.0 with 2N NaOH, freshly prepared on the day needed.

10. Sperm dilution buffer (SDB): 250 mM sucrose, 75 mM KCl, 0.5 mM spermidine trihydrochloride, 0.2 mM spermine tetrahydrochloride; titrated to pH 7.4 with NaOH.

11. Ficoll solutions: 0.1× MMR+6% Ficoll 400, and 0.4× MMR+6% Ficoll 400, filter sterilized.

12. Gentamycin stock solution: 10 mg/ml gentamycin.

13. Agarose injection plates: 2% agarose dissolved in dH$_2$O and autoclaved. Pour into 50 mm petri dishes and float 2×2 cm pieces of autoclaved silicone (cut from a silicone baking sheet or a similar product) in the center of the dish. Once the agarose has set, cover the surface with sterile 1× MMR, replace lids, and seal with parafilm for storage at 4°C.

2.2. Antibiotic Selection of Transgenic Embryos

1. Translucent or transparent flat-bottomed plastic bins suitable for rearing tadpoles, such as Nasco Flex-tanks. Glass tanks can also be used.

2. G418 (Geneticin) (Gibco-BRL).

2.3. Blot Analysis of Retinal Degeneration

1. Dot blot apparatus (for example Biorad Bio-Dot).

2. LI-COR Odyssey imaging system.

3. Nylon membrane (e.g., Immobillon-P, Millipore).

4. Miniature homogenizer (e.g., Kontes Pellet Pestle).

5. Mini-scalpel and forceps or similar dissection tools (e.g., Beaver Microsharp or a similar one).

6. Tricaine (MS-222) anesthetic.

7. Modified SDS-PAGE loading buffer (standard SDS-PAGE loading buffer diluted 2× with phosphate-buffered saline (PBS), and containing 1 mM PMSF and 2 mM EDTA). For 1 ml, combine 0.5 ml of PBS, 0.5 ml of SDS-PAGE loading buffer (5% SDS, 0.1 M Tris HCl pH 6.8, 40% sucrose, and 0.1% Bromophenol blue), 40 μl of 2-mercaptoethanol, 4 μl of 0.5 M EDTA pH 8.0, and 10 μl of 100 mM PMSF.

8. 20 mM Sodium Phosphate pH 7.5.

9. Hybridoma B630N cell culture supernatant (a monoclonal anti-rod opsin antibody with broad cross-reactivity available from Dr. W. Clay Smith, University of Florida).

10. IR-Dye 800 conjugated goat anti-mouse secondary antibody (LICOR).

11. PBS, powdered milk, Tween-20, and SDS.

3. Methods

3.1. Generation of Transgenic X. laevis Embryos

1. Prepare linearized transgene DNA.

2. Two days prior to experiment: late in the day, inject three or more female *X. laevis* with 50 units of human chorionic gonadotropin (subcutaneous injection). The females are subsequently kept in 18°C dH$_2$O containing 10 mM NaCl.

3. One day prior to experiment: Late in the day, reinject the female *X. laevis* with 700 units of human chorionic gonadotropin.

4. On the day of the experiment—Prepare fresh cysteine solution, and dilute the restriction enzyme (the same enzyme used for linearization of the transgene construct) to 0.1 unit/μl with SDB. Thaw aliquots of egg extract and sperm nuclei and store with diluted restriction enzyme on ice (see Note 2).

5. Ensure that the female *X. laevis* are laying eggs, and transfer them to clean tanks.

6. Steps 7–14 are conveniently split between two researchers. One researcher can carry out steps 7–9 while the second carries out steps 10–14. An experienced individual can perform all steps simultaneously. However, the goal is for steps 9 and 14 to be completed simultaneously.

7. Squeeze eggs into a 10 cm petri dish containing 1× MMR. Squeezing frogs correctly requires some instruction and practice, and should not cause any injury to the frogs. Do not use eggs that have been previously laid into the tank water. Try to obtain on the order of 800–1,600 eggs.

8. Replace the 1× MMR solution covering the eggs with 2% cysteine solution, and agitate the dish until the jelly coating is removed. Wash the eggs repeatedly in 1× MMR, removing any abnormal or lysing eggs in the process (at least three washes).

9. Remove the 1× MMR solution and silicone square from a sufficient number of agarose dishes (typically 2–4) and replace with 0.4× MMR+6% Ficoll solution. Transfer the de-jellied eggs into the wells formed by the silicone squares, carefully forming a single layer of tightly packed eggs, while transferring as little solution as possible.

10. Add 2.5 μl of the linearized DNA constructs to two Eppendorf tubes (if two different constructs will be injected by the two researchers) (Fig. 1a).

11. Add 2 μl of sperm nuclei to each tube, and incubate for 5 min at 18°C.

12. Add 0.5 μl of diluted restriction enzyme, 3.5 μl egg extract, and 10 μl of SDB, mix gently, and incubate for 10 min at 18°C.

13. Dilute the reaction in SDB to give a final concentration of 0.3 nuclei/nl (see Note 3). Back-load two injection needles with the reactions, connect the needles to the syringe pump, and mount them in the micromanipulators. The injection needles should be mounted at an angle of 45° from horizontal. Set the syringe pump to deliver 36 μl/h (10 nl/s) (see Note 4).

14. Inject the eggs as quickly as possible, making sure to leave the needle in each egg for a total of 1 s. Eggs should be injected half way between the pole and equator, such that the needle enters perpendicularly, doing as little damage as possible (Fig. 1d–e). An experienced injector can inject at a rate of 40 eggs/minute, so two individuals can inject 1,600 eggs in approximately 20 min. After this point, both the eggs and reactions will begin to deteriorate in quality.

15. After the first set of injections are complete, set the plates aside, and resume the procedure at step 6 to perform another set of injections (if desired).

16. Monitor the injected eggs and watch for the start of cell division—this should be reasonably synchronized across the plate. At the second cell division, use a fire-polished Pasteur pipette to remove all the correctly dividing eggs (four cells) that can be identified (Fig. 1f), and place them in a dish of 0.1× MMR+6% Ficoll containing 50 μg/ml gentamycin antibiotic. Under optimal conditions, 1/3 of the injected eggs will divide correctly, 1/3 will not divide, and 1/3 will divide abnormally due to receiving more than one sperm nucleus. Assess the numbers in each category, and adjust the dilution factor or quantity of nuclei added in further reactions accordingly.

17. After 24 h, transfer the surviving embryos to tadpole ringer for rearing (Fig. 1g), or proceed with the antibiotic selection protocol below if desired. Under optimal conditions, the majority of the correctly dividing embryos will survive the first 24 h, and the yield after 14 days will be reduced by approximately 1/3—the attrition is likely due to genomic damage. Approximately 1/3 of the embryos will be transgenic.

3.2. Antibiotic Selection of Transgenic Embryos

1. On the day following fertilization (gastrula or neurula stage), transfer the surviving embryos to 0.1× MMR containing 20 µg/ml G418. Place no more than 200 embryos per liter of antibiotic solution in a suitable container such as a Nasco Flex Tank, and maintain the tanks at 18°C.

2. Monitor the embryos, continuously removing any dead embryos—after 120 h, a significant proportion of the embryos will be developmentally delayed, arrested, or dead. For the purposes of troubleshooting it may be useful to divide initial experiments into selected and nonselected groups so that the effects of the G418 treatment can be differentiated from those due to normal attrition. Occasionally shorter treatments (96 h) or longer treatments (up to 144 h) are necessary before selection effects are apparent.

3. When healthy and developmentally delayed embryos can be clearly differentiated (Fig. 1h, i), the healthy embryos can be separated manually (regardless of whether the selection has progressed to completion), transferred to 0.1× MMR or 1× tadpole ringer, and allowed to develop to the stage required for analysis (e.g., stage 49–50, 14 days following fertilization). At this point, the animals are transferred to normal housing conditions (clear plastic tanks containing tadpole ringer, 18°C, with daily feeding of powdered frog chow). Typically, 20% of the embryos subjected to G418 selection will survive, and >90% of these will be transgenic.

4. Although this protocol usually results in >90% transgenic animals, it is still critical to confirm that the majority of animals are transgenic. This can be done by a variety of methods, the simplest being to screen the animals visually for fluorescence if the transgene encodes a fluorescent product such as a GFP fusion protein. Other suitable methods include PCR of genomic DNA, southern blot (15), co-injection of a transgene encoding a fluorescent protein (3), immuno-labeling of frozen sections from the contralateral eye with an antibody specific for the transgene product (5–7), or a dot- or western blot assay similar to that described below using an antibody specific for the transgene product (5–7) (we have used antibodies 1D4 and 2B2 for labeling our rhodopsin transgene products, as these antibodies do not label the endogenous X. laevis rhodopsin; we have also used anti-HA for HA-tagged transgene products (3)).

3.3. Dot Blot Analysis of Retinal Degeneration

The following procedures are optimized for a time point of 14 days post fertilization.

1. Sacrifice the transgenic tadpoles by an overdose of Tricaine anesthetic (0.1% in 0.1× MMR).

2. Enucleate one eye from each animal to be analyzed and place in an Eppendorf tube containing 100 μl of modified SDS-PAGE loading buffer. (The remaining eye can be used for other assays such as histology or RNA isolation. For histology, fix overnight in 4% paraformaldehyde in 0.1 M sodium phosphate buffer pH 7.5.)

3. Homogenize for 30 s, rinsing the homogenizer in dH$_2$O between samples.

4. Once all samples are homogenized, centrifuge for 5 min at maximum speed in a benchtop microfuge (see Note 5).

5. Dilute each sample 300× using 20 mM sodium phosphate pH 7.5 (use a 96-well plate to aid organization) (see Notes 3 and 6).

6. Load the dot blot apparatus with a sheet of membrane prepared according to the manufacturer's instructions, and add 270 μl of sodium phosphate buffer per well (see Note 7).

7. Add 30 μl of each sample prepared in step 6 to each well prepared in step 7 (i.e., each sample is further diluted on loading into the apparatus, for a combined dilution of 3,000×) (see Notes 3 and 6).

8. Draw the samples through the membrane using vacuum, followed by several rinses of dH$_2$O.

9. Remove the membrane from the apparatus, rinse with dH$_2$O, and air-dry.

10. Prepare the membrane for immunoblotting according to the manufacturer's instructions (see Note 7).

11. Block with PBS containing 1% powdered milk for 30 min.

12. After rinsing with PBS/0.5% Tween, label overnight with B630N cell culture supernatant diluted 20× in PBS/0.5% Tween/0.1% powdered milk (see Notes 3 and 6).

13. After rinsing with PBS/0.5% Tween, label with IRDye800 secondary antibody diluted 10,000× in PBS/0.1% powdered milk/0.5% Tween/0.02%SDS for 2–4 h. This antibody must be protected from all light exposure (see Notes 3 and 6).

14. Image the dot blot using a LI-COR Odyssey imaging system. Quantify the signal from each sample—these measurements can be used for comparative purposes between animals and between groups of animals. In general, a low B630N signal (i.e., low rod opsin levels) is likely to be a result of missing or abnormal rod photoreceptors, and indicates RD—however this should be confirmed by a second assay (for example, histology performed on contralateral eyes) (Fig. 2).

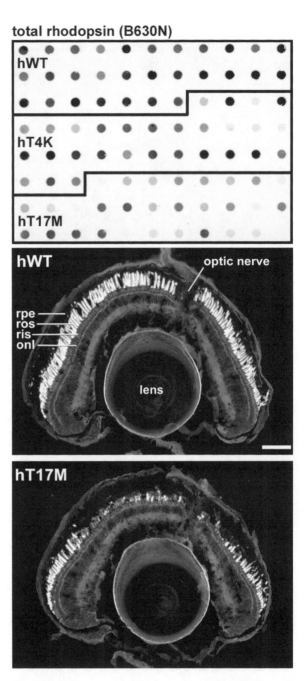

Fig. 2. Analysis of transgenic *Xenopus laevis*. *Top*: B630N dot blot for total rod opsin from an experiment involving three different transgene constructs (wild-type human rhodopsin, human T4K rhodopsin, and human T17M rhodopsin). On average, animals expressing the hT17M mutant show the lowest intensity rod opsin signals, likely indicating RD. *Lower panels*: Confocal microscopy of representative contralateral eyes (cryosections stained with wheat germ agglutinin) confirms RD in the hT17M mutant animals. Panels reproduced with permission from Fig. 1 of Tam et al. (5) (Bar = 100 μm).

Alternatives to the Odyssey imaging system (such as chemiluminescence-based detection) could be employed. The Odyssey imaging system gives a broad linear response and is ideal for this purpose. However, nonparametric statistical methods (necessitated by the non-normal distribution of the resulting data; see introduction) require only ordinal data, and therefore a completely linear response is not critical, although every effort should be made to ensure that the assay response is as linear as possible. The assay can be easily optimized using serial-diluted samples obtained from non-transgenic eyes.

4. Notes

1. For troubleshooting purposes, it may be useful to use a GFP transgene with expression driven in all tissues by a promoter such as CMV.

2. From this point onward, it is advisable (but not critical) to carry out further steps in an 18°C cold room.

3. Dilutions and concentrations may need to be optimized.

4. Theoretically, it is optimal to inject an average of one sperm nucleus per egg, whereas we typically inject three. This number was arrived at empirically, and may reflect a tendency for sperm nuclei to leak from the injection site, and for a portion of the sperm nuclei to be nonviable.

5. These samples are also suitable for analysis by standard western blot.

6. The concentrations given result in the majority of samples lying within a linear response range of the assay in our hands.

7. For Immobilon-P, wet with methanol, and then rinse with dH_2O.

Acknowledgments

This research was funded by the Canadian Institutes for Health Research, and the Foundation Fighting Blindness (Canada).

References

1. Moritz OL, Tam BM (2010) Recent insights into the mechanisms underlying light-dependent retinal degeneration from X. laevis models of retinitis pigmentosa. Adv Exp Med Biol 664:509–515. doi:10.1007/978-1-4419-1399-9_58

2. Tam BM, Qazalbash A, Lee HC, Moritz OL (2010) The dependence of retinal degeneration

caused by the rhodopsin P23H mutation on light exposure and vitamin A deprivation. Invest Ophthalmol Vis Sci 51(3):1327–1334

3. Hamm LM, Tam BM, Moritz OL (2009) Controlled rod cell ablation in transgenic Xenopus laevis. Invest Ophthalmol Vis Sci 50(2):885–892. doi:iovs.08-2337 (pii)

4. Tam BM, Qazalbash A, Lee HC, Moritz OL (2010) The dependence of retinal degeneration caused by the rhodopsin P23H mutation on light exposure and vitamin a deprivation. Invest Ophthalmol Vis Sci 51(3):1327–1334. doi:iovs.09-4123 (pii)

5. Tam BM, Moritz OL (2009) The role of rhodopsin glycosylation in protein folding, trafficking, and light-sensitive retinal degeneration. J Neurosci 29(48):15145–15154. doi:29/48/15145 (pii)

6. Tam BM, Moritz OL (2007) Dark rearing rescues P23H rhodopsin-induced retinal degeneration in a transgenic Xenopus laevis model of retinitis pigmentosa: a chromophore-dependent mechanism characterized by production of N-terminally truncated mutant rhodopsin. J Neurosci 27(34):9043–9053. doi:27/34/9043 (pii)

7. Tam BM, Xie G, Oprian DD, Moritz OL (2006) Mislocalized rhodopsin does not require activation to cause retinal degeneration and neurite outgrowth in Xenopus laevis. J Neurosci 26(1):203–209. doi:26/1/203 (pii)

8. Tam BM, Moritz OL (2006) Characterization of rhodopsin P23H-induced retinal degeneration in a Xenopus laevis model of retinitis pigmentosa. Invest Ophthalmol Vis Sci 47(8):3234–3241. doi:47/8/3234 (pii)

9. Moritz OL, Tam BM, Hurd LL, Peranen J, Deretic D, Papermaster DS (2001) Mutant rab8 Impairs docking and fusion of rhodopsin-bearing post-Golgi membranes and causes cell death of transgenic Xenopus rods. Mol Biol Cell 12(8):2341–2351

10. Mazelova J, Astuto-Gribble L, Inoue H, Tam BM, Schonteich E, Prekeris R, Moritz OL, Randazzo PA, Deretic D (2009) Ciliary targeting motif VxPx directs assembly of a trafficking module through Arf4. EMBO J 28(3):183–192. doi:emboj2008267 (pii)

11. Tam BM, Moritz OL, Papermaster DS (2004) The C terminus of peripherin/rds participates in rod outer segment targeting and alignment of disk incisures. Mol Biol Cell 15(4):2027–2037. doi:10.1091/mbc.E03-09-0650

12. Ritter LM, Boesze-Battaglia K, Tam BM, Moritz OL, Khattree N, Chen SC, Goldberg AF (2004) Uncoupling of photoreceptor peripherin/rds fusogenic activity from biosynthesis, subunit assembly, and targeting: a potential mechanism for pathogenic effects. J Biol Chem 279(38):39958–39967. doi:10.1074/jbc.M403943200

13. Peterson JJ, Tam BM, Moritz OL, Shelamer CL, Dugger DR, McDowell JH, Hargrave PA, Papermaster DS, Smith WC (2003) Arrestin migrates in photoreceptors in response to light: a study of arrestin localization using an arrestin-GFP fusion protein in transgenic frogs. Exp Eye Res 76(5):553–563

14. Loewen CJ, Moritz OL, Tam BM, Papermaster DS, Molday RS (2003) The role of subunit assembly in peripherin-2 targeting to rod photoreceptor disk membranes and retinitis pigmentosa. Mol Biol Cell 14(8):3400–3413. doi:10.1091/mbc.E03-02-0077

15. Moritz OL, Tam BM, Papermaster DS, Nakayama T (2001) A functional rhodopsin-green fluorescent protein fusion protein localizes correctly in transgenic Xenopus laevis retinal rods and is expressed in a time-dependent pattern. J Biol Chem 276(30):28242–28251. doi:10.1074/jbc.M101476200

16. Tam BM, Moritz OL, Hurd LB, Papermaster DS (2000) Identification of an outer segment targeting signal in the COOH terminus of rhodopsin using transgenic Xenopus laevis. J Cell Biol 151(7):1369–1380

17. Baker SA, Haeri M, Yoo P, Gospe SM 3rd, Skiba NP, Knox BE, Arshavsky VY (2008) The outer segment serves as a default destination for the trafficking of membrane proteins in photoreceptors. J Cell Biol 183(3): 485–498

18. Kizhatil K, Baker SA, Arshavsky VY, Bennett V (2009) Ankyrin-G promotes cyclic nucleotide-gated channel transport to rod photoreceptor sensory cilia. Science 323(5921):1614–1617

19. Luo W, Marsh-Armstrong N, Rattner A, Nathans J (2004) An outer segment localization signal at the C terminus of the photoreceptor-specific retinol dehydrogenase. J Neurosci 24(11):2623–2632

20. Langmann T, Lai CC, Weigelt K, Tam BM, Warneke-Wittstock R, Moritz OL, Weber BH (2008) CRX controls retinal expression of the X-linked juvenile retinoschisis (RS1) gene. Nucleic Acids Res 36(20):6523–6534. doi:gkn737 (pii)

21. Moritz OL, Peck A, Tam BM (2002) Xenopus laevis red cone opsin and Prph2 promoters allow transgene expression in amphibian cones, or both rods and cones. Gene 298(2):173–182

22. Mani SS, Besharse JC, Knox BE (1999) Immediate upstream sequence of arrestin directs rod-specific expression in Xenopus. J Biol Chem 274(22):15590–15597

23. Zhu X, Ma B, Babu S, Murage J, Knox BE, Craft CM (2002) Mouse cone arrestin gene

characterization: promoter targets expression to cone photoreceptors. FEBS Lett 524(1–3):116–122

24. Lerner LE, Gribanova YE, Whitaker L, Knox BE, Farber DB (2002) The rod cGMP-phosphodiesterase beta-subunit promoter is a specific target for Sp4 and is not activated by other Sp proteins or CRX. J Biol Chem 277(29):25877–25883. doi:10.1074/jbc.M201407200

25. Babu S, McIlvain V, Whitaker SL, Knox BE (2006) Conserved cis-elements in the Xenopus red opsin promoter necessary for cone-specific expression. FEBS Lett 580(5):1479–1484. doi:S0014-5793(06)00150-5 (pii)

26. Whitaker SL, Knox BE (2004) Conserved transcriptional activators of the Xenopus rhodopsin gene. J Biol Chem 279(47):49010–49018. doi:10.1074/jbc.M406080200

27. Viczian AS, Verardo M, Zuber ME, Knox BE, Farber DB (2004) Conserved transcriptional regulation of a cone phototransduction gene in vertebrates. FEBS Lett 577(1–2):259–264. doi:S0014579304012281 (pii)

28. Kroll KL, Amaya E (1996) Transgenic Xenopus embryos from sperm nuclear transplantations reveal FGF signaling requirements during gastrulation. Development 122(10):3173–3183

29. Moritz OL, Biddle KE, Tam BM (2002) Selection of transgenic Xenopus laevis using antibiotic resistance. Transgenic Res 11(3):315–319

30. Wen XH, Shen L, Brush RS, Michaud N, Al-Ubaidi MR, Gurevich VV, Hamm HE, Lem J, Dibenedetto E, Anderson RE, Makino CL (2009) Overexpression of rhodopsin alters the structure and photoresponse of rod photoreceptors. Biophys J 96(3):939–950. doi:S0006-3495(08)00054-4 (pii)

31. Tan E, Wang Q, Quiambao AB, Xu X, Qtaishat NM, Peachey NS, Lem J, Fliesler SJ, Pepperberg DR, Naash MI, Al-Ubaidi MR (2001) The relationship between opsin overexpression and photoreceptor degeneration. Invest Ophthalmol Vis Sci 42(3):589–600

32. Chung JH, Whiteley M, Felsenfeld G (1993) A 5′ element of the chicken beta-globin domain serves as an insulator in human erythroid cells and protects against position effect in Drosophila. Cell 74(3):505–514. doi:0092-8674(93)80052-G (pii)

33. Allen BG, Weeks DL (2006) Using phiC31 integrase to make transgenic Xenopus laevis embryos. Nat Protoc 1(3):1248–1257. doi:nprot.2006.183 (pii)

34. Allen BG, Weeks DL (2005) Transgenic Xenopus laevis embryos can be generated using phiC31 integrase. Nat Methods 2(12):975–979. doi:nmeth814 (pii)

35. Ogino H, McConnell WB, Grainger RM (2006) High-throughput transgenesis in Xenopus using I-SceI meganuclease. Nat Protoc 1(4):1703–1710. doi:nprot.2006.208 (pii)

36. Ogino H, McConnell WB, Grainger RM (2006) Highly efficient transgenesis in Xenopus tropicalis using I-SceI meganuclease. Mech Dev 123(2):103–113. doi:S0925-4773(05)00191-7 (pii)

37. Lee DC, Xu J, Sarunic MV, Moritz OL (2010) Fourier domain optical coherence tomography as a noninvasive means for in vivo detection of retinal degeneration in Xenopus laevis tadpoles. Invest Ophthalmol Vis Sci 51(2):1066–1070. doi:iovs.09-4260 (pii)

38. Amaya E, Kroll K (2010) Production of transgenic Xenopus laevis by restriction enzyme mediated integration and nuclear transplantation. J Vis Exp (42). doi:10.3791/2010

39. Chesneau A, Sachs LM, Chai N, Chen Y, Du Pasquier L, Loeber J, Pollet N, Reilly M, Weeks DL, Bronchain OJ (2008) Transgenesis procedures in Xenopus. Biol Cell 100(9):503–521. doi:BC20070148 (pii)

40. Murray AW (1991) Cell cycle extracts. Methods Cell Biol 36:581–605

Chapter 9

Analysis of Photoreceptor Degeneration in the Zebrafish *Danio rerio*

Holger Dill, Bastian Linder, Anja Hirmer, and Utz Fischer

Abstract

Disturbances in the general mRNA metabolism have been recognized as a major defect in a growing number of hereditary human diseases. One prominent example of this disease group is Retinitis pigmentosa (RP), characterized by selective loss of photoreceptor cells. RP can be caused by dominant mutations in key factors of the pre-mRNA processing spliceosome. In these cases, the complex events leading to the RP phenotype can only insufficiently be analyzed in rodents or other model organisms due to the essential functions of these splice factors. Here we introduce the zebrafish *Danio rerio* as a valuable vertebrate model system to study RP and related diseases.

Key words: Retinitis pigmentosa, Photoreceptor degeneration, mRNA metabolism, Spliceosome, Genetic analysis, Zebrafish

1. Introduction

Mutations that affect pre-mRNA processing are a frequent cause of genetic diseases. Depending on the mutated component, these diseases can be grouped into two major classes. The first and major group encompasses diseases where mutations affect regulatory sequences in distinct mRNAs and hence interfere with their accurate maturation. In contrast to this group stands the second class of diseases, which is characterized by mutations in general trans-acting factors involved in pre-mRNA processing. Because in the latter case, a more widespread defect in mRNA metabolism can be anticipated, the etiology of these diseases is expected to be rather complex and difficult to analyze at the molecular level.

One prominent example for a hereditary disease caused by mutations in general pre-mRNA processing factors is Retinitis pigmentosa (RP). This neurodegenerative disease is characterized by a severe rod–cone dystrophy leading to blindness (for review see ref. 1).

Bernhard H.F. Weber and Thomas Langmann (eds.), *Retinal Degeneration: Methods and Protocols*, Methods in Molecular Biology, vol. 935, DOI 10.1007/978-1-62703-080-9_9, © Springer Science+Business Media, LLC 2013

The vast majority of RP cases is caused by mutations in genes with specific functions in visual perception (2). However, approximately 11% of autosomal dominant RP cases result from mutations in one of the three general splice factor genes PRPF3, PRPF8, and PRPF31 (3–5). Their gene products are part of the U4/U6.U5 tri-snRNP, a particle that is formed by an intricate network of interactions between more than 30 proteins and 3 snRNAs ((6) and references therein). This snRNP contributes substantially to the active center of the spliceosome and contains essential components for the dynamic rearrangements that occur during its assembly and activation (for a recent review, see ref. 7 and references therein).

The question arises: How can mutations in general splice factors transform into a highly tissue-specific phenotype as observed in RP patients? To answer this question, a valuable disease model is required. The zebrafish *Danio rerio* offers several advantages for this type of investigation over other common model organisms. First, using a morpholino-based knockdown approach allows fine-tuned gene-silencing (8), an important condition when analyzing essential proteins such as splice factors. Second, effects on photoreceptor cell morphology and function can be directly studied in a functionally cone-dominated retina that is similar to its human counterpart (9). Finally, it allows for the expression profiling of eye-specific transcripts and is thus advantageous over cell culture systems (10).

In this chapter we summarize strategies and methods that have recently been used to investigate retina histology and vision-controlled behavior of zebrafish larvae deficient in RP-associated splice factors (11). After a general introduction of zebrafish maintenance and manipulation by microinjection, protocols for the immunohistochemical and immunological analysis of the eye are provided. The last part describes the analysis of the visuomotor behavior of manipulated larvae and provides an easy-to-use computer program for its analysis.

2. Materials

2.1. Zebrafish Maintenance and Breeding

1. Zebrafish Tu (Tübingen Zebrafish stock collection; http://www.eb.tuebingen.mpg.de).
2. Danieau's embryo medium stock: 58 mM NaCl, 0.7 mM KCl, 0.4 mM $MgSO_4 \times 7H_2O$, 0.6 mM $Ca(NO_3)_2$, 0.5 mM HEPES, 1 mM Methylene blue in water.

2.2. Microinjection of Zebrafish Embryos

1. Morpholino antisense oligos (Gene Tools, Philomath USA). Morpholino stocks (3 mM in water) are stored at –80°C.
2. Glass capillaries GC100F-10 (Cat No. 30-0019, Harvard Apparatus, Hamden, USA).

3. P-97 Flaming/Brown micropipette puller (Cat No. 1B150F-3, Sutter Instrument Company, Novato, USA).

4. Microinjector FemtoJet (Cat No. 920010504, Eppendorf, Hamburg, Germany).

5. SMZ 800 stereomicroscope (Nikon, Melville, USA).

6. Microloader tips (Cat No. 5242 956.003, Eppendorf, Hamburg, Germany).

7. 100× 1-phenyl-2-thiourea (PTU) stock (Cat No. P7629, Sigma-Aldrich, St. Louis, USA), 0.02 M in water.

2.3. Analysis of the Zebrafish Retina by Immunofluorescence Staining

2.3.1. Fixation of Zebrafish Larvae

1. Zebrafish larvae (age depending on the experiment).

2. Forceps.

3. Small lockable glass tubes (~8 ml).

4. Shaker.

5. PBST washing buffer: 0.1% Tween 20 in PBS (0.14 M NaCl, 2.7 mM KCl, 3.2 mM $Na_2HPO_4 \times 12H_2O$, 1.5 mM KH_2PO_4, pH 7.4).

6. Fixative solution: 4% paraformaldehyde in PBST.

2.3.2. Embedding of Fixed Larvae

1. 30% Aqueous saccharose solution.

2. Aluminum foil.

3. Tissue-Tek O.C.T. Compound (Sakura, Zoeterwoude, The Netherlands).

4. Stemi SV6 stereomicroscope (Zeiss, Jena, Germany).

5. Styrofoam-box filled with liquid nitrogen.

6. Plastic beaker filled with isopentane.

2.3.3. Cryosectioning

1. Jung Frigocut 2800N Cryomicrotome (Leica Mycrosystems, Wetzlar, Germany).

2. SuperFrost Plus microscope slides (Cat No. J3800AMNZ, Menzel, Braunschweig, Germany).

2.3.4. Immunofluorescence Staining of Cryosections

1. Cuvette for microscope slides.

2. Humid chamber.

3. Blocking solution: 2% goat serum (Cat No. CL1200-100, Cedarlane, Burlington, Canada) in PBS.

4. Primary antibody in PBS with 0.3% Triton X-100 and 5% goat serum.

5. Secondary antibody in PBS with 0.3% Triton X-100 and 5% goat serum.

6. Vectashield Mounting Medium with DAPI (Cat No. H-1200, Vector Laboratories, Burlingame, USA) diluted 1:1 with H_2O

and 2.5% DAKO fluorescent mounting medium (Cat No. S3023, Dako Deutschland GmbH, Hamburg, Germany).

7. Square coverslips (24 × 60 mm).

8. Axiovert 200 M microscope (Zeiss, Jena, Germany).

9. Axiocam MRm digital camera (Zeiss, Jena, Germany).

2.4. Single Larvae Western Blotting

1. SDS loading dye (100 mM Tris pH 6.8, 1% SDS, 50% Glycerine, Bromophenol blue, Xylene cyanol) mixed 1:1 with Buffer B (8 M Urea, 100 mM NaH_2PO_4, 10 mM Tris pH 8.0); add 1/20 volume 14.3 M β-Mercaptoethanol before usage.

2. SDS-PAGE equipment and Western blot apparatus.

3. Biotrace NT Nitrocellulose transfer membrane (Cat No. 66485, Pall, Pensacola, USA).

4. Primary and secondary antibodies in 1× NET-gelatine buffer (150 mM NaCl, 5 mM EDTA, 50 mM Tris pH 7.5, 0.05% Triton X-100, 2.5 g/l gelatine).

5. TBT (150 mM NaCl, 6 mM Tris, 19 mM Tris/HCl, 0.5% Tween 20 (v/v)).

2.5. Analysis of Visuomotor Behavior

1. Apparatus to measure OKN and stereomicroscope with Axiocam MRc5 digital camera (Zeiss, Jena, Germany).

2. 3% (w/v) methyl cellulose in 0.3× Danieau's embryo medium without Methylene blue.

3. NIH ImageJ with "Excel_Writer.jar" plug-in and "fish_eye_analysis.txt" macro toolset (available at http://www.biochem. biozentrum.uni-wuerzburg.de/protocols/).

4. Microsoft Excel with "fishtab.xlt" in the default template folder (available at http://www.biochem.biozentrum.uni-wuerzburg. de/protocols/).

3. Methods

3.1. Zebrafish Maintenance and Breeding

Adequate keeping conditions are essential to sustain health and fertility of zebrafish. Adult male and female fish are kept separated in a recirculation system at ~28.5°C and conditioned water. The light–dark cycle is adjusted to 14 h of light and 10 h of darkness. If used for continuous egg production, feed fish three times a day with dry food flakes or *baby brine shrimp (small artemia)*.

The following procedure ensures constant spawning of fertilized eggs.

1. In the late evening, set up mating crosses in a mating container separated by a sieve.

2. At the beginning of the light period, put males and females together in fresh fish water. Laid eggs will fall through the sieve and be protected from being eaten by the adult fish.

3. Collect eggs with a plastic pipette and store them in 0.3× Danieau's embryo medium in a Petri dish for subsequent microinjection.

3.2. Microinjection of Zebrafish Embryos

To transiently knock down genes of interest in reverse genetic approaches, morpholino antisense oligos are injected into zebrafish zygotes. To avoid harsh disturbance of embryonic development or off-target effects, it is advisable to titrate morpholinos down to a sublethal or nontoxic concentration in a preliminary test. This is especially important when analyzing essential genes, like splice factors.

1. Prepare a Petri dish filled with 1.5% agarose dissolved in 0.3× Danieau's embryo medium. Place a mold with rectangular strips on the agarose surface and let the agarose cool down to room temperature (see Note 1).

2. Produce micropipettes for injection from glass capillaries by using a micropipette puller.

3. Dilute morpholino stocks to an appropriate concentration with deionized, UV-sterilized water directly before injection. Heat morpholino solutions to 65°C for 10 min to make them soluble and afterwards keep them at room temperature (RT).

4. For microinjection only embryos at the one-cell stage should be used. To prepare newly fertilized eggs for injection, place them into the agarose slots with forceps and orientate them with yolk opposite to the micromanipulator. Remove the remaining embryo medium with a glass pipette.

5. Transfer ~1 μl morpholino solution to a micropipette with a microloader tip.

6. Adjust injection pressure to finally inject a volume of ~0.5 nl directly into the yolk. Morpholino oligos will be transported to the overlaying cells by ooplasmic streaming.

After injection, embryos are raised in an incubator at ~28.5°C and same illumination conditions as adult fish (see Subheading 3.1 and Note 2). Developmental stages are determined according to (12). For histological analyses at stages beyond 31 hours post fertilization (hpf) pigmentation is perturbing. To inhibit melanization, embryos can be treated with PTU after gastrulation. Knockdown efficiency needs to be controlled for every individual experiment by standard Western blot procedures (see Subheading 3.4).

3.3. Analysis of the Zebrafish Retina by Immunofluorescence Staining

To make the retinal tissue accessible for histological analysis, eyes of the larvae need to be prepared by cryosectioning. Immunofluorescence staining with appropriate primary antibodies and adequate fluorochrome-conjugated secondary antibodies allows for the analysis of photoreceptor morphology by fluorescence microscopy. Carry out all steps at RT, unless otherwise indicated.

3.3.1. Fixation of Zebrafish Larvae

1. Remove chorion with forceps if necessary (embryonic stages beyond 24 hpf).

2. Transfer larvae into a glass tube.

3. Remove the embryo medium and rinse larvae once in PBST.

4. Fix larvae with fixative solution overnight at 4°C or for 1 h.

5. To remove the remaining fixative solution wash three times in PBST for 5 min each on a shaker.

3.3.2. Embedding of Fixed Larvae

1. For cryoprotection incubate fixed embryos in 30% saccharose in a glass tube overnight at 4°C.

2. Make a cylinder using aluminum foil, height approximately 1.5 cm, diameter approximately 1.0 cm (see Note 3).

3. Fill the cylinder with Tissue-Tek.

4. Grab the tail of a larva with forceps and put it head-down into the cryomatrix (see Fig. 1a).

5. Put a maximum of five larvae into one cylinder and check if all larvae are directed parallel. Binocular usage is optional for this.

6. Precool a plastic beaker filled with isopentane in a Styrofoam-box with liquid nitrogen.

7. Pick the cylinder with forceps and put its bottom into the iso-pentane until the matrix is completely frozen (see Fig. 1b). Take care that no isopentane flows into the cylinder.

8. Store the frozen blocks at −80°C.

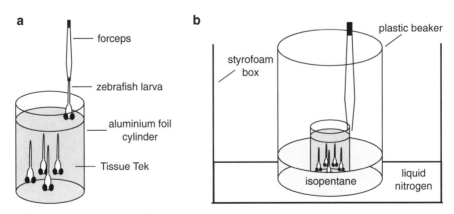

Fig. 1. Preparation of zebrafish larvae for cryosectioning. (**a**) PFA fixed larvae are positioned head-down in an aluminum cylinder filled with Tissue-Tek cryomatrix. Semifluid texture of the cryomatrix keeps larvae in a vertical position. (**b**) Samples are frozen with liquid nitrogen-cooled isopentane.

3.3.3. Cryosectioning

1. Precool the cryomicrotome to –20°C.

2. Remove the aluminum foil of a frozen block.

3. Fix the block with a drop of Tissue-Tek on the microtome specimen holder.

4. Adjust thickness of the slices to approximately 8 μm and the angle between blade and block in a way that larvae are cut in a 90° angle to the body axis.

5. Cut one or more slices. Take care that they do not overlap.

6. Absorb the slices onto a room tempered SuperFrost Plus microscope slide.

7. Store slides in a slide case at –20°C.

3.3.4. Immunofluorescence Staining of Retinal Sections

1. Wash slides three times in a cuvette with PBS for 10 min each.

2. Put slides on a holder in a humid chamber (see Fig. 2).

3. Block unspecific binding sites by pipetting 1 ml of 2% goat serum in PBS on each slide and incubate it for 20 min.

4. Remove the blocking solution by soaking it up with a paper towel.

5. Apply primary antibody solution onto the slides (~150 μl per slide), cover each slide with plastic foil, and incubate overnight at 4°C.

6. Remove unbound primary antibody by washing the slides three times with PBS in a cuvette for 15 min each.

7. Repeat steps 5 and 6 with the secondary antibody solution. For example, use Texas Red dye-conjugated goat anti-mouse

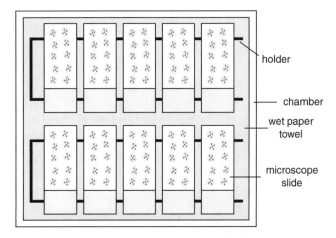

Fig. 2. Microscope slides are put on a holder in a humid chamber and incubated with antibody solution. To avoid drying-out of specimens, even when applying minute amounts of antibody solution, microscope slides are covered with plastic foil.

IgG + IgM (Jackson ImmunoResearch, Baltimore, USA) (see Notes 4 and 5).

8. Put a few drops of mounting medium on the slide and place a square coverslip on it. The contained DAPI stains the nucleus. Subject the stained cryosections to analysis by fluorescence microscopy.

3.4. Single Larvae Western Blotting

Transfer individual embryos into Eppendorf-caps (0.5 ml) with a plastic Pasteur pipette. If larvae are older than 2 days post fertilization (dpf), anesthetize larvae first by keeping them on ice for 30 min.

1. Remove embryo medium completely using a 200 µl pipette.

2. Add 22 µl SDS/Urea loading dye.

3. Heat at 95°C for 10 min.

4. Homogenize by trituration with a 20 µl pipette.

5. Spin down at $16,100 \times g$ for 15 min in a standard benchtop microcentrifuge to remove yolk debris.

6. Load 20 µl lysate on a polyacrylamide gel and follow standard SDS-PAGE/Western blot procedure.

3.5. Analysis of Visuomotor Behavior

Even if retinal morphology appears in a wild-type manner, processing of visual input within the retina can be disturbed. To detect these subtle effects, behavioral assays are applicable. We routinely measure the optokinetic nystagmus (OKN) to analyze visual capacity of zebrafish larvae. Therefore a rotating pattern of bright and dark stripes is presented to the larva (Fig. 3 and see Note 6).

1. Prepare 6 cm Petri dish filled with 3% methyl cellulose, and calibrate OKN grating (adjust speed).

2. Place individual larvae into the center of camera view, embed with methyl cellulose (see Note 7), and form an air bubble to monitor rotation (see Note 8).

3. Orient in a way that allows convenient separation of eyes by semi-automated image processing (see Note 8).

4. Simultaneously start image acquisition and rotation of grating (switch direction after 10 s; stop at 20 s); for quantitative analysis count the number of saccades presented; for qualitative analysis save video as avi-file (uncompressed) (see Note 9).

5. In ImageJ, switch toolset to "fish_eye_analysis" and import the avi-file as image sequence ("fish_avi_import" button: ▣).

6. Adjust brightness/contrast in a way that separates eyes and body axis (for a preset, use the "fish_image_adjust" button:).

7. Convert to binary image (process/binary/make binary).

8. Perform particle analysis to create ellipses corresponding to eyes and body axis ("fish_particle_analysis" button:).

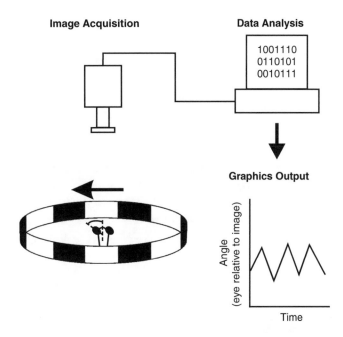

Fig. 3. Graphical representation of the OKN test workflow. A rotating striped pattern is presented to immobilized larvae. Eye movements are recorded and angles of the eye relative to the image plotted over time.

9. Consecutively measure the ellipses corresponding to left eye, body, and right eye, respectively: use the "fish_measure_eye" tool (✖) and click into the center of the corresponding ellipse; when prompted save Excel file (write all results to the same file, select "replace file" and "create new worksheet" when prompted).

10. Open the results file in Excel, insert new worksheet ("fishtab" template), and then click "plot eye movement."

4. Notes

1. To fix eggs in an appropriate position for microinjection also deepenings in synthetic resin can be used. These molds are more difficult to prepare but can be reused.

2. Unfertilized eggs have to be removed from developing embryos after first cell divisions, as they provide a source for growth of bacteria and mold fungus.

3. Aluminum cylinders can easily be produced by winding aluminum foil around a thick permanent marker and fixing it with autoclave tape.

4. Avoid the use of secondary antibodies coupled to fluorochromes with excitation wavelengths similar to green fluorescent protein (395 nm). Retinal tissues show autofluorescence at this wavelength.

5. Incubation time with the secondary antibody solution can be reduced to 2 h at RT.

6. Our OKN response apparatus is custom designed and built in-house. It uses a backlit cylindrical metal grating (6 cm diameter, 12° stripes) that is driven by an electric motor (6 rpm) and illuminated by a neon tube. To enhance contrast of the pigmented fish eyes in the image recordings, the fish tray is illuminated from below by dim LEDs.

7. To prepare methyl cellulose embedding medium, dissolve methyl cellulose powder in 0.3× Danieau's embryo medium. This takes some time and is best done by shaking/rotating overnight in a Falcon tube. To remove air bubbles from the highly viscous solution, spin down in a standard benchtop centrifuge ($3,500 \times g$/30 min).

8. When embedding larvae in methyl cellulose, arrange them in a way that allows good separation of the eyes from the trunk in the subsequent image analysis. For this, it is important that the head is oriented horizontally in both, the anterior/posterior and left/right axis. While all other steps of the digital image analysis can be performed automatically, separation of eyes needs to be optimized manually for each video recording. To help monitoring the pattern of movement presented, an air bubble can be formed in the methyl cellulose that mirrors the grating. If placed sideways of the body of the larvae, this does not influence OKN behavior. The eyes of the larvae are analyzed as particles whose angle relative to the image is then measured. This is achieved by converting each frame of the video to a binary image (black and white) and a subsequent analysis of the black particles present in each frame. It is important that the eyes can be identified as individual black particles automatically in each frame, i.e., they are separated by white space in the binary image. For this, use manual contrast adjustment (image/adjust/brightness/contrast) before conversion to binary image (process/binary/make binary). After conversion, the tool "erode" (process/binary/erode) can be used to further facilitate particle separation.

9. We routinely use the Axiovision software (rel. 4.8) to record a time-lapse image series that is exported as uncompressed avi-file. Nevertheless, for subsequent analysis in ImageJ, any format that can be imported as image stack is feasible (for detailed information, see ImageJ documentation).

References

1. Hartong DT, Berson EL, Dryja TP (2006) Retinitis pigmentosa. Lancet 368(9549): 1795–1809

2. Daiger SP, Bowne SJ, Sullivan LS (2007) Perspective on genes and mutations causing retinitis pigmentosa. Arch Ophthalmol 125(2): 151–158

3. Chakarova CF, Hims MM, Bolz H, Abu-Safieh L, Patel RJ, Papaioannou MG, Inglehearn CF, Keen TJ, Willis C, Moore AT, Rosenberg T, Webster AR, Bird AC, Gal A, Hunt D, Vithana EN, Bhattacharya SS (2002) Mutations in HPRP3, a third member of pre-mRNA splicing factor genes, implicated in autosomal dominant retinitis pigmentosa. Hum Mol Genet 11(1): 87–92

4. McKie AB, McHale JC, Keen TJ, Tarttelin EE, Goliath R, van Lith-Verhoeven JJ, Greenberg J, Ramesar RS, Hoyng CB, Cremers FP, Mackey DA, Bhattacharya SS, Bird AC, Markham AF, Inglehearn CF (2001) Mutations in the pre-mRNA splicing factor gene PRPC8 in autosomal dominant retinitis pigmentosa (RP13). Hum Mol Genet 10(15):1555–1562

5. Vithana EN, Abu-Safieh L, Allen MJ, Carey A, Papaioannou M, Chakarova C, Al-Maghtheh M, Ebenezer ND, Willis C, Moore AT, Bird AC, Hunt DM, Bhattacharya SS (2001) A human homolog of yeast pre-mRNA splicing gene, PRP31, underlies autosomal dominant retinitis pigmentosa on chromosome 19q13.4 (RP11). Mol Cell 8(2):375–381

6. Liu S, Rauhut R, Vornlocher HP, Luhrmann R (2006) The network of protein-protein interactions within the human U4/U6.U5 tri-snRNP. RNA 12(7):1418–1430

7. Wahl MC, Will CL, Luhrmann R (2009) The spliceosome: design principles of a dynamic RNP machine. Cell 136(4):701–718

8. Nasevicius A, Ekker SC (2000) Effective targeted gene 'knockdown' in zebrafish. Nat Genet 26(2):216–220

9. Bilotta J, Saszik S (2001) The zebrafish as a model visual system. Int J Dev Neurosci 19(7):621–629

10. Leung YF, Dowling JE (2005) Gene expression profiling of zebrafish embryonic retina. Zebrafish 2(4):269–283

11. Linder B, Dill H, Hirmer A, Brocher J, Lee GP, Mathavan S, Bolz HJ, Winkler C, Laggerbauer B, Fischer U (2011) Systemic splicing factor deficiency causes tissue-specific defects: a zebrafish model for retinitis pigmentosa. Hum Mol Genet 20(2):368–377

12. Kimmel CB, Ballard WW, Kimmel SR, Ullmann B, Schilling TF (1995) Stages of embryonic development of the zebrafish. Dev Dyn 203(3):253–310

Chapter 10

Analysis of Optokinetic Response in Zebrafish by Computer-Based Eye Tracking

Sabina P. Huber-Reggi, Kaspar P. Mueller, and Stephan C.F. Neuhauss

Abstract

Large-field movements in the visual surround trigger spontaneous, compensatory eye movements known as optokinetic response (OKR) in all vertebrates. In zebrafish (*Danio rerio*) the OKR is well developed at 5 days post fertilization and can be used in the laboratory for screening of visual performance following genetic manipulations or pharmaceutical treatments. Several setups for measurement of the zebrafish OKR have been described. All of them are based on the presentation of moving gratings to the larva or to the adult fish. However, they differ in the way of presenting gratings and in the method of analysis. Here, we describe a detailed protocol for our newest software that enables computer-generation of the moving stripes and automatic tracking of eye movement. This protocol makes it possible to quantitatively measure OKR in both larvae and adult fishes in a fast and reliable way.

Key words: Zebrafish larvae, Adult zebrafish, Optokinetic response, Eye movements, Vision, Visual behavior testing, Oculomotor

1. Introduction

Eye movements occur in all vertebrates and in some invertebrates and are thought to be required for high-resolution vision. Two main groups of eye movements exist. Gaze shifting eye movements aim at shifting of the eyes toward an object of interest and include saccadic movements, smooth pursuit, and vergence movements. Gaze stabilizing eye movements include the vestibular ocular reflex (VOR) and the optokinetic response (OKR) and aim at stabilization of a relative movement of the image on the retina, the retinal slip. Retinal slip is caused by either self-motion or motion of the surround and results in a blurred image. VOR and OKR are involuntary compensatory eye movements restoring high visual acuity. When the environment is continuously moving in one direction, the OKR produces a nystagmus composed of cycles of a slow eye

Bernhard H.F. Weber and Thomas Langmann (eds.), *Retinal Degeneration: Methods and Protocols*, Methods in Molecular Biology, vol. 935, DOI 10.1007/978-1-62703-080-9_10, © Springer Science+Business Media, LLC 2013

movement in the direction of the stimulus and a fast resetting movement, called saccade, in the opposite direction. The OKR is triggered by a velocity and direction input coming from the retina and encoded by a neural circuit involving pretectal nuclei (1, 2).

In a laboratory setting, an OKR can be easily elicited by a striped drum rotating around the subject. The OKR has been measured in a number of model organisms, incl. monkey, rabbit, mouse, and fish (e.g., goldfish, medaka, and zebrafish) (3–8). The combination of high-fecundity, extracorporally developing embryos and rapid development of most functions, incl. the visual system, has made zebrafish a model organism of increasing importance for studying visual function. Zebrafish are afoveate animals and therefore, in contrast to humans, do not display gaze shifting eye movements. Another difference between the human and fish visual system is the position of the eyes and the anatomy of the optic nerve. Zebrafish are lateral eyed, and binocular overlap is minimal since all axons from the optic nerve cross at the optic chiasm and project to the contralateral brain side. Humans have frontally positioned eyes and binocular vision, since around half of the axons project to the ipsilateral brain side (2). These differences allow us to study the OKR in zebrafish without the complications of smooth pursuit and binocular vision.

Several setups for measurement of the zebrafish OKR have been described. All of them are based on the presentation of moving gratings to the larva or, more recently, to the adult fish. However, different approaches exist for presenting the gratings and analyzing data. In initial experiments, the larva was placed inside a rotating drum equipped with vertical black-and-white stripes. The rotational speed of the drum was changed mechanically (9). In order to change the properties of the visual stimulus, different drums with stripes of different contrast or width can be used. Although this method is still widely used (10), computer-generated moving gratings are to our mind more convenient, since they allow to continuously change different parameters, such as contrast, spatial frequency and/or angular velocity, direction of rotation, and any other stimulus parameter of choice. In order to project the gratings onto the drum, a digital light projector is placed either on the plane of the subject (linear projection) or below the subject. Using linear projection, only monocular stimulation is possible (11). When the projector is placed below the subject, the gratings are projected via a mirror to the whole drum enabling binocular stimulation (12, 13). In order to avoid visible light from the projector influencing the recording, the animal is illuminated from below with infrared-emitting diodes. An infrared-pass filter in front of the camera ensures selective transmission of the infrared light to the camera.

In initial experiments, analysis of eye movement was performed by visual inspection and by counting the number of saccades occurring. Although this qualitative method—first described for zebrafish by

Clark (14)—has been very convenient for a rapid screening of vision mutants, a quantitative approach is needed for uncovering more subtle oculomotor defects. This has been achieved by computer-based tracking of eye position and subsequent quantitative analysis of changes in eye position over time. For this method—first described by Roeser and Baier (12)—image series are acquired by an infrared-sensitive CCD camera mounted onto a dissecting microscope. Custom-made tracking software extracts information about eye position from the acquired images.

Most OKR setups described in the literature are built for measurement of eye movements in larvae. OKR testing in adult fishes is more challenging, mainly because of the difficulty of restraining body movements of the fish. We were able to solve this problem and published a working method for OKR measurement in the adult (13). In the same year, an alternative setup has been described by Zou et al. (15). In this paper, however, eye movements are only qualitatively analyzed through visual inspection instead of software-based tracking of eye position.

Here, we describe a detailed protocol for the custom-made setup currently used in our laboratory. The animal is stimulated binocularly by computer-generated gratings and the eye position over time is automatically tracked. The resulting eye velocity is calculated in real time. We describe the detailed procedure for recording OKR in larvae as well as in adult fishes. We then describe our standard eye movement quantification approach which allows for detection of subjects with vision defects as well as for investigation of the OKR behavior itself. Since our system is under continuous development (1, 2, 11, 13, 16, 17), some of the details described in the protocol may change over time. However, our detailed protocol should enable the reader to apply the methodology of quantitative OKR measurements. Recently a commercial instrument based on the described setup has become available (VisioTracker by TSE-Systems).

Additionally, we present here a simple assay that enables a nonautomated qualitative analysis of OKR performance in larvae without the need of a computer-based setup. This methodology is suited for those researchers that do not have access to a computer-based setup and are interested in a rapid qualitative screening of vision mutants.

2. Materials

2.1. Reagents

1. 3% methylcellulose in water: Boil 100 ml ddH$_2$O in a beaker, then start stirring. Add 3 g methylcellulose (while the hot water is stirring vigorously). Continue to stir till the methylcellulose is dispersed into the liquid. Pour the dispersion quickly into two 50 ml Falcon Tubes and rotate (360°) at 4°C overnight. The day after, spin the clear viscous solution at 4°C, 179×g for ca.

10 min, in order to remove air bubbles. Store at 4°C for long-term use. Incubate the solution at 28°C for about a day before use (see Note 1).

2. Tricaine methanesulfonate solution (MS-222; Sigma E10521): Dissolve 300 mg Tricaine methanesulfonate in 1 L fish system water.

2.2. Equipment for OKR Recording

1. Serum pipette.

2. Dissecting needle.

3. Forceps.

4. Thin wooden stick.

5. OKR setup for larvae comprising (Fig. 1):

   (a) A dissecting microscope (e.g., SZH-10, *Olympus Corporation*, Japan).

   (b) An infrared-sensitive CCD-camera (e.g., Guppy F-038B NIR, *Allied Vision Technologies*, Germany) equipped

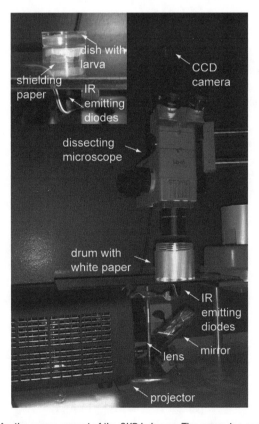

Fig. 1. Setup for the measurement of the OKR in larvae. The computer-generated stimulus pattern is projected via a wide-angle conversion lens to a mirror placed below the larva. The stimulus is reflected in the mirror and directed onto a drum surrounding the larva. A cluster of 15 infrared-emitting diodes illuminates the larva from below and is shielded by a piece of wax paper in a 35 mm Petri dish (see inset on the *left*). An infrared-sensitive CCD camera on the top of a dissecting microscope records the movement of the eyes.

with an infrared-pass filter (e.g., RG715, *Olympus Corporation*, Japan).

(c) A glass plate as a stand for the animal and the drum.

(d) A stimulus computer running the open source Python library Vision Egg (18).

(e) An LCD projector (e.g., PLV-Z3000, *Sanyo*, Japan) (see Note 2).

(f) A wide-angle conversion lens (e.g., HD-4500PRO, *Raynox*, Japan).

(g) A mirror.

(h) A control computer running custom-made software based on NI LabView 2009 and NI-Vision Development Module 2009 (*National Instruments*, USA).

(i) A cluster of infrared-emitting diodes ($\lambda_{peak} = 940$ nm) (e.g., BL0106-15-28, *Kingbright*, Taiwan) shielded by a piece of wax paper in a 35 mm Petri dish.

(j) 35 mm Petri dish containing the larva embedded in 3% methylcellulose and aligned to lay dorsal side up.

(k) A transparent plastic drum containing a white blotting paper on its internal wall.

6. OKR setup for adult fishes: (a) to (i) are identical to the setup for larvae. Additionally, the setup for adult fishes comprised the following:

(j) A custom-made glass chamber ($W \times H \times L = 12$ mm $\times 12$ mm $\times 65$ mm) (Fig. 2) containing the fish restrained by two pieces of sponge and two plastic half pipes. Two inlets attached to both sides of the chamber allow for fish water inflow. A third tube attached at the end of the chamber allows for water outflow back to the supply tank.

(k) A support stand.

(l) A peristaltic pump (e.g., SR25, 65 rpm, 24 VDC, novo-prene tube N 4.8 mm $\times 1.6$ mm, *Gardner Denver Thomas*, USA).

(m) A 24 V power supply for the pump (e.g., FSP 2405, *Voltcraft*, Germany).

(n) A USB-Relais to switch ON/OFF the pump (e.g., USBREL8, *Quancom Informationssysteme GmbH*, Germany).

(o) A water bath equipped with an aquarium heater (e.g., 50 W, *Jäger*, Germany).

(p) An air pump (e.g., R301, *Rena*, USA).

(q) A white plastic drum ($d = 12.5$ cm; e.g., cut from a chemical drum) with three small openings at the bottom edge for the tubes of the flow-through chamber.

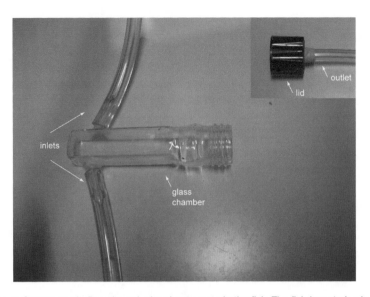

Fig. 2. Custom-made flow-through chamber to restrain the fish. The fish is restrained as described in methods. Fish water—maintained at 28°C in a water bath and oxygenated by an air pump (not shown)—flows at max 40 ml/min on the gills through two inlets attached to both sides of the chamber. The flow rate is generated by a peristaltic pump (not shown). The water effuses back to the supply tank via a third tube attached on the lid of the chamber.

2.3. Equipment for Manual OKR Measurements (Fig. 3)

1. Dissecting microscope (e.g., SV8, *Zeiss*, Germany).

2. Light source with light guides (e.g., KL 750, *Leica*, Germany).

3. 35 mm Petri dish containing the larva embedded in 3% methylcellulose and aligned to lay dorsal side up.

4. Turntable (turning can be done manually or by a motorized drive).

5. Paper with stripes of the desired color and width. The paper has to fit in the turntable.

6. Serum pipette.

7. Dissecting needle.

3. Methods

3.1. Recording of the OKR in Larvae

Protocols for fish breeding can be found online in the Zebrafish book (http://zfin.org/zf_info/zfbook/zfbk.html) or in *Zebrafish: A practical approach* (19).

3.1.1. Embedding the Larva (See Note 3)

1. Pour pre-warmed (28°C) 3% methylcellulose solution in a 35-mm Petri dish. Be careful not to produce air bubbles (see Note 4).

2. Suck a larva with a serum pipette and put it on the methylcellulose together with as little E3 medium as possible. To achieve

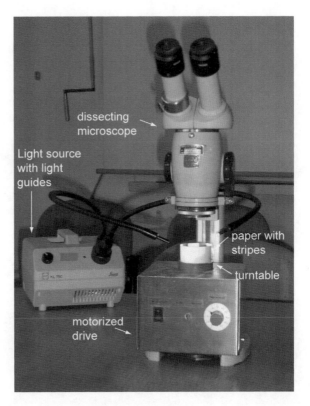

Fig. 3. Setup for manual measurement of the OKR in larvae. The larva is placed on a turntable inside of a paper with a striped pattern. Rotation of the drum is driven by a motorized drive. The larva is illuminated from above by a light source with light guides. The eye movement is observed through the dissecting microscope.

this, we tap the side of the pipette so that the larva swims to the bottom. Suck off any remaining E3 medium around the larva in order to avoid dilution of the methylcellulose solution.

3. Embed the larva dorsal up in the center of the dish. To orient the larva use a dissecting needle (see Note 4).

4. Allow the larva to get used to the methylcellulose for about 10 min before starting recording.

3.1.2. Starting the Setup

1. Start up the whole setup:

    (a) Switch on both the stimulus and the control computer.

    (b) Plug in the infrared LED-cluster

    (c) Switch on the projector.

2. Write the Configuration File containing the stimulus parameters (see Notes 5–7).

3. Stimulus computer: Start the stimulus program and wait for a message-box. Press "Bind port and listen for connections."

4. Control Computer: Start the OKR program. Press "New set up larvae." The OKR user interface will appear on the screen (Fig. 4).

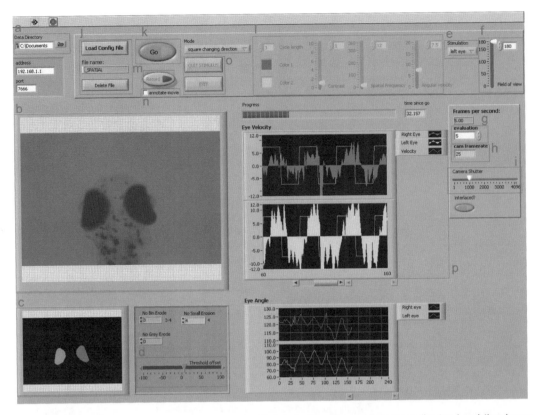

Fig. 4. OKR user interface for eye movement measurement in larvae. Recording controls are on the *top*. A real-time image of the larva is displayed on the *left*. Tracking and eye velocity data are shown in the *center*. The angle and the velocity of the right and left eye are displayed, the velocity of the rotating pattern is shown with a *white line*. On the *bottom left* are the particle detection parameters. On the *right* is the control of frame-rate. Letters (a) to (p) refer to the steps described in the main text.

3.1.3. Recording Eye Movement

1. Choose the data folder where you want to save your data (a). Then press "Current folder."

2. Place the larva under the dissecting microscope and center it in the visual field of the camera (b). The larva should be oriented in the same direction as the light beam. On the screen the larva is seen as in Fig. 4 (see Note 8). Choose the highest possible magnification. Pay attention that the eyes are visible on the screen. When the larva is in focus, place the plastic drum around the animal.

3. The software recognizes the dark pigmented eyes based on the pixel intensity. Check if the eyes are recognized well (c), and adjust the "threshold offset" (d) if necessary (e.g., if body pigmentation spots are close to the eye).

4. Choose between a binocular stimulation (field of view = 360°), a monocular stimulation of the right eye, and a monocular stimulation of the left eye (e). In the case of a monocular stimulation, the field of view can be regulated (between 0° and 180°) (f).

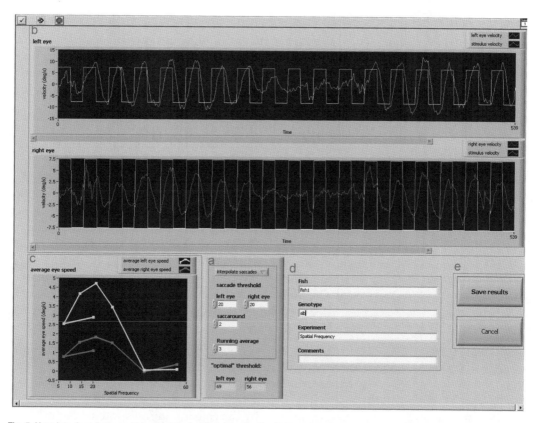

Fig. 5. User interface for smoothing and saving the data. On the *bottom right* the parameters to filter saccades and smoothen the velocity curves can be set. The effect of these changes is seen on the velocity curves on the *top* and on the velocity averaged over the same stimulus conditions (*bottom left*). Letters (a) to (e) refer to the steps described in the main text.

5. Choose the frame rate at which the images from the camera are processed by the software (g). We use 5 frames/s for screening of mutants and 25 frames/s for quantitative analysis of the OKR behavior itself. This frame rate has to be lower than the frame rate of the camera (h). Change the opening time of the camera shutter if necessary (i). Lowering the opening time reduces image brightness but increases the frame rate (h).

6. Load the Configuration File (j).

7. Press the "Go"-button (k) to start the experiment (see Notes 9 and 10). The experiment can be aborted by pressing "Go" again. If "Go" is pressed without having loaded a Configuration File, the stimulus will run with the parameters shown in (l). These parameters (colors, contrast, spatial frequency, and angular velocity) can be changed here. However, without a Configuration File the eye position over time will not be recorded.

8. When the end of the Configuration File is reached, a window appears (Fig. 5). Here, the parameters to filter saccades and smooth the velocity curves—saccade threshold, saccaround,

and running average—can be set (a) (see Note 11). The velocity curve of each eye after smoothing is shown in (b) and the velocity averaged over the same stimulus conditions is indicated in (c). Enter subject information (fish number, genotype, experiment, and, optionally, any comments) (d). Save the results (e).

9. After the first run as well as after having changed the Configuration File, a window pops up with the request to enter the name for a results-file or to choose an already existing one. Enter a name or choose an existing file. As long as the Configuration File is not changed, the following recordings will be saved in the same results-file. The results-file contains values for the average slow-phase velocity for each fish and for each measured conditions. For each fish recorded, an additional tab-file containing the raw data is automatically saved. Each line represents a frame. Columns A and B contain values for the angular eye position of the right and the left eye, respectively. Columns C and D contain values for the eye velocity in degree per second of the right and the left eye, respectively. The further columns contain information about the stimulus parameters.

10. Continue with step 4 to measure the same larva with a new paradigm. Go back to step 2 to measure a different larva.

3.1.4. Recording a Movie

All the frames imaged by the camera during stimulus presentation can be recorded and visualized later on.

1. Before starting the stimulus, press the button "Record" (see Fig. 4, (m)).

2. Enter the name under which the movie has to be saved. Movies are automatically saved in AVI-format.

3. Activate "annotate movie" (n) if it is wished that the current stimulus properties are written in the lower right corner of each frame.

4. Start the stimulus as described above.

5. Press "Record" (m) again to stop recording of the movie.

3.1.5. Shutting Down the Setup

1. Press "Quit Stimulus" and "Exit" (see Fig. 4, (o)).

2. Shut down both computers.

3. Unplug the IR LED-Cluster.

4. Switch off the projector.

3.2. Recording of the OKR in Adult Fishes

3.2.1. Starting the Setup

1. Step 1 is identical as for the setup for larvae (see Subheading 3.1.2).

2. Write the Configuration File containing the stimulus parameters (see Note 12).

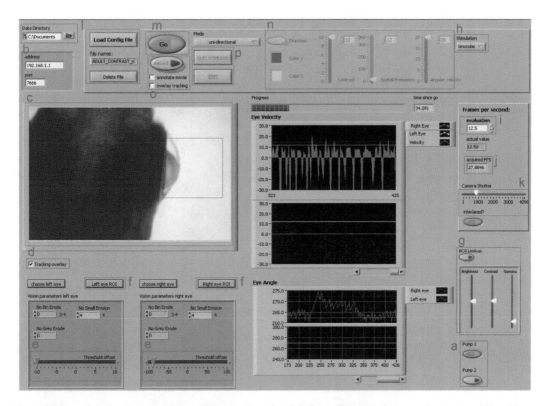

Fig. 6. OKR user interface for eye movement measurement in adult. Recording controls are on the *top*. A real-time image of the fish including particle detection is displayed on the *left*. On the *bottom left* are the particle detection parameters. Tracking and eye velocity data are shown in the *center*. On the *right* is the control of frame rate. Letters (a) to (p) refer to the steps described in the main text.

3. Stimulus computer: Start the stimulus program and wait for a message-box. Press "Bind port and listen for connections."

4. Control Computer: Start the OKR program. Press "New set up adults." The OKR user interface will appear on the screen (Fig. 6).

3.2.2. Restraining the Fish

1. Warm up fish water in the supply tank using a water bath set at 28°C. Oxygenate the fish water with an air pump.

2. Turn the flow-through chamber to a vertical position (front end down) and fill it with fish water by switching the pump on the user interface (see Fig. 6 (a)) until the water level reaches the upper rim.

3. Briefly anesthetize the fish in 300 mg/l MS-222 (see Note 13).

4. Prepare a half plastic pipe and insert a humid piece of sponge.

5. As soon as the fish stops swimming, gently lay the body on the piece of sponge, leaving the head incl. the gills free (Fig. 7a).

6. Cover with a second humid piece of sponge (Fig. 7b) and stabilize the sponges with a second half plastic pipe (Fig. 7c).

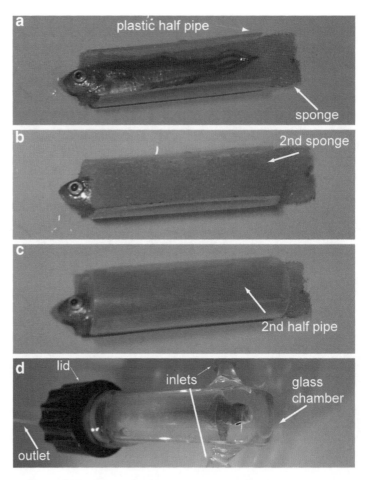

Fig. 7. Steps for restraining an adult fish. (a) The anesthetized fish is laid on a humid piece of sponge, which had been inserted into a plastic half pipe. (b) The fish is covered with a second humid piece of sponge. (c) Everything is covered with the second half of the plastic pipe. (d) The restrained fish is inserted into the glass chamber that had been connected to the two inlets and filled with fish water. The head of the fish looks to the bottom of the chamber. The chamber is then closed with the lid, which is attached to the outlet.

Again, pay attention to leave the head and the gills free (see Note 14).

7. Fit everything into the flow-through chamber which is fixed on a support stand. The fish has to look toward the bottom of the chamber (Fig. 7d). Use a thin wooden stick to push the fish together with the pieces of sponge and plastic half pipes down until the gills are on the height of the water inlets. Take care that no air bubbles are present in the front end of the chamber, i.e., around the head of the fish.

8. Close the lid of the flow-through chamber with the water outlet attached.

9. Switch on the peristaltic pump.

The setup for the adult is similar to the larval one.

1. Choose the data folder where you want to save your data (Fig. 6, (b)). Then press "Current folder."

2. Turn the flow-through chamber containing the fish into horizontal position, place it under the dissecting microscope, and center it in the visual field of the camera (c) (see Note 15). The fish should be oriented in the same direction as the light beam. Choose an appropriate magnification (the eye to be recorded from should be as large as possible to still fit into the image) (see Note 16). Place the plastic drum around the fish such that the three tubes of the chamber can exit the drum through its openings.

3. In the setup for adults the particle detection is directly overlaid on the live image (c) if "Tracking overlay" is activated (d). Select a ROI around the lens of the eye to be recorded from by pressing "Right eye ROI" or "Left eye ROI" (f). Check if the rim of the eye is recognized well (c) and adjust the "threshold offset" for the eye to be recorded (e).

4. Contrast, brightness, and gamma of the image can be adjusted after having activated the button "BCG Lookup" (g).

5. We usually stimulate adult fishes binocularly (field of view = 360°). However, it is possible to choose a monocular stimulation of the right eye and a monocular stimulation of the left eye (h). In the case of a monocular stimulation, the field of view can be regulated as in larval experiments.

6. Choose the frame rate at which the images from the camera are processed by the software (i). We typically use 12.5 frames/s. This frame rate has to be lower than the frame rate of the camera (j). Change the opening time of the camera shutter if necessary (k).

7. Load the desired Configuration File (l).

8. Press the "Go"-button (m) to start the experiment. The experiment can be aborted by pressing "Go" again (see Notes 17–19). If "Go" is pressed without a Configuration File loaded, the stimulus will run with the parameters shown in (n) as in the setup for larvae.

9. When the end of the Configuration File is reached, the data can be filtered and saved as in the setup for larvae (Fig. 8 and Note 20).

10. The same fish can be measured again with a new paradigm. Fishes easily survive for 30 min in the chamber without consequences on their health.

11. After successful measurement, turn the chamber back to a vertical position, switch off the pump, and remove the fish together with the sponge and plastic half pipes using forceps. Release

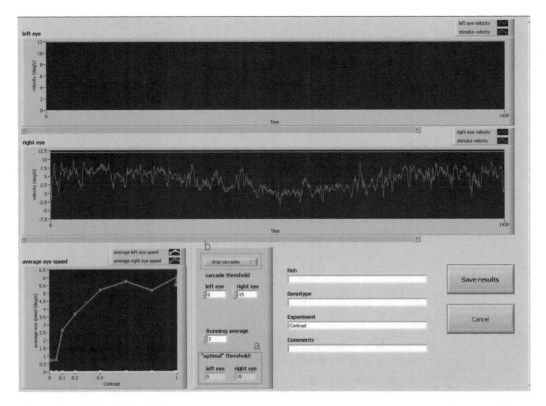

Fig. 8. User interface for smoothing and saving the data in the adult fish. On the *bottom right* the parameters to filter saccades and smoothen the velocity curves can be set. The effect of these changes is seen on the velocity curves on the *top* and on the velocity averaged over the same stimulus conditions (*bottom left*). Letters (a) and (b) refer to the steps described in the main text.

the fish into a tank with fish water. Fill the chamber with fish water again by switching the pump on until the water level reaches the upper rim. Continue with Subheading 3.2.2, step 3, to measure the next fish.

3.2.4. Recording a Movie

A movie of the live image can be recorded as with larvae (see Fig. 6, (o)). Activate "overlay tracking" to overlay the eye tracking on each frame.

3.2.5. Shutting Down the Setup

1. Switch off the peristaltic pump.

2. Remove the fish from the chamber and put it back to its tank.

3. Shut down the aquarium heater, the power supply of the pumps, and the air pump.

4. Press "Quit Stimulus" and "Exit" (see Fig. 6, (p)).

5. Shut down both computers.

6. Unplug the IR LED-Cluster.

7. Switch off the projector.

3.3. Quantification of Eye Movement

Here, we describe the quantification method currently most used in our laboratory. This method is well suited for screening of vision defects. A more precise method for investigation of the OKR itself has been recently developed in our laboratory (16) (see Note 21). However, since investigation of the OKR itself is probably not the aim of most readers, we do not go through the details at this place.

3.3.1. Plotting the Average Eye Velocity over an Experimental Condition

We usually plot the average slow-phase eye velocity over an experimental condition, e.g., varying contrast. For this, we use the automatically generated results-file which contains the average slow-phase velocity for each condition and for each subject. This value has been calculated after filtering and smoothing of the raw data. Data analysis can be performed with any statistics software.

1. Open the results-file with the statistical program of preference.
2. Plot a line graph with the varying condition on the *x*-axis and the average eye velocity on the *y*-axis. If different groups need to be compared (e.g., different genotypes or different treatments), plot them as different series in one graph.

3.4. Manual OKR Measurements

3.4.1. Embedding the Larva

Larvae are embedded in 3% methylcellulose as described for OKR recording (see Subheading 3.1.1).

3.4.2. Measuring of the OKR

1. Insert the striped pattern of choice in the turntable to form a drum.
2. Place the larva inside the drum.
3. Switch on the light source.
4. Rotate the drum and watch eye movements through the microscope.
5. Score the direction of slow-phase movements (with the drum or reverse to the drum movement). Count the number of saccades per given time interval as a readout of performance (see Note 22).

4. Notes

1. Methylcellulose is difficult to solubilize. When methylcellulose is added to hot stirring water, a cloudy dispersion is formed. This takes 1–2 min. Afterwards, the dispersion has to be poured very quickly into Falcon tubes to avoid sedimentation of the methylcellulose on the bottom of the beaker. This would give rise to aliquots of different concentrations. The Falcon

tubes need to rotate as soon as they are at 4°C because the methylcellulose starts to solubilize quickly at this temperature. The day after, the solution has to be centrifugated till all air bubbles disappear. We recommend to keep the solution at 4°C for long-term storage. However, the methylcellulose has to be warmed up to 28°C before use. This is the protocol used currently in our laboratory and is based on Brockerhoff et al. (10). However, other protocols exist and may work as well (19).

2. Resolution of the projector should be as high as possible (preferably use an HD-projector) to enable presentation of narrow stripes necessary to determine spatial resolution. In addition, the projector should have a high contrast ratio and a deep black level.

3. We embed our larvae in a 3% methylcellulose solution in order to restrain body movement with only minimal effect on eye movements. Zebrafish larvae survive in methylcellulose since this is a nontoxic viscous medium that allows oxygenation through the skin. Alternatively, the body of the larva can be embedded in low-melting agarose with the head and gills exposed to water as described by Beck et al. (20). However, this method is more time consuming.

   Dishes containing methylcellulose can be reused several times, as long as the quality is intact (air bubbles should not be present; the solution should not be diluted or too sticky). In order to recycle them, dishes can be stored at 28°C in a humidified chamber for later use.

4. Avoid production of air bubbles at any time point by gently pouring the methylcellulose solution into the dish and by gently positioning the larva inside the solution.

5. To write a Configuration File, open an empty excel datasheet. Each column represents one parameter, and each line one sequence. A new sequence needs to be started as soon as one parameter changes. Enter the parameters as described below and save the file as a tab-file (see Fig. 9 for an example):

   (a) Column A: Write "Contrast" in the first line. For sine-wave grating choose values between 0 and 1. If you want sharp stripes with sharp borders, choose 10. Write a new line for each new sequence.

   (b) Column B: Write "Spatial Frequency" in the first line. The Spatial Frequency (SF) is given in cycles/360° and determines how many patterns of two different stripes are displayed in 360° (e.g., a value of 1 means that 2 stripes with two different colors are shown). Choose the desired value for each sequence. To determine the visual acuity of a larva, we normally run sequences with values between 7 and 56.

	A	B	C	D	E	F	G	H	I	J	K
1	Contrast	Spatial Frequency	angular velocity	Color1 red	Color1 green	Color1 blue	Color2 red	Color2 green	Color2 blue	No. Cycles	Cycle duration
2	0.7	20	7.5	0.6	0.6	0.6	0	0	0	3	3
3	0.7	7	7.5	0.6	0.6	0.6	0	0	0	3	3
4	0.7	14	7.5	0.6	0.6	0.6	0	0	0	3	3
5	0.7	21	7.5	0.6	0.6	0.6	0	0	0	3	3
6	0.7	28	7.5	0.6	0.6	0.6	0	0	0	3	3
7	0.7	42	7.5	0.6	0.6	0.6	0	0	0	3	3
8	0.7	56	7.5	0.6	0.6	0.6	0	0	0	3	3
9	0.7	42	7.5	0.6	0.6	0.6	0	0	0	3	3
10	0.7	28	7.5	0.6	0.6	0.6	0	0	0	3	3
11	0.7	21	7.5	0.6	0.6	0.6	0	0	0	3	3
12	0.7	14	7.5	0.6	0.6	0.6	0	0	0	3	3
13	0.7	7	7.5	0.6	0.6	0.6	0	0	0	3	3

Fig. 9. Example of Configuration File. In this example SF is changed in each sequence, contrast and angular velocity are constant. The first line represents the calibration sequence (see Note 7).

(c) Column C: Write "angular velocity" in the first line. This parameter determines the angular velocity of the stimulus and is given in degree per second. Choose the desired value for each sequence. To determine temporal resolution, we typically run sequences with values between 5 and 30.

(d) Column D–F: Always in the first line, write "color1 red" in column D, "color1 green" in column E, and "color1 blue" in column F. Choose values between 0 and 1. Each value specifies the intensity of the respective color-channel. For grey stripes choose the same value for all channels, whereby the value has to be higher than 0 and smaller than 1. We routinely use a value of 0.6. For completely white stripes use a value of 1 for all channels.

(e) Column G–I: Analog to column D–F but for color 2. For black stripes choose the value 0 for all channels. For pure red set green and blue to 0 and red to 1.

(f) Column J: Write "nr Cycles" in the first line. Choose the number of cycles needed for each sequence. A value of 2 means that the stimulus will change the direction of rotation once during the specific sequence.

(g) Column K: Write "Cycle duration" in the first line. It defines the duration of each cycle in seconds. Choose the value wanted for each sequence.

6. We normally change only one parameter in each Configuration File, e.g., we measure the contrast sensitivity and therefore vary the contrast value but leave all other parameters constant.

In the case of contrast, we start with the highest contrast, reduce it stepwise, and increase it again. Note that the contrast values from 0 to 1 are relative with 1 being the maximal contrast chosen. The real contrast has to be determined by measuring the luminance from the drum with a photometer.

In the case of SF and angular velocity, we start with the lowest value, enhance it stepwise, and reduce it again.

7. At the beginning of recording, the eyes are pre-stimulated with a standard stimulus (typically contrast = 0.99, SF = 20 cycles/360°, and angular velocity = 7.5°/s for larvae). This avoids artifacts from starting the experiment. This pre-stimulation is written as the first sequence in the Configuration File and should last typically for 9 s. Data from this sequence will be deleted before analysis.

8. Sometimes the larva is not immobilized properly. In this case it may help to wait longer till the start of the recordings. The larva will eventually calm. A drift of the larval position over time could be due to movement of the viscous solution because of handling. Also in this case the drift should reduce over time. It also helps to use light-adapted larvae if this is compatible with the experiment as light-adapted larvae tend to be calmer. If the larva is still moving, please check the following:

    (a) Make sure that the larva is embedded dorsal side up.

    (b) Check the texture of the methylcellulose solution. If it is too diluted, try with a new solution.

    (c) If the mutation/treatment analyzed causes a higher motor activity, it may be necessary to increase the methylcellulose concentration.

9. If the eye movement is low or absent check the following:

    (a) Make sure that the larva is still alive by checking its blood flow.

    (b) Make sure that the stimulus is running properly. If the stimulus shuts down unexpectedly, close the software and the python program and restart both (first the python program and then the OKR software).

    (c) Make sure that the projector lamp is working properly and not getting weaker. Measure the luminance from the drum during stimulus presentation using a photometer. We recommend to do this on a regular basis, at least every 6 months, in order to assure that contrast and brightness stay constant over time.

    (d) Look for light sources in the room that could interfere. Maintain the room as dark as possible.

    (e) Check the quality of the methylcellulose solution.

    (f) Make sure that the larva is embedded dorsal side up.

    (g) Measure a healthy and untreated wild-type larva as a control. If this larva shows a normal OKR and you have checked all points from (a) till (f), you may have found a larva with impaired OKR. Congratulation!

10. Sometimes eye movement does not seem to be matched to movement of the stimulus (see Fig. 4, (p)). If this happens, make sure that the stimulus runs stably. Check for irregularities

in stimulus pattern velocity and check for any deviance from the parameters determined in the Configuration File. If deviances are present, restart the python file and then the OKR software.

11. The eye velocity is determined from the eye position over time. We usually consider the eye velocity during the slow phase of the OKR (SPV) as a readout for OKR performance. In order to calculate the SPV, we need to filter out the saccades (fast resetting movements in the opposite direction than the stimulus) and to smooth the curve. We usually do this with the help of an empirically tested formula (17): If eye velocity (v) in a certain frame (f) exceeds a determined saccade threshold (default: $20°/s$), eye velocity of this frame as well as of a defined amount of preceding frames (saccaround) is replaced with the eye velocity of the frame preceding the saccaround. Analogously, the eye velocity of the defined amount of following frames is replaced by the value 1 frame after the saccaround. By a frame rate of 5 frames/s, we usually set the saccaround to 2 (($vf...f-2$) is set to $v(f-3)$ and ($vf+1...f+2$) is set to $v(f+3)$). The velocity curve is further smoothened by a running average. At a frame rate of 5 frames/s, we usually set a running average of 7 frames ($v(f) = (\Sigma v(f-3...f+3))/7$). It is also possible to drop the saccades without saccaround. This can be defined in (a) on the top (see Fig. 5). See Subheading 3.3 and Note 21 for more details on data analysis.

12. Write the Configuration File following the guidelines for experiments with larvae (see Notes 5–7). For recordings in adult fish, we typically stimulate binocularly and in one direction only. Therefore, each sequence consists of only one cycle. The length of the sequences can be set as preferred. We usually record with sequences lasting for 9 s. As for recordings in larvae, eyes are pre-stimulated with a standard stimulus typically lasting 9 s with contrast = 0.99, SF = 36 cycles/360°, and angular velocity = 12°/s. This pre-stimulation is not considered in data analysis.

    To determine the visual acuity of an adult fish, we usually run sequences with SF values between 18 and 180 cycles/360°. To determine the temporal resolution, we usually run sequences with angular velocity values between 5 and 55°/s.

13. Always use a freshly prepared solution of MS-222, since tricaine is light sensitive and quickly loses its activity, and toxic by-products may be formed.

14. In case fishes strongly vary in size, use different pieces of sponge with different sizes, or add additional small pieces for smaller fish.

15. Before initiating an experiment, leave the fish in the flow-through chamber for 1–2 min with running water supply in order to let it recover from anesthesia and calm down.

16. Since temporal-to-nasal eye velocity has been shown to be much higher and more stable (13), we usually evaluate only the eye stimulated in temporal-to-nasal direction. This way we can also control the position of that eye more precisely.

17. If eye movements are jerky and not correlated to visual stimulation, stop presentation of gratings and wait for 30 s. Restart the stimulation with optimal parameters, i.e., high contrast (1 or higher), medium spatial frequency (ca. 36 cycles/360°), and high angular velocity (ca. 20°/s). Repeat this until eye movements are stable and well correlated to visual stimulation.

18. If the fish does not show any eye movements at all, make sure that the pump is running. Oxygenation may be insufficient if the gills are covered by the sponge. In this case, immediately release the fish and let it recover in a tank with fresh fish water. Turn the chamber back to a vertical position, switch off the pump, and remove the fish together with the sponge and plastic half pipes using forceps.

19. If the fish manages to disengage itself from the restraining system, shut down the pump, turn the chamber back to a vertical position, open the lid, remove sponge and plastic half pipes using forceps, position a tank with fish water below the chamber, and remove the fish by turning the chamber by 180°.

20. In contrast to the method used for larvae, the threshold for saccade filtering is not fixed but an ideal threshold is searched for each eye in an iterative process. The ideal threshold is the one that results in the highest sum of average eye velocities and it is displayed below the smoothing settings (see Fig. 8, (a)). Moreover, saccades are usually dropped and saccaround is not performed. Nevertheless, it is possible to use the saccaround method. To define the method of choice, press (b). The curve is smoothened by a running average as in recordings of larvae. At a frame rate of 12.5 frames/s, we typically use a running average of 7 (see Note 11 for details about the smoothing algorithm).

21. In our laboratory, different processing methods have been applied in the past depending on the research question (11, 13, 16, 17). Here, we describe in detail the method of choice for a rapid screening of vision defects. However, for a quantitative analysis of the OKR behavior itself—e.g., for analysis of the eye movement waveform—a higher frame rate is needed and the method described here is not precise enough. For this kind of quantitative analysis, we refer to our work on the mutant *belladonna* (16). A fraction of the homozygous *belladonna* larvae displays a reversed OKR and spontaneous eye oscillations in the absence of a moving stimulus. In order to quantitatively analyze those eye movements, a more precise quantification software was developed using the R statistical computing language. Briefly, the eye movement was recorded

with a frame rate of 12.5 frames/s (nowadays we record with 25 frames/s). The eye position trace was smoothened with a Gaussian smoothing kernel. Slow-phase segments were determined by setting acceleration thresholds. The slow-phase velocity was defined by taking the maximum eye velocity across all slow-phase segments within a condition.

22. If the eye movement is low or absent check the following:

   (a) Make sure that the larva is still alive by checking its blood flow.

   (b) Check the light intensity from the light source and try to vary it.

   (c) Look for light sources in the room that could interfere. Maintain the room as dark as possible.

   (d) Check the quality of the methylcellulose solution.

   (e) Make sure that the larva is embedded dorsal side up and calm.

   (f) Make sure that the drum is rotating smoothly.

   (g) Measure a healthy and untreated wild-type larva as a control. If this larva shows a normal OKR and you have checked all points from (a) till (f), you may have found a larva with impaired OKR.

References

1. Huang YY, Neuhauss SC (2008) The optokinetic response in zebrafish and its applications. Front Biosci 13:1899–1916

2. Maurer CM, Huang YY, Neuhauss SC (2011) Application of zebrafish oculomotor behavior to model human disorders. Rev Neurosci 22:5–16

3. Henderson JW, Crosby EC (1952) An experimental study of optokinetic responses. AMA Arch Ophthalmol 47:43–54

4. Bergmann F et al (1963) Optokinetic nystagmus and its interaction with central nystagmus. J Physiol 168:318–331

5. Mitchiner JC, Pinto LH, Vanable JW Jr (1976) Visually evoked eye movements in the mouse (*Mus musculus*). Vision Res 16:1169–1171

6. Easter SS Jr (1972) Pursuit eye movements in goldfish (*Carassius auratus*). Vision Res 12:673–688

7. Carvalho P, Noltie D, Tillitt D (2002) Ontogenetic improvement of visual function in the medaka oryzias latipes based on an optomotor testing system for larval and adult fish. Anim Behav 64:1–10

8. Easter SS Jr, Nicola GN (1997) The development of eye movements in the zebrafish (*Danio rerio*). Dev Psychobiol 31:267–276

9. Brockerhoff SE et al (1995) A behavioral screen for isolating zebrafish mutants with visual system defects. Proc Natl Acad Sci USA 92:10545–10549

10. Brockerhoff SE (2006) Measuring the optokinetic response of zebrafish larvae. Nat Protoc 1:2448–2451

11. Rinner O, Rick JM, Neuhauss SC (2005) Contrast sensitivity, spatial and temporal tuning of the larval zebrafish optokinetic response. Invest Ophthalmol Vis Sci 46:137–142

12. Roeser T, Baier H (2003) Visuomotor behaviors in larval zebrafish after GFP-guided laser ablation of the optic tectum. J Neurosci 23:3726–3734

13. Mueller KP, Neuhauss SC (2010) Quantitative measurements of the optokinetic response in adult fish. J Neurosci Methods 186:29–34

14. Clark DT (1981) Visual responses in the developing zebrafish (*Brachydanio rerio*). University of Oregon Press, Eugene

15. Zou SQ et al (2010) Using the optokinetic response to study visual function of zebrafish. J Vis Exp. doi:10.3791/1742

16. Huang YY et al (2006) Oculomotor instabilities in zebrafish mutant belladonna: a behavioral model for congenital nystagmus caused by axonal misrouting. J Neurosci 26:9873–9880

17. Haug MF et al (2010) Visual acuity in larval zebrafish: behavior and histology. Front Zool 7:8

18. Straw AD (2008) Vision egg: an open-source library for realtime visual stimulus generation. Front Neuroinformatics 2:4

19. Nüsslein-Volhard C, Dahm R (2002) Zebrafish. Oxford University Press, New York

20. Beck JC et al (2004) Quantifying the ontogeny of optokinetic and vestibuloocular behaviors in zebrafish, medaka, and goldfish. J Neurophysiol 92:3546–3561

Chapter 11

Analysis of the *Drosophila* Compound Eye with Light and Electron Microscopy

Monalisa Mishra and Elisabeth Knust

Abstract

The *Drosophila* compound eye is a regular structure, in which about 750 units, called ommatidia, are arranged in a highly regular pattern. Eye development proceeds in a stereotypical fashion, where epithelial cells of the eye imaginal discs are specified, recruited, and differentiated in a sequential order that leads to the highly precise structure of an adult eye. Even small perturbations, for example in signaling pathways that control proliferation, cell death, or differentiation, can impair the regular structure of the eye, which can be easily detected and analyzed. In addition, the *Drosophila* eye has proven to be an ideal model for studying the genetic control of neurodegeneration, since the eye is not essential for viability. Several human neurodegeneration diseases have been modeled in the fly, leading to a better understanding of the function/misfunction of the respective gene. In many cases, the genes involved and their function are conserved between flies and human. More strikingly, when ectopically expressed in the fly eye some human genes without a *Drosophila* counterpart can induce neurodegeneration, detectable by aberrant phototaxis, impaired electrophysiology, or defects in eye morphology. These defects are often rather subtle alteration in shape, size, or arrangement of the cells, and can be easily scored at the ultrastructural level. This chapter aims to provide an overview regarding the analysis of the retina by various means.

Key words: *Drosophila melanogaster*, Light microscopy, Deep pseudopupil, Electron microscopy, Cryolabeling, Whole mount, Compound eye

---

1. Introduction

1.1. The Structure of the Drosophila Compound Eye

The *Drosophila* compound eye is a highly ordered structure composed of about 750 functional units called ommatidia, which are regularly arranged in a hexagonal pattern, visible from the outside by the facets, which are formed by the lenses (Fig. 1a). Each ommatidium is an elongated, barrel-like structure of about 100 μm in length, the distal 10% of which is occupied by the cornea and the crystalline cone, which together form the dioptric apparatus (Fig. 2a). Below, the eight, highly elongated photoreceptor cells (PRCs) follow, which are associated with pigment and cone cells. The cell bodies

Bernhard H.F. Weber and Thomas Langmann (eds.), *Retinal Degeneration: Methods and Protocols*, Methods in Molecular Biology, vol. 935, DOI 10.1007/978-1-62703-080-9_11, © Springer Science+Business Media, LLC 2013

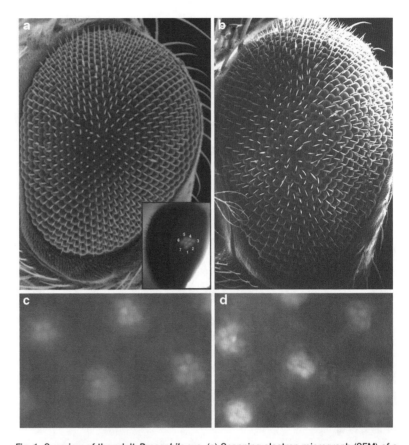

Fig. 1. Overview of the adult *Drosophila* eye. (**a**) Scanning electron micrograph (SEM) of a wild-type *Drosophila* compound eye showing the highly regular arrangement of facets. Each lens has a diameter of approx. 18 µm. Inset: Light micrograph of a wild-type eye revealing the deep pseudopupil in the form of a trapezoid rhabdom. (**b**) Overexpression of the cytoplasmic domain of *Crumbs* in all cells of the eye results in a rough eye phenotype. (**c**) Optical neutralization of the wild-type eye showing the trapezoid arrangement of the rhabdomeres. (**d**) Optical neutralization of a fly expressing *crb* RNAi shows the loss of the trapezoid arrangement of the rhabdomeres (**c** and **d** kindly provided by N. Gurudev).

of the outer PRCs R1–R6 span the entire length of the retina and project axons to the lamina, the first optic neuropile. The axons of the central R7 and R8 cell synapse in the medulla, the second neuropile of the optic lobe.

All eight PRCs of an individual ommatidium point their apical membrane towards the center (Fig. 2c). The apical membrane itself is subdivided into the most apical rhabdomere and the stalk, which connects the rhabdomere with the zonula adherens (ZA), and which corresponds to the inner segment of the vertebrate PRC (Fig. 2d). The rhabdomere, the light-sensing organelle, is composed of an array of densely packed microvilli of 1.5 µm in length and about 60 nm in width, which accounts for about 90% of the cell's plasma membrane and harbors the visual pigment rhodopsin. The eight rhabdomeres within each ommatidium are arranged in a

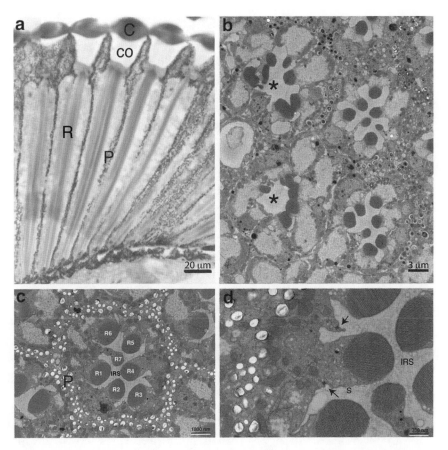

Fig. 2. General organization of the compound eye. (**a**) Light micrograph of a longitudinal section illustrating the cornea (C), the cone (co), the rhabdom (R), and the pigment in the pigment cells (P). Note that pigment cells separate ommatidia from each other. (**b**) Electron micrograph of a transverse section of a mosaic eye, carrying wild-type ommatidia and *crb* mutant clones (*asterisks*) in the same eye. Loss of *crb* results in photoreceptor cells (PRCs) with defective shapes (compare Fig. 1c). (**c**) Electron micrograph of a transverse section of an ommatidia representing the seven PRCs (R1–R7), which are well separated by the interrhabdomeral space (IRS). (**d**) Higher magnification of a PRC, showing the rhabdomere, the adherens junctions (*arrows*), and the stalk membrane(s).

highly stereotype, trapezoid pattern. The outer PRCs R1–R6 are located in the periphery, while the R7 and R8 cells occupy the distal and the proximal portion of the center, respectively. Therefore, each cross section shows only seven PRCs. In contrast to many other insects, such as the honeybee, *Drosophila* has an open rhabdom, in which the rhabdomeres of the PRCs are well separated from each other by the interrhabdomeral space (Fig. 2c). The diameter of the rhabdomeres of the central R7 and R8 is ~1 µm, whereas that of the peripheral rhabdomeres R1–R6 measures about 2 µm (ref. 1). The microvilli of the rhabdomeres of the outer R1–R6 cells are slightly tilted towards one side in the distal portion of the retina and towards the other side in the proximal portion (2). This feature, termed rhabdomere twisting, decreases the sensitivity of the PRCs to polarized light.

The rhabdomeres are functionally equivalent to the outer segments of vertebrate PRCs, as both contain the components of the phototransduction machinery. R1–R6 contain Rhodopsin1 (Rh1) as visual pigment, which is encoded by the *ninaE* gene (3, 4). R7 expresses either Rh3 or Rh4 (5, 6), responsible for ultraviolet sensitivity (7), and R8 expresses either Rh5 or Rh6, which have blue and green sensitivity, respectively (8).

1.2. Various Phenotypes Associated with Distinct Mutations

The highly stereotypic organization of the cells within each ommatidium is essential for proper functioning of the eye. In the last decades, many genes have been characterized, mutations in which effect different aspects of this organization, such as the number of PRCs per ommatidium, their proper arrangement, their morphology and/or function, the shape of the rhabdomere, including the length and/or alignment of the microvilli, or changes in the length of stalk membrane. Some mutations are described below. Mutations that affect cell fate specification of PRCs result in the lack of individual PRCs or a change in their identity. For example, in *sevenless* (*sev*) or *bride of sevenless* (*boss*) mutant flies, the R7 cell is absent (9–12). In eyes lacking *rough* the identity of R2 and R5 is affected, which impairs the specification of R3 and R4 (13). Mutations in genes affecting the number or arrangement of PRCs are often manifested in a rough eye phenotype, such as in Ellipse, a dominant mutation in the EGF-receptor homologue (14), in loss-of-function mutations of *canoe* (15), in gain-of-function mutations of *sevenless* (*sev^{S11}*) (16), or upon overexpression of the membrane-bound cytoplasmic domain of Crumbs (17) (Fig. 1b). The rough-eye phenotype of some *calphotin* alleles is the result of misoriented rhabdomeres and PRC death (18). Mutations associated with genes like *orthodenticle* (*otd*) and *PpH13* alter the shape of the rhabdomeres by changing the length/size of the microvilli, but keep photoreceptor number unaltered (19, 20). In hypomorphic alleles of the gene encoding *Myosin Va* or upon early expression of the membrane-bound cytoplasmic domain of Crumbs ectopic rhabdomeres form (21, 22). In rhabdomeres mutant for *canoe* and *cofilin* rhabdomeres are confined to only the distal third of the retina, similar as in PRCs lacking *crumbs*, *stardust*, or *DPATJ*, which additionally exhibit a reduction in stalk membrane length and undergo light-dependent retinal degeneration (23–29). Mutations in *spacemaker/eyes shut* prevent the separation of rhabdomeres, thus leading to a closed rhabdom without any interrhabdomeral space (30, 31). Finally, mutations leading to defective organelles like endosomes, multivesicular bodies, or lysosomes result in defective photoreceptors by affecting the transportation of pigments (32, 33). Other mutations affect the function of PRCs without changing their morphology. Such defects can be easily detected by measuring the electroretinogram (ERG). The ERG reflects the summed activity of all PRCs and a superimposed, "evoked potential" from the first optic ganglion, the lamina. Mutants with altered ERGs can be classified according to these two components (34) (reviewed in (35, 36)).

1.3. Various Approaches to Study *Drosophila* Photoreceptors

Pioneering work of Benzer and his collaborators identified mutants in the visual system based on a modified phototactic behavior. This phototactic behavioral test is the simplest way for detecting visual system impairment (37, 38). Shortly later, Heisenberg employed an optomotor response approach to study photoreceptor function (39) (reviewed in (40)). In the same year, a novel screening approach was developed, called deep pseudopupil (DPP), which allows to rapidly uncover defects in ommatidial and PRC morphology. DPP is an optical phenomenon based on the highly stereotypic arrangement of PRCs and the superposition of the virtual images of several rhabdomeres (41) (Fig. 1a, inset). Any gross disruption that affects retinal organization and hence the stereotypic arrangement of the rhabdomeres causes a loss of DPP, e.g., in *rdgC* mutants (42). A further development of this method, called optical neutralization of the cornea, uses either the autofluorescent of rhodopsin or the fluorescence induced upon illumination of eyes expressing green fluorescent protein (GFP) from transgenes under the control of PRC-specific promoters. This assay allows to easily screen large numbers of flies and provides additional information, such as defects in morphogenesis, planar polarity, or cell death (43, 44) (Fig. 1c, d). Once a defect has been detected using either DPP or optical neutralization, a more detailed analysis of the mutant phenotype has to follow, such as histological analysis under light and electron microscope, which provides information on the fine structure of the PRCs, such as the length of microvilli or stalk membranes, the presence of pigment granules and various other organelles, or the integrity of the base of the rhabdomere or the adherens junction. Eyes with morphological defects can be further analyzed by immunohistochemistry to search for defects in the localization of marker proteins. This can be achieved by either cryo-sectioning/labeling or whole mount labeling. Table 1 lists several antibodies, which label different compartments of adult PRCs. Mutants having structural defects and/or impaired protein localization can be further analyzed with electrophysiological methods for their visual response (36).

1.4. *Drosophila* Genetics in Vision Research

The genetic tools available in *Drosophila* research have allowed studying the function of many genes required for development and function of the eye in great detail. The genome sequences revealed not only that many genes are conserved between flies and human, but in addition that mutations in homologous genes can cause similar diseases/phenotypes in human and *Drosophila*. Strikingly, nearly 75% of human disease-causing genes are believed to have a functional homolog in flies (45). Therefore, and due to the fact that the

Table 1
Some useful markers to label different compartments of adult PRCs

Protein	Localization	Antibody	References[a]
F-actin	Rhabdomere	Phalloidin[b]	
Crumbs	Stalk membrane	Cq4[c] (mouse, monoclonal)	(27, 69, 70)
Stardust	Stalk membrane	Anti-Sdt[pep153] (rabbit)	(72)
		Anti-C-terminus	(73)
		Anti-PDZ (rabbit and mouse monoclonal mAB B8-1)	(26, 74)
		Anti-N-terminus (rat)	(75)
DPATJ	Stalk membrane	Anti-DPATJ	(23)
		Anti-Dlt[d] (mouse and rabbit)	(71)
DE-Cadherin	Adherens junction	DCAD2 (mouse monoclonal[c])	(76)
β-Catenin/Armadillo	Adherens junction	Anti-Arm N2 7A1[c]	(77)
Unconventional myosin, P-Moesin	Rhabdomere base		(78, 79)
Na+-K+-ATPase α-subunit	Baso-lateral membrane	α5 (mouse monoclonal, raised against the chicken protein)[c]	(80, 81)
Cut	Nucleus	2B10 (mouse monoclonal)[c]	(82)
Spacemaker/eyes shut	Interrhabdomeral space	mAb21A6[c]	(31, 83)
Chaoptin	Lateral sides of rhabdomeres	mAB24B10[c]	(83)
Carbohydrate epitopes	Rhabdomere outline	Anti-HRP (Dianova)	M. Mishra (unpublished)

[a]Indicates the origin of the antibody and/or the first publication showing staining in the eye
[b]Phalloidin is a bicyclic peptide isolated from the mushroom *Amanita phalloides* that selectively binds F-actin. Several variants are available, conjugated to different fluorophores (e.g., FITC, Alexa dyes, etc.)
[c]Monoclonal antibodies can be obtained from DSHB (http://dshb.biology.uiowa.edu/)
[d]DPATJ was initially supposed to be *discs lost* (*dlt*) (71), but was later correctly mapped (84)

eye is a nonessential organ in flies, the *Drosophila* eye has become an ideal model to study the function of human genes involved in neurodegeneration, even of those genes that do not have a *Drosophila* counterpart (*see*, for example, (46, 47) for *Drosophila* as a model for polyglutamine disorders). Using the various techniques established over the years, it is easy to address biological questions concerning the function of genes in the *Drosophila* eye. By extensive mutagenesis screens using chemicals, e.g., ethyl methanesulfonate, ionizing radiation, e.g., X-rays, or transposons (e.g., P-elements) (reviewed in (48)), many mutations affecting eye development and function have been collected (35, 49). Besides detecting novel genes, mutagenesis screens can be used to identify additional components of a given signaling pathway active in the *Drosophila* eye. This approach was first applied to identify mutations that enhance or suppress the phenotype induced by mutations in *sevenless*, which encodes a receptor tyrosine kinase required for the specification of the R7 cells. In this screen *Son of sevenless* (*Sos*) was uncovered, which acts downstream of Sevenless and encodes a Ras guanine nucleotide exchange factor (GEF) (50, 51). Since then, this kind of screen has been frequently used as an unbiased approach, for example to identify modifiers of Tau-induced neurodegeneration in a *Drosophila* model for Alzheimer's disease (52).

While initially only viable mutations with a function in the eye could be detected in genetic screens, the induction of genetic mosaics using mitotic recombination allowed the identification and characterization of homozygous mutant tissues/cells in otherwise heterozygous animals. Thereby, the analysis of the later function of a gene, whose mutations result in lethality when the whole animal is mutant, is possible (53–55). This method was also used in screens aimed to identify novel genes with functions in the eye (56). Initially, X-ray irradiation was used to induce somatic recombination, but the number of clones achieved was very low. The development of the yeast FLP/FRT system tremendously increased the frequency of mosaicism. This system is based on the introduction of the yeast flip recombinase (FLP) gene and its target sequences FRT (*fl*ip recombinase *r*ecognition *t*argets) into the fly genome (57). Upon activation of the FLP recombinase by a tissue- and/or stage-specific promoter, homozygous mutant cells are induced (Fig. 2b), which, depending on the proliferation capacity, give rise to large areas of mutant tissues. The introduction of an additional, lethal mutation on the chromosome bearing the wild-type allele makes it possible to produce eyes that are almost completely composed of mutant tissues (58). One of the promoters used to activate FLP recombinase is the heat-shock promoter, which activates FLP randomly in all tissues upon raising the temperature for a short period of time to 37°C. Alternatively, *ey*-FLP, in which expression of FLP is under the control of the eye-specific *eyeless* (*ey*) promoter, efficiently generates flies in which almost all eye cells are mutant, while the rest of the animal is wild type, and thus permits the performance of simple F1 screens, aimed to identify eye-specific phenotypes (59). The possibility to mark either the mutant or the wild-type cells by GFP is a further advantage of this assay (60). With this method it can be determined whether a given gene is required in those cells, where it is active (cell autonomous function), or whether it exerts its function onto neighboring cells (nonautonomous function), e.g., if it encodes a signaling molecule.

Methods described above provide possibilities to study phenotypes obtained upon loss of function of a gene of interest. A useful complement to these strategies is the GAL4–UAS system, designed to induce stage- and tissue-specific (over)expression of a gene of interest (61). It is a bipartite system, in which one transgenic line, the activator or driver line, expresses the yeast transcription factor Gal4 in a known temporal and/or spatial pattern. The second transgenic line, the responder or effector line, carries the gene of interest (often only its coding region, obtained by cloning a cDNA) under the control of *u*pstream *a*ctivating *s*equences (UAS), the target sites of Gal4. To activate gene expression, activator and effector lines are crossed. The resulting progenies carry both transgenes and express the gene of interest under the control of the desired regulatory sequence (62). Further refinement of this method was achieved by the combination of the UAS/GAL4 system with a temperature-sensitive variant of the GAL4 repressor GAL80, called the *t*emporal *a*nd *r*egional *g*ene *e*xpression *t*argeting (TARGET) technique, in which GAL80ts is expressed under the control of the ubiquitous *tubulin 1α* promotor (62). By a simple temperature shift, GAL80 becomes inactivated and allows GAL4 to activate the UAS-gene of interest ((63); reviewed in (64)).

To summarize, *Drosophila* photoreceptors are accessible in vivo to a variety of genetic and cell biological techniques, including mosaic analysis, overexpression studies, immunohistochemistry, transmission and scanning electron microscopy, and confocal microscopy. Development, morphology, and function of photoreceptors are relatively invariant from animal to animal and well studied. Since the eye is not an essential tissue and not required for an animal's viability and fertility, it is a great system to study genes involved in neurodegeneration, including human genes not encoded in the fly's genome. For example, the overexpression of human ataxin-1, a gene associated with Spinocerebellar ataxia type 1 (SCA1), in the fly retina causes neurodegeneration similar to that observed in humans expressing a disease-inducing version of the ataxin protein characterized by expansion of a polyglutamine (polyQ) tract. More interesting, screening for genes that modify this phenotype in the fly uncovered genes that are involved in transcriptional regulation, RNA processing, and cellular detoxification (65), and are thus possible candidates as targets for future therapy. This and other examples demonstrate that the *Drosophila* eye is an ideal model to study the function of human genes involved in neurodegeneration (reviewed in (66–68)).

2. Materials

2.1. Cryofixation Reagents and Equipment

1. 4% Paraformaldehyde in phosphate-buffered saline (PBS) (obtained by dilution of 16% (EM grade; from Electron Microscopy Sciences (EMS)).

2. PBS pH 7.4 and PBST (PBS + 1% Tween20) at room temperature.

3. 10 and 25% Sucrose (AppliChem, Cat no: 57-5-1) solution, diluted in PBS.

4. 5% Normal horse serum (NHS) blocking solution (dilute 30% NHS (ABD Serotec, Co9SA) with PBT).

5. Tissue embedding media NEG50™ (Thermo Scientific).

6. Vectashield mounting media (Vector lab).

7. Coverslips (24 × 50 mm).

8. 1.5 ml Eppendorf tubes.

9. Dry ice.

10. Embedment molds for embedment (or cap of 1.5 ml Eppendorf tube).

11. 1 ml transfer pipettes.

12. Razor blade, glass slide, and sample holder.

13. Light microscope and cryostat.

2.2. Fixation for Light and Electron Microscopy

1. 50% Glutaraldehyde (EMS #16320) diluted to 2.5% with Phosphate Buffer (PB) (EMS #11600-05) and 16% paraformaldehyde (EMS #15700) diluted to 2% with PB for primary fixation in a 1.5 ml Eppendorf tube (see Note 1).

2. 2% OsO_4 for secondary fixation: Mix 2 parts 4% OsO_4 (EMS #19150) with one part 2% $KMnO_4$ solution ($KMnO_4$ in distilled water) and one part distilled water.

3. Ethanol, absolute, and diluted to 50, 70, 90, and 100% (see Note 2).

4. Propylene oxide (EMS #20410) for dehydration.

5. Rocking platform for agitation.

6. EPON: Mix the components of the Epon 812 kit (EMS #14120) in a fresh plastic beaker according to the supplier's instruction: EMbed 812 (20 ml), DDSA (16 ml), MNA (8 ml), DMP-30 (0.66 ml). Mix it for 1 h with a magnetic stirrer at room temperature (see Note 3).

7. Embedding mold (EMS #70907) to embed the sample in resin.

8. Maintain an oven at 60°C for polymerization.

2.3. Sectioning and Staining of Samples for Light Microscopy

1. Ultramicrotome, razor blade, and Diamond Histo Knife.

2. To prepare glass knifes, break the glass (EMS #71012) with a knife maker. Melt wax, dip a small container called the boat (to collect sections on water) into it, and immediately press it against the edge of the glass knife to fix it to the boat (Fig. 3).

3. To collect sections, mount an eyelash at one end of a toothpick by means of nail polish.

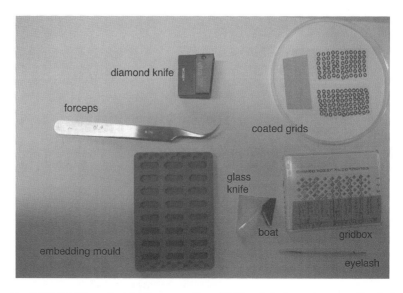

Fig. 3. Equipment required for the preparation of light and electron microscopy. See text for further explanation.

4. The toluidine blue solution (0.25% Toluidine blue (EMS #14950) and 0.25% Sodium borate (EMS #21130)) is prepared and mixed on a magnetic stirrer for 30 min. Filter the solution and store it at room temperature (see Notes 4 and 5).

5. DPX (Sigma #44581) for mounting the slide.

2.4. Sectioning and Staining of Samples for Electron Microscopy

2.4.1. Coating of Grids

1. Wash single-slot grids (EMS #G200F1-Cu) with acetone and let them dry.

2. For making formvar solution, dilute formvar (EMS #15810) in 100% $CHCl_3$, to make a final concentration of 1%.

3. Prepare glass slides by cleaning with a Kimwipe to remove fat and dust.

4. To coat the slides with a film of formvar, dip them into the formvar solution using the casting device (EMS #71305-01) (Fig. 4a).

5. Take out the slides and let them dry inside the fume hood.

6. Cut out the film from the slide with a razor blade (Fig. 4b).

7. Prepare a rectangular cuvette filled with distilled water. Dip the slide with the film still attached to it into the water in an angle of 45° (Fig. 4c). The film will detach from the slide and float on the water (Fig. 4d). A silvery appearance of the side of the film that was in contact with the slide indicates that it has the right thickness of 20–30 nm.

8. Put the grids on the floating film with forceps so that the dull surface of the grid is oriented towards you (Fig. 4e). Once the

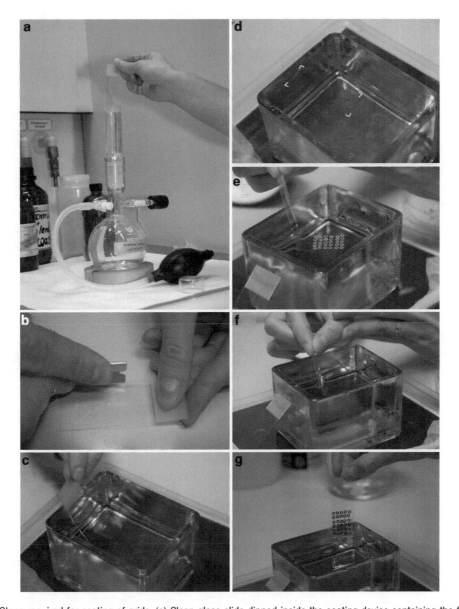

Fig. 4. Steps required for coating of grids. (**a**) Clean glass slide dipped inside the coating device containing the formvar solution. (**b**) Slide coated with formvar, cut by a razor blade to separate the film. (**c**) Slide with cut film dipped inside the water-containing cuvette to separate the film from the glass slide. (**d**) *Grey* film floating on top of the clean water (corners marked by *white angles*). (**e**) Grids are arranged on top of the thin film and the free end is used to pick up the grid along with the film. (**f**) Grids with the film are now sticking to the coverslip inside water. (**g**) Lifting of the grids from the water.

grids are attached to the formvar film, put a dust-free coverslip (24 × 50 mm) on the free side of the film and press it against the water. This will lift the film with the grids from the water and attach them on the coverslip (Fig. 4f, g).

9. Put the coverslip on a petri dish with a filter paper (grids upside). After drying, grids are ready to be used.

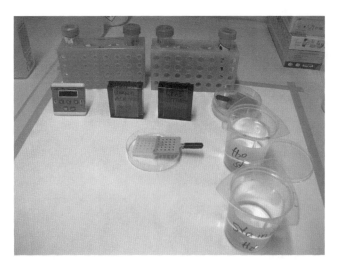

Fig. 5. Picture of grid-staining area showing the required tools. See text for further explanation.

2.4.2. Sectioning and Staining of Grids

1. Diamond knife, fine forceps, and filter paper cut into small triangular shape.

2. Lead citrate solution: Boil 500 ml of water for 30 min (this will help to take out CO_2 from water) and allow it to cool down to room temperature. Dissolve 0.2 g lead citrate (EMS #27800) in 50 ml CO_2-free water in a Falcon tube. Add 500 µl 10N sodium hydroxide. Shake the tube a bit. Let it stand overnight at room temperature to clear the solution. It is best when freshly prepared, but can be used up to 1 month stored at room temperature (see Note 6). Uranyl acetate (UA) solution: Dissolve UA (EMS #22400) in 70% methanol to make a final concentration of 2% and mix it for 1 h in the dark. Fill the UA solution into a syringe and attach a filter (Millipore 0.22) at the tip. After filtering, the UA solution is ready for use. It is best when freshly prepared, but can be used up to 1 month when stored at 4°C.

3. Grid-staining chamber (PELCO™22510) and grid box (EMS #71140) to store your samples with appropriate label (Fig. 5).

3. Methods

3.1. Dissection of the Compound Eye

1. Put the flies on a CO_2 pad.

2. Cut off the head with a razor blade and pull out the proboscis with forceps without smashing the eyes.

3. The whole head can be used for cryo-, light-, and electron microscopy preparation.

3.2. Methods to Score for Rhabdomere Phenotypes in the Intact Head

3.2.1. Deep Pseudopupil Analysis to Score for Defective Rhabdomeres

DPP analysis can be performed in living flies (41). Here it is described for isolated heads. Put the dissected heads with the "neck" on a slide. Shine blue light from the top (in the case of white-eyed flies) or white light from below (in the case of red-eyed flies) through the compound eye. The rhabdomeres efficiently absorb the light. Due to the precise architecture of the retina, the superposition of the pictures of several ommatidia appears as one single pseudopupil in the postero-dorsal quadrant of the eye (Fig. 1, inset). Any gross disruption of the regular retinal organization affects the stereotypic arrangement of rhabdomeres, and ultimately results in a loss of DPP (41, 42). The pseudopupil itself is best viewed using a low power (10×) objective with a large optical aperture. Adjust the light source in order to maximize the contrast between the pseudopupil and the surrounding eye surface. Tilting the head can blur the image.

3.2.2. Optical Neutralization of the Cornea

While the absence of a DPP demonstrates defects in the structure of the rhabdomeres, optical neutralization gives additional information on the nature of the defects. Dissected fly heads are mounted on a slide. If flies express a GFP-tagged protein, fluorescence can be used. Otherwise, one can make use of bright light microscopy for flies with pigmented eye.

Fluorescence microscopy using a water immersion objective can be performed with living flies (43, 44). Alternatively, heads are cut off from the flies and immersed in oil on a slide, covered with a coverslip, and viewed using an oil immersion objective (63×) (N. Gurudev, personal communication).

3.3. Clonal Analysis

Here we describe the clonal analysis of *crumbs* (*crb*) as an example of how to score a phenotype in the *Drosophila* eye of a mutant allele that leads to earlier lethality, using established methods essentially as described (58, 59). The mitotic recombination event is induced in heterozygous animals, where one chromosome carries a wild-type allele of *crb*, and the other one a mutant allele. Upon mitotic recombination, followed by mitosis, two cell clones are formed, in which the cells are either homozygous for the wild-type allele or homozygous for the mutant allele. The sizes of the clones depend on the time point of induction, but also on the viability of mutant tissues. *crb* mutant clones will cover approximately 20–30% of the adult eye. They are scattered on the entire eye and can be recognized as white patches, since they are additionally marked by the recessive marker *white* (*w*). To induce large eye clones, in which most of the eye is mutant for *crb*, the FLP/FRT system is combined with a recessive lethal marker (e.g., *lethal* (3) *cell lethal R3* (*cl3R3*) in the example below) so that those cells, which are homozygous for the wild-type allele, are at the same time homozygous for the lethal marker, thus undergoing apoptosis (60). Large *crb* mutant clones are obtained by setting up the following cross.

P: *yw* P{*ey*-FLP.N}/*yw* P{*ey*-FLP.N} ; ; P{neoFRT}82B *clR3* P{*white⁺-un1*}90E/*TM6B* **X**

w/Y ; ; P{neoFRT}82B *crb^11A22*/*TM6B*

F1: *yw* P{*ey*-FLP.N}/*w* ; ; P{neoFRT}82B *clR3* P{*white⁺-un1*}90E/ P{neoFRT}82B *crb^11A22*

Eyes of adult F1 animals are mosaic, with the mutant clones being white and the few and small wild-type clones being red (Fig. 2b).

3.4. Light Microscopy Approach

3.4.1. Tissue Fixation and Embedding for Light and Electron Microscopy

1. Fix the heads in an Eppendorf tube with 2% paraformaldehyde and 2.5% glutaraldehyde in PB (pH 7.2) at 4°C overnight as primary fixation (see Note 1).

2. Wash the heads thoroughly with PBS three times for 10 min each wash (solvent exchange).

3. The heads are subjected to secondary fixative for 2 h at room temperature in darkness with the secondary fixative (0.2% OsO4 and 1% KMnO$_4$ in PB). This step can be eliminated if the fixation is only for light microscopy.

4. Wash the heads with distilled water three times for 10 min each wash.

3.4.2. Dehydration and Embedding

1. Dehydration is performed with a series of ethanol solutions (50, 70, 90, 95, 2×100% for 10 min each), followed by two washes with Propylene oxide (absolute) for 10 min each. Each step of dehydration should be carried out in a closed tube with shaking. After these steps heads are ready for infiltration with resin (see Note 2).

2. Infiltrate Epon mixture into the head with resin and propylene oxide according to Table 2. All steps must be performed at room temperature with shaking under the fume hood (see Note 3).

3. Embed the heads in pure resin in an embedding mold. You can add a small label with the genotype written on it into the mold. Fill the mold with pure resin and put the head in the mold

Table 2
Infiltration with resin and propylene oxide

Steps	Propylene oxide: Epon	Ratio	Duration	Options
1.	Propylene oxide: Epon resin	3:1	2 h	Cap closed
2.	Propylene oxide: Epon resin	1:1	Overnight	Cap closed
3.	Propylene oxide: Epon resin	1:3	3 h	Cap closed
4.	Pure epon		3 h	Cap open

perpendicular to the edge of the mold so that one eye is next to the edge. Keep the mold in the oven at 60°C and allow the block to polymerize for 12–24 h (see Note 7).

3.4.3. Sectioning and Staining of the Eye for Light Microscopy

1. Trim the block to take out extra resin from the top of the eye if there is any. Trim the side of the block containing the specimen into a trapezoid and start collecting sections of 500 nm thickness. Trim ~16 μm from the cornea to reach the rhabdom.

2. Pick up the sections with a toothpick and collect them on a water droplet put onto a slide. Allow the droplet to dry on top of a hot plate (temperature 60–65°C). This will help to stick the section properly on the slide. After the sections are dry put a little droplet of Toluidine blue solution to the sections. Allow it to stay on the hot plate for a few minutes, depending on the temperature of the plate, allowing the stain to dry. Wash the sections with distilled water and dry them over a hot plate. The rhabdom shape can be visualized with a 20× or a 40× objective under a light microscope (see Note 4). For the comparison of rhabdom size of several genotypes, it is necessary to take sections from the same depth of the rhabdom. The rhabdomere size diminishes and the interrhabdomeral space increases from the distal to the proximal part of the rhabdom. It is better to check for the rhabdom phenotype always at the level of the photoreceptor nuclei. The same block can be trimmed and used to check for the rhabdom phenotype under the electron microscope.

3. Another block should be used for the analysis of the phenotype in longitudinal sections. Take a perfect longitudinal section so that you can see the cornea, cone, rhabdom column, and basal lamina clearly under the light microscope (see Fig. 2a).

4. After sectioning and staining, add DPX to the slide and mount the specimens with a coverslip. For the rhabdom phenotype, take images under 63× or 100× magnification under an oil immersion objective. Pictures from the same magnification can be compared with the wild type to check for any mutant phenotype.

3.5. Electron Microscopy Approach

1. Flies having defective rhabdomeres as revealed by light microscopy can also be subjected for analysis at high resolution under the electron microscope. For this, the plastic block needs to be cut into 70 nm sections by means of a diamond/glass knife. Trim the block closer to the eye with a new razor blade in a trapezoid form, which will allow to get a "ribbon" of serial sections easily.

2. Collect the sections on formvar-coated single-slot grids. Ultrathin sections (<70 nm) should look grey or silver due to their reflection in water. Collect only those sections, which show a homogenous reflection on a silver surface. Align the sections

with an eyelash. Dip the grids into the water of the knife boat with forceps to collect the sections and collect the sections on the grid with the eyelash. Soak excess water with a filter paper, cut in a triangular shape. Store the grids in a grid box with appropriate label.

3. Put the sections on the grid into the grid-staining holder and slide the cover (Fig. 5). They are now ready for staining with uranyl acetate and lead citrate to give contrast under the electron microscope. Uranyl acetate stains the negative background like cytoplasm and lead stains membranous structures.

4. Put the grid-staining holder into a staining vessel. Fill the staining vessel with 70% methanol in order to keep the grids wet. Exchange the 70% methanol with UA solution in the staining box and keep for at least 10 min. Wash the grids three times with 70% methanol (solvent exchange) in the staining vessel. Thereafter, wash it three times in 50% methanol followed by three times in 30% methanol and finally three times in distilled water.

5. To give better contrast the grids are counterstained with lead citrate. Add lead citrate solution to the staining vessel and allow it to incubate for 5 min. Wash three times with distilled water inside the chamber followed by three more washes inside the beaker filled with water. Allow the grids inside the grid chamber to dry. Transfer the grids into the grid box with appropriate label. Grids are ready for examination under the electron microscope.

6. To get an overall idea about the phenotype it is necessary to take images covering at least 6–8 ommatidia. In red-eyed flies, ommatidia are well separated from each other by pigment cells, which are filled with pigment granules (Fig. 2a, c). In white-eyed flies, the outlining of the ommatidia can still be recognized despite the lack of pigments. The lower magnification picture will give a first impression about the rhabdom phenotype. The next step is to zoom in and take picture of individual ommatidia, which will allow, for example, to measure the length of microvilli and stalk membranes, to detect defective junctions or changes in the size or shape of organelles.

3.6. Cryofixation and Immunolabeling of Eye Sections for Confocal Microscopy

1. Place the fly heads in an Eppendorf tube with 4% PFA for 30 min at room temperature in shaking condition. Wash the heads three times with PBS for 15 min each time.

2. Infiltrate the heads with 10% sucrose in PBS for 2 h on a rocker in a cold room. Transfer the heads to 25% sucrose solution and incubate them overnight in a cold room with gentle rocking.

3. Transfer the heads to the embedment mold filled with mounting media. Align the heads under a microscope in such a way that the eyes are looking towards the base of the mold/downwards.

Put at least 12 heads in each boat, arranged in two rows. Place the boat over dry ice and allow it to freeze. The blocks are ready for sectioning or can be stored at –80°C at this point for future use.

3.6.1. Cryosectioning

1. The key instrumentation for cryosection is the cryostat, which is essentially a microtome inside a freezer. Take the cryo sample holder and add a drop of mounting media to it. Take out the frozen block with forceps and stick it to the mounting media (see Note 8). Freeze the sample holder inside the cryostat until it is hard. Fix the sample holder to the cryostat and the eyes are ready for sectioning.

2. Trim the block in the form of a trapezoid with a thick razor blade. Adjust the cryotome to section at a thickness of 10–15 μm. Adjust the temperature of the cryostat to –21°C for the blade and –18°C for the object temperature (there should be always a temperature difference of 2–3° between the object and the blade). Align the glass spacer and the blade properly so that there is a distance of 0.5 mm between the glass blade and the spacer; the spacer should be always ahead of the blade (see Note 9). Sections are picked up with a glass slide and stored inside the cryotome until you are done with the sectioning.

3.6.2. Cryolabeling

1. Wash the slides with PBS twice followed by one wash with PBST and incubate for 10 min at room temperature.

2. Block the slides with 5% NHS diluted in PBST for 1 h at room temperature. Add the primary antibody diluted with blocking solution. Keep it overnight at 4°C in a moist chamber to avoid drying.

3. Wash the slide three times with PBST, 10 min each wash. Add the secondary antibody diluted with blocking solution and keep the slide inside a wet chamber for at least 2 h at room temperature in the dark. At this step it is wise to add fluorescently labeled phalloidin along with the secondary antibody. Phalloidin binds to F-actin and provides a good staining for the overall shape and organization of the PRCs, in particular the rhabdomere.

4. Wash the slide with PBS, followed by two more washes with distilled water. Mount the slide with Vectashield with a cover-slip and seal it with nail polish.

5. Slides are ready for examination under the confocal microscope. Take first an overview picture covering 6–8 rhabdoms. Then zoom in and adjust for one rhabdom to view the labeling more clearly.

3.7. Whole Mount Staining for Confocal Microscopy

Whole mount staining allows to study photoreceptors without cryosectioning. This is a good method to study the localization of proteins at various developmental stages.

1. Dissect the eyes (take out the brain and the lamina) and place them in an Eppendorf tube containing 4% PFA. Fix the eyes for 30 min at room temperature in shaking conditions.

2. Wash the eyes three times with PBS (20 min each wash).

3. Block the sample for 1 h with 5% NHS diluted with PBST.

4. Incubate with the antibody (diluted with blocking solution) by shaking overnight at 4°C. If the antibody dilution has been used successfully on cryosections, then the antibody should work for whole mount staining with the same concentration.

5. Wash the eyes with PBST three times (20 min each wash) at room temperature. Add the appropriate secondary antibody along with phalloidin (this will allow you to see the rhabdom) and incubate at room temperature for 2 h in the dark.

6. Wash the eyes with PBS for 10 min followed by two more washes with water. Eyes are ready for mounting.

7. Remove the cornea with a needle. Make a bridge on the slide (by spacers) and add 100 μl of Vectashield. Align the eyes under a dissecting microscope so that they face downwards. Add a coverslip. Mounting of the eye is a critical point. If properly done, z-stacks collected under the confocal microscope will allow to see every layer of photoreceptors.

4. Notes

Preparation of eye sections and their examination under the electron microscope is a lengthy process, where each and every step might cause poor quality or artifacts. The following steps help to reduce that.

1. Concentrations of glutaraldehyde and paraformaldehyde used for the primary fixation should be measured accurately. Higher fixative concentration dissolves the ultrastructure, resulting in poor-quality pictures.

2. Dehydration steps are very crucial and should be maintained as indicated. The tissue has to be properly and perfectly dehydrated, as resin is incompatible with water. Presence of water might induce holes in the resin-embedded blocks, making sectioning difficult.

3. Timing for infiltration steps has to be accurately maintained, because poor infiltration causes defective resin blocks and consequently difficulties in sectioning. In most red-eyed flies, the

pigment granules seem to be washed away due to poor infiltration process. To avoid this, polymerization of the block should be allowed for more than 24 h. If the problem persists, increase the time of step 3 (Table 1) to 12 h.

4. Perfect staining of the sample is essential for examination of the rhabdom under the light microscope. Do not dry the stain completely (on the hot plate), which might result in overstaining of your sample. As a consequence, the rhabdom phenotype and/or the structure cannot be observed clearly. If this is the case, just wash your sample with 70% ethanol and stain it again.

5. If wrinkles are forming after staining increase the temperature of the hot plate.

6. Proper staining of specimens is essential for electron microscopy. Poor staining induces the formation of lead crystals, which spoil the quality of the image. To avoid lead crystal formation during staining, the first wash after lead citrate staining should be done rapidly. Few more washes should be carried out in order to remove lead citrate completely.

7. Chemicals used for fixation and staining for light/electron microscopy are highly toxic and should be handled under a fume hood. All materials in contact with the resin must be polymerized (60°C, 24 h) before disposed to the regular waste.

8. When cryosectioning, do not section the block immediately after taking it out from –80°C. Bring the block temperature to –20°C before sectioning. This will result in smooth sectioning.

9. Look for the golden reflection with the blade and the glass spacer in the cryostat. A better alignment will help to get smooth sections.

Acknowledgments

We thank Michaela Rentsch for help with the electron micrographs, Franziska Friedrich for help in preparing Figs. 3, 4, and 5, and Nagananda Gurudev for the figure of the optical neutralization. Work of E. K. is supported by the Max-Planck Society (MPG) and a grant from the EC (HEALTH-F2-2008-200234).

References

1. Wolff T, Ready DF (1991) Cell death in normal and rough eye mutants of *Drosophila*. Development 113:825–839

2. Baumann O, Lutz K (2006) Photoreceptor morphogenesis in the *Drosophila* compound eye: R1–R6 rhabdomeres become twisted just before eclosion. J Comp Neurol 498:68–79

3. Zuker CS, Cowman AF, Rubin GM (1985) Isolation and structure of a rhodopsin gene from *D. melanogaster*. Cell 40:851–858

4. O'Tousa JE, Baehr W, Martin RL, Hirsh J, Pak WL, Applebury ML (1985) The *Drosophila ninaE* gene encodes an opsin. Cell 40: 839–850

5. Montell C, Jones K, Zuker C, Rubin G (1987) A second opsin gene expressed in the ultraviolet-sensitive R7 photoreceptor cells of Drosophila melanogaster. J Neurosci 7:1558–1566

6. Zuker CS, Montell C, Jones K, Laverty T, Rubin GM (1987) A rhodopsin gene expressed in photoreceptor cell R7 of the Drosophila eye: homologies with other signal-transducing molecules. J Neurosci 7:1550–1557

7. Feiler R, Bjornson R, Kirschfeld K, Mismer D, Rubin GM, Smith DP, Socolich M, Zuker CS (1992) Ectopic expression of ultraviolet-rhodopsins in the blue photoreceptor cells of Drosophila: visual physiology and photochemistry of transgenic animals. J Neurosci 12:3862–3868

8. Salcedo E, Huber A, Henrich S, Chadwell LV, Chou WH, Paulsen R, Britt SG (1999) Blue- and green-absorbing visual pigments of Drosophila: ectopic expression and physiological characterization of the R8 photoreceptor cell-specific Rh5 and Rh6 rhodopsins. J Neurosci 19:10716–10726

9. Harris WA, Stark WS, Walker JA (1976) Genetic dissection of the photoreceptor system in the compound eye of Drosophila melanogaster. J Physiol 256:415–439

10. Reinke R, Krantz DE, Yen D, Zipursky SL (1988) Chaoptin, a cell surface glycoprotein required for Drosophila photoreceptor cell morphogenesis, contains a repeat motif found in yeast and human. Cell 52:291–301

11. Tomlinson A, Bowtell DD, Hafen E, Rubin GM (1987) Localization of the sevenless protein, a putative receptor for positional information, in the eye imaginal disc of Drosophila. Cell 51:143–150

12. Campos-Ortega JA, Jürgens G, Hofbauer A (1979) Cell clones and pattern formation: studies on sevenless, a mutant of Drosophila melanogaster. Wilhelm Roux's Arch Dev Biol 186:27–50

13. Tomlinson A, Kimmel BE, Rubin GM (1988) Rough, a Drosophila homeobox gene required in photoreceptors R2 and R5 for inductive interactions in the developing eye. Cell 55:771–784

14. Baker NE, Rubin GM (1989) Effect on eye development of dominant mutations in Drosophila homologue of the EGF receptor. Nature 340:150–153

15. Miyamoto H, Nihonmatsu I, Kondo S, Ueda R, Togashi S, Hirata K, Ikegami Y, Yamamoto D (1995) Canoe encodes a novel protein containing a GLGF/DHR motif and functions with Notch and scabrous in common developmental pathways in Drosophila. Genes Dev 9:612–625

16. Basler K, Christen B, Hafen E (1991) Ligand-independent activation of the sevenless receptor tyrosine kinase changes the fate of cells in the developing Drosophila eye. Cell 64:1069–1081

17. Grzeschik N, Knust E (2005) IrreC/rst-mediated cell sorting during Drosophila pupal eye development depends on proper localisation of DE-cadherin. Development 132:2035–2045

18. Yang Y, Ballinger D (1994) Mutations in calphotin, the gene encoding a Drosophila photoreceptor cell-specific calcium-binding protein, reveal roles in cellular morphogenesis and survival. Genetics 138:413–421

19. Mishra M, Oke A, Lebel C, McDonald EC, Plummer Z, Cook TA, Zelhof AC (2010) Pph13 and orthodenticle define a dual regulatory pathway for photoreceptor cell morphogenesis and function. Development 137:2895–2904

20. Zelhof AC, Koundakjian E, Scully AL, Hardy RW, Pounds L (2003) Mutation of the photoreceptor specific homeodomain gene Pph13 results in defects in phototransduction and rhabdomere morphogenesis. Development 130:4383–4392

21. Li BX, Satoh AK, Ready DF (2007) Myosin V, Rab11 and dRip11 direct apical secretion and cellular morphogenesis in Drosophila photoreceptor cells. J Cell Biol 177:659–669

22. Muschalik N, Knust E (2011) Increased levels of the cytoplasmic domain of Crumbs repolarise developing Drosophila photoreceptors. J Cell Sci 124:3715–3725

23. Richard M, Grawe F, Knust E (2006) DPATJ plays a role in retinal morphogenesis and protects against light-dependent degeneration of photoreceptor cells in the Drosophila eye. Dev Dyn 235:895–907

24. Johnson K, Grawe F, Grzeschik N, Knust E (2002) Drosophila Crumbs is required to inhibit light-induced photoreceptor degeneration. Curr Biol 12:1675–1680

25. Hong Y, Ackerman L, Jan LY, Jan Y-N (2003) Distinct roles of Bazooka and Stardust in the specification of Drosophila photoreceptor membrane architecture. Proc Natl Acad Sci U S A 100:12712–12717

26. Berger S, Bulgakova NA, Grawe F, Johnson K, Knust E (2007) Unravelling the genetic complexity of Drosophila stardust during photoreceptor morphogenesis and prevention of light-induced degeneration. Genetics 176:2189–2200

27. Pellikka M, Tanentzapf G, Pinto M, Smith C, McGlade CJ, Ready DF, Tepass U (2002) Crumbs, the Drosophila homologue of human CRB1/RP12, is essential for photoreceptor morphogenesis. Nature 416:143–149

28. Pham H, Yu H, Laski FA (2008) Cofilin/ADF is required for retinal elongation and morphogenesis of the *Drosophila* rhabdomere. Dev Biol 318:82–91

29. Matsuo T, Takahashi K, Suzuki E, Yamamoto D (1999) The Canoe protein is necessary in adherens junctions for development of ommatidial architecture in the *Drosophila* compound eye. Cell Tissue Res 298:397–404

30. Husain N, Pellikka M, Hong H, Klimentova T, Choe K-M, Clandinin TR, Tepass U (2006) The Agrin/perlecan-related protein eyes shut is essential for epithelial lumen formation in the Drosophila retina. Dev Cell 11:483–493

31. Zelhof AC, Hardy RW, Becker A, Zuker CS (2006) Transforming the architecture of compound eyes. Nature 443:696–699

32. Cheli VT, Daniels RW, Godoy R, Hoyle DJ, Kandachar V, Starcevic M, Martinez-Agosto JA, Poole S, DiAntonio A, Lloyd VK, Chang HC, Krantz DE, Dell'Angelica EC (2010) Genetic modifiers of abnormal organelle biogenesis in a Drosophila model of BLOC-1 deficiency. Hum Mol Genet 19:861–878

33. Pulipparacharuvil S, Akbar MA, Ray S, Sevrioukov EA, Haberman AS, Rohrer J, Kramer H (2005) *Drosophila* Vps16A is required for trafficking to lysosomes and biogenesis of pigment granules. J Cell Sci 118:3663–3673

34. Wu CF, Wong F (1977) Frequency characteristics in the visual system of *Drosophila*: genetic dissection of electroretinogram components. J Gen Physiol 69:705–724

35. Hardie RC, Postma M (2008) Phototransduction in microvillar photoreceptors of Drosophila and other invertebrates. In: Basbaum AI, Kaneko A, Shephard GM, Westheimer G (eds) The senses: a comprehensive reference. Academic, San Diego, pp 77–130

36. Pak WL (2010) Why *Drosophila* to study phototransduction? J Neurogenet 24:55–66

37. Pak WL, Grossfield J, Whiten V (1969) Non-phototactic mutants in a study of vision of *Drosophila*. Nature 222:351–354

38. Hotta Y, Benzer S (1969) Abnormal electroretinograms in visual mutants of *Drosophila*. Nature 222:354–356

39. Heisenberg M (1971) Isolation of mutants lacking the optomotor response. Drosoph Inf Serv 112:65–93

40. Heisenberg M (1997) Genetic approach to neuroethology. Bioessays 19:1065–1073

41. Franceschini N (1972) Pupil and pseudopupil in the compound eye of *Drosophila*. In: Wehner R (ed) Information processing in the visual systems of arthropods. Springer, Berlin, pp 75–82

42. Steele F, O'Tousa JE (1990) Rhodopsin activation causes retinal degeneration in *Drosophila* rdgC mutant. Neuron 4:883–890

43. Pichaud F, Desplan C (2001) A new visualization approach for identifying mutations taht affect differentiation and organization of the *Drosophila* ommatidia. Development 128:815–826

44. Meyer NE, Joel-Almagor T, Frechter S, Minke B, Huber A (2006) Subcellular translocation of the eGFP-tagged TRPL channel in *Drosophila* photoreceptors requires activation of the phototransduction cascade. J Cell Sci 119:2592–2603

45. Pandey UB, Nichols CD (2011) Human disease models in *Drosophila melanogaster* and the role of the fly in therapeutic drug discovery. Pharmacol Rev 63:411–436

46. Whitworth AJ (2011) *Drosophila* models of Parkinson's disease. Adv Genet 73:1–50

47. Ambegaokar SS, Roy B, Jackson GR (2010) Neurodegenerative models in *Drosophila*: polyglutamine disorders, Parkinson disease, and amyotrophic lateral sclerosis. Neurobiol Dis 40:29–39

48. St. Johnston D (2002) The art and design of genetic screens: *Drosophila melanogaster*. Nat Rev Genet 31:176–188

49. Wang T, Montell C (2007) Phototransduction and retinal degeneration in *Drosophila*. Pflugers Arch 454:821–847

50. Rogge RD, Karlovich CA, Banerjee U (1991) Genetic dissection of a neurodevelopmental pathway: son of sevenless functions downstream of the sevenless and EGF receptor tyrosine kinases. Cell 64:39–48

51. Bonfini L, Karlovich CA, Dasgupta C, Banerjee U (1992) The son of sevenless gene product: a putative activator of Ras. Science 255:603–606

52. Shulman JM, Feany MB (2003) Genetic modifiers of tauopathy in *Drosophila*. Genetics 165:1233–1242

53. Garen SH, Kankel DR (1983) Golgi and genetic mosaic analyses of visual system mutants in *Drosophila melanogaster*. Dev Biol 96:445–466

54. Becker HJ (1957) Über Röntgenmosaikflecken und Defektmutationen am Auge von *Drosophila* und die Entwicklungsphysiologie des Auges. Z Indukt Abstamm Vererbungsl 88:333–373

55. Stern C (1936) Somatic crossing over and segregation in *Drosophila melanogaster*. Genetics 21:625–730

56. Thaker HM, Kankel DR (1992) Mosaic analysis gives an estimate of the extent of genomic involvement in the development of the visual system in *Drosophila melanogaster*. Genetics 131:883–894

57. Golic KG, Lindquist S (1989) The FLP recombinase of yeast catalyzes site-specific recombination in the Drosophila genome. Cell 59:499–509

58. Stowers RS, Schwarz TL (1999) A genetic method for generating *Drosophila* eyes composed exclusively of mitotic clones of a single genotype. Genetics 152:1631–1639

59. Xu T, Rubin GM (1993) Analysis of genetic mosaics in developing and adult Drosophila tissues. Development 117:1223–1237

60. Newsome TP, Asling B, Dickson BJ (2000) Analysis of *Drosophila* photoreceptor axon guidance in eye-specific mosaics. Development 127:851–860

61. Brand AH, Perrimon N (1993) Targeted gene expression as a means of altering cell fates and generating dominant phenotypes. Development 118:401–415

62. Elliott DA, Brand AH (2008) The GAL4 system: a versatile system for the expression of genes. Methods Mol Biol 420:79–95

63. McGuire SE, Le PT, Osborn AJ, Matsumoto K, Davis RL (2003) Spatiotemporal rescue of memory dysfunction in *Drosophila*. Science 302:1765–1768

64. McGuire SE, Deshazer M, Davis RL (2004) Gene expression systems in *Drosophila*: a synthesis of time and space. Trends Genet 20:384–391

65. Fernandez-Funez P, Nino-Rosales ML, de Gouyon B, She WC, Luchak JM, Martinez P, Turiegano E, Benito J, Capovilla M, Skinner PJ, McCall A, Canal I, Orr H, Zoghbi HY, Botas J (2000) Identification of genes that modify ataxin-1-induced neurodegeneration. Nature 408:101–106

66. Cook T, Zelhof A, Mishra M, Nie J (2011) 800 facets of retinal degeneration. Prog Mol Biol Transl Sci 100:331–368

67. Lu B (2009) Recent advances in using *Drosophila* to model neurodegenerative diseases. Apoptosis 14:1008–1020

68. Bonini NM, Fortini ME (2002) Applications of the *Drosophila* retina to human disease modeling. In: Moses K (ed) Drosophila eye development. Springer, Heidelberg, pp 257–271

69. Tepass U, Knust E (1993) *Crumbs* and *stardust* act in a genetic pathway that controls the organization of epithelia in *Drosophila melanogaster*. Dev Biol 159:311–326

70. Izaddoost S, Nam S-C, Bhat MA, Bellen HJ, Choi K-W (2002) *Drosophila* crumbs is a positional cue in photoreceptor adherens junctions and rhabdomeres. Nature 416:178–183

71. Bhat MA, Izaddoost S, Lu Y, Cho KO, Choi KW, Bellen HJ (1999) Discs lost, a novel multi-PDZ domain protein, establishes and maintains epithelial polarity. Cell 96:833–845

72. Bachmann A, Schneider M, Grawe F, Theilenberg E, Knust E (2001) *Drosophila* Stardust is a partner of Crumbs in the control of epithelial cell polarity. Nature 414:638–643

73. Hong Y, Stronach B, Perrimon N, Jan LY, Jan YN (2001) Drosophila Stardust interacts with Crumbs to control polarity of epithelia but not neuroblasts. Nature 414:634–638

74. Bulgakova NA, Rentsch M, Knust E (2010) Antagonistic functions of Two stardust isoforms in *Drosophila* photoreceptor cells. Mol Biol Cell 21:3915–3925

75. Bulgakova NA, Kempkens Ö, Knust E (2008) Multiple domains of *Drosophila* Stardust differentially mediate localisation of the Crumbs/Stardust complex during photoreceptor development. J Cell Sci 121:2018–2026

76. Oda H, Uemura T, Harada Y, Iwai Y, Takeichi M (1994) A *Drosophila* homolog of cadherin associated with armadillo and essential for embryonic cell–cell adhesion. Dev Biol 165:716–726

77. Riggleman B, Schedl P, Wieschaus E (1990) Spatial expression of the Drosophila segment polarity gene armadillo is posttranscriptionally regulated by wingless. Cell 63:549–560

78. Karagiosis SA, Ready DF (2004) Moesin contributes an essential structural role in *Drosophila* photoreceptor morphogenesis. Development 131:725–732

79. Satoh AK, Li BX, Xia H (2008) Calcium-activated myosin V closes the drosophila pupil. Curr Biol 18:951–955

80. Lebovitz RM, Takeyasu K, Fambrough DM (1989) Molecular characterization and expression of the (Na$^+$ + K$^+$)-ATPase alpha-subunit in *Drosophila melanogaster*. EMBO J 8:193–201

81. Yasuhara JC, Baumann O, Takeyasu K (2000) Localization of Na/K-ATPase in developing and adult *Drosophila melanogaster* photoreceptors. Cell Tissue Res 300:239–249

82. Blochlinger K, Bodmer R, Jan LY, Jan YN (1990) Patterns of expression of cut, a protein required for external sensory organ development in wild-type and cut mutant Drosophila embryos. Genes Dev 4:1322–1331

83. Zipursky SL, Venkatesh TR, Teplow DB, Benzer S (1984) Neuronal development in the *Drosophila* retina: monoclonal antibodies as molecular probes. Cell 36:15–26

84. Pielage J, Stork T, Bunse I, Klämbt C (2003) The cell survival gene *discs lost* encodes a cytoplasmic Codanin-1 like protein, not a homolog of the tight junction PDZ-protein Patj. Dev Cell 5:841–851

Part IV

In Situ Analyses

Chapter 12

Cell-Specific Markers for the Identification of Retinal Cells by Immunofluorescence Microscopy

Christiana L. Cheng, Hidayat Djajadi, and Robert S. Molday

Abstract

Identification and visualization of specific cells and cellular structures in the retina are fundamental for understanding the visual process, retinal development, disease progression, and therapeutic intervention. The increased usage of transgenic and naturally occurring mutant mice has further emphasized the need for retinal cell-specific imaging. Immunofluorescence microscopy of retinal cryosections and whole mount tissue labeled with cell-specific markers has emerged as the method of choice for identifying specific cell populations and mapping their distribution within the retina. In most cases indirect labeling methods are employed in which lightly fixed retinal samples are first labeled with a primary antibody targeted against a cell-specific protein of interest and then labeled with a fluorescent dye-tagged secondary antibody that recognizes the primary antibody. The localization and relative abundance of the protein can readily be imaged under a conventional fluorescent or confocal scanning microscope. Immunofluorescence labeling can be adapted for imaging more than one protein antigen through the use of multiple antibodies and different, nonoverlapping fluorescent dyes. A number of well-characterized immunochemical markers are now available for detecting photoreceptors, bipolar cells, amacrine cells, horizontal cells, Müller cells, and retinal pigment epithelial cells in the retina of mice, and other mammals.

Key words: Mouse, Retina, Immunofluorescence labeling, Retinal cell-specific markers, Antibodies, Fixation, Cryosections, Retinal whole mount, Fluorescence microscopy

1. Introduction

Identification and visualization of specific retinal cell types are fundamental in the study of their role in vision, retinal development, disease progression, and therapeutic intervention. In the past, the structural and cellular organization of mammalian retinas was investigated preferentially in primates (monkeys), cows, cats, rabbits, and rats. In recent years mice have emerged as the main animal model for research as the rapidly advancing transgenic and knockout technologies are being applied in mice, and naturally occurring mutant mice are being recognized as relevant models for

Bernhard H.F. Weber and Thomas Langmann (eds.), *Retinal Degeneration: Methods and Protocols*, Methods in Molecular Biology, vol. 935, DOI 10.1007/978-1-62703-080-9_12, © Springer Science+Business Media, LLC 2013

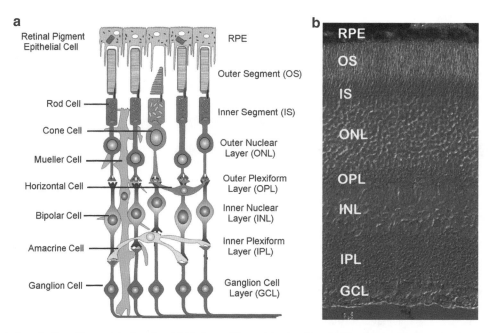

Fig. 1. Organization of the vertebrate retina. (**a**) Diagram of the vertebrate retina showing the organization of various retinal cell types and retinal layers. (**b**) Mouse retinal cryosection stained with DAPI to identify nuclear layers and imaged with DIC and DAPI fluorescence. *RPE* retinal pigment epithelial, *OS* outer segment, *IS* inner segment, *ONL* outer nuclear layer, *OPL* outer plexiform layer, *INL* inner nuclear layer, *IPL* inner plexiform layer, *GCL* ganglion cell layer.

studying human diseases. In the retinal field, mice serve as a powerful tool to investigate mechanisms underlying retinal function and development, and to explore the pathogenesis of retinal degeneration. This chapter of immunohistochemical marker analysis will focus on the mouse retina, but the techniques described are generally applicable to other vertebrate species.

The capability of efficient yet highly complicated communication between neurons in the retina is attributed to the intelligent organization of various retinal cell types (Fig. 1). Communication between neurons occurs within two plexiform layers where the residing dendrites and axons of neighboring neurons make their synaptic connections, achieving a wide network of vertical and lateral contacts simultaneously. The cell bodies of the neurons in the retina are located within the outer and inner nuclear layer (INL); this allows for maximum number of cells in a compacted space in a highly ordered fashion. The back of the retina consists of a layer of phagocytotic retinal pigmented epithelial (RPE) cells whose apical processes intercalate between the photoreceptor outer segments in which the visual transduction components reside. The inner segments of photoreceptors containing the energy-producing and biosynthetic machinery lie in between the outer segments and the cell bodies. Situated between the inner segments and the cell bodies of photoreceptors is the outer limiting membrane characterized as having numerous occluding junctions and serving as a blood-retinal barrier sealing off the remaining retina from potentially harmful material present in the blood circulation.

The photoreceptor cell bodies are positioned in the outer nuclear layer (ONL), below which is the outer plexiform layer (OPL) where the numerous synapses of photoreceptors make contacts with the dendrites of bipolar cells and horizontal cells. The cell bodies of bipolar cells, horizontal cells, and amacrine cells are located in the INL, and these cells network with the processes of ganglion cells in the inner plexiform layer (IPL). The nuclei of ganglion cells reside in the ganglion cell layer (GCL). This layer has far fewer nuclei than the inner or ONLs. The axons of ganglion cells bundle into tracts that run radially and form the nerve fiber layer. The inner limiting membrane, another barrier that separates the retina from vitreous chamber, is formed by the direct contact of cell processes of the Müller cells. These glial cells, which protect and support the neurons, span the retina vertically with their radial processes terminating at the outer and inner limiting membrane and their cell bodies present in the INL.

As with other vertebrates, mice have two types of photoreceptors, rods and cones. Like most animals, the mouse retina is rod-dominated with about 1–3% of the photoreceptors being cones (1, 2). However the average cone density in a mouse retina (3,500 cones per mm^2) (1) is still comparable to that of extrafoveal primate retina (2,000–4,000 cones per mm^2) (3) and that of cat and rabbit retinas. Two types of cone photoreceptors are present in the mouse retina, short-wavelength (blue-light sensitive) S cones and mid-wavelength (green-light sensitive) M cones, distributed in a dorsoventral gradient (2, 4). Only one type of horizontal cell is found in the mouse retina (5), while there are at least ten cone bipolar cell types and one rod bipolar cell type (6). The bipolar cells produce processes extending into distinct regions of the IPL, with the OFF-cone bipolar cells in the outer IPL and the ON-cone bipolar cells in the inner IPL (7). The 20–30 different subtypes of amacrine cells in mammalian retinas (8) can be subdivided into two major categories, the glycinergic and γ-aminobutyric acidergic. In mouse, most amacrine cells form a narrow layer that is two-cell bodies thick in the inner part of INL (1), and some amacrine cells are found displaced in the GCL. The density of ganglion cells is higher in the central retina with a gradual decline towards the peripheral retina (9).

With the incredible diversity of retinal cell types, one can imagine the degree of difficulty to study the retina at a cellular level. Over the years many researchers have characterized specific proteins that are expressed uniquely in a given cell type. These proteins have become defined as cell-specific markers providing a mean for reliable identification of a given population of cells.

To visualize an individual cell type, the indirect fluorescence method is most often employed. This method involves a primary

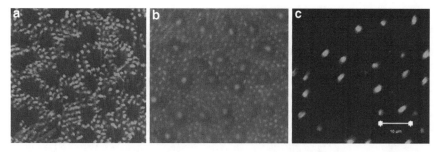

Fig. 2. Human (**a**, **b**) and mouse (**c**) retina whole mounts. (**a**) Fluorescence image of rhodopsin (Rho 1D4) labeling of rods surrounding unlabeled cones depicted as holes. (**b**) Fluorescence image of ABCA4 (Rim 3F4) labeling of cones surrounded by labeled rods (25). (**c**) Fluorescence image of cone opsin (blue and red/green opsin) labeling of cone photoreceptors in a mouse retinal whole mount.

antibody that recognizes the cell-specific protein of interest, and a secondary antibody that is targeted to the primary antibody and that is conjugated to a fluorophore. The signal from the fluorophore is amplified because of the potential for at least two secondary antibodies to bind to each primary antibody. The specificity conferred by the primary antibody and the signal amplification from the secondary antibody make this method the ideal choice for immunohistochemistry. Furthermore, a single secondary antibody can be used to detect different primary antibodies generated in a given species adding versatility to the method. Most primary antibodies work better with cryosections rather than paraffin-embedded sections mostly due to the difficulties in retrieving accessible antigen in the latter. Therefore this chapter focuses on immunofluorescence staining of retinal cryosections. The chapter also describes the method for labeling whole-mount retinas (Fig. 2), as many informative advantages are associated with studying whole-mount retinas, such as the distribution of cell types or the differential expression level of proteins across the entire retina.

In addition, this chapter is directed towards the more widely used fixation and labeling methods. There are many more cell-specific markers available than those described here; most of the markers used in this chapter are commercially available (Table 1). In general, a good marker should be specific to only one cell type or a limited number of cell types, should be expressed over a defined time of the development, should be relatively insensitive to common fixation, and should have known cross-species reactivity. A marker that possesses these qualities is hard to find, especially for bipolar cells, which have been shown to be very species specific. A few molecular markers have been recognized for their cellular and subcellular specificity and have been widely used as specific markers. Examples include antibodies to rhodopsin (Rho1D4 and Rho4D2) as rod photoreceptor markers and more specifically rod outer segment markers (10, 25), blue opsin and red/green opsin for blue and red/green cone photoreceptors (11, 12), postsynaptic density

Table 1

Examples of immunochemical markers for the identification of retinal cells and analysis of cellular and subcellular structures

Cell type	Antigen	Antibody	Source	References
RPE	Ezrin	Rabbit anti-ezrin	Abcam	(26)
Rod photoreceptor	Rhodopsin	Mouse anti-rhodopsin clone 1D4 or 4D2	Millipore or StressMarq	(10, 25)
Cone photoreceptor	Red/green-sensitive opsin	Rabbit anti-red/green opsin	Chemicon	(11)
Cone photoreceptor	Blue-sensitive opsin	Rabbit anti-blue opsin	Chemicon	(12)
Cilium/axoneme	Retinitis pigmentosa 1 protein (RP1)	Chicken anti-RP1 clone EAP15A	Liu et al. 2004	(27)
Photoreceptor inner segment	Sodium/potassium ATPase α3	Mouse anti-Na/K ATPase clone XVIF9-G10	ABR	(25)
Synapses	Postsynaptic density protein (PSD95)	Mouse anti-PSD95 clone 7E3-1B8	ABR	(14)
Synapses	Synaptophysin (SVP38)	Mouse anti-SVP38	Santa Cruz	(28)
Rod bipolar cell	Protein kinase C (PKCα)	Mouse anti-PKCα clone MC5	Sigma	(7, 15)
Cone bipolar cell	Excitatory amino acid transporter (EAAT5)	Rabbit anti-EAAT5	Alpha Diagnostic	(29, 30)
Horizontal cell	Calbindin	Mouse anti-calbindin-D-28 K clone CB955	Sigma	(7)
Amacrine cell	Syntaxin-1A	Rabbit anti-syntaxin 1A	Synaptic Systems	(31)
Müller cell and RPE cell	Cellular retinaldehyde-binding protein	Rabbit anti-CRALBP	Bunt-Milam and Saari 1983	(21)

protein (PSD95) for cone and rod synaptic terminals (13, 14), protein kinase C (PKCα) for rod bipolar cells (7, 15), calbindin for horizontal cells (7, 16), choline acetyltransferase (ChAT) for amacrine cells (17), Thy-1 for ganglion cells (18, 19), and vimentin (20) and CRALBP (21) for Müller cells. A list of widely used cell-specific markers is given in Table 1. Examples of mouse cryosections labeled with various cell-specific markers for immunofluorescence microscopy are given in Figs. 2–4.

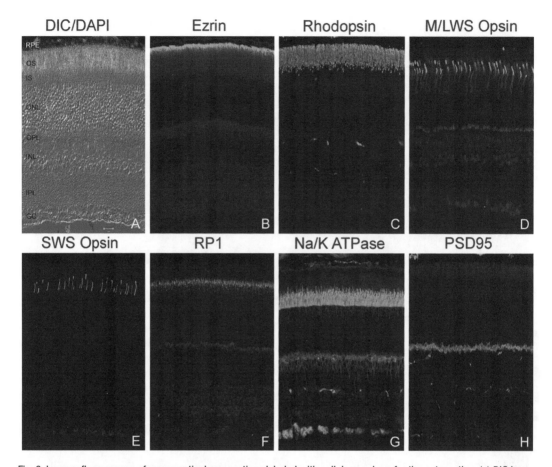

Fig. 3. Immunofluorescence of mouse retinal cryosections labeled with cellular markers for the outer retina. (**a**) DIC image of the retina stained with DAPI as a reference for the location of labeling in the following images. (**b**) Section Imunno-stained for ezrin. Apical microvilli of RPE that intercalate the photoreceptor outer segments are labeled. (**c**) Section immuno-stained for rhodopsin (Rho 1D4). The outer segments of rod photoreceptors are labeled. (**d**) Section immunostained for red/green-sensitive opsin. Cone outer segments are intensely labeled and the cell body faintly labeled. (**e**) Section immuno-stained for blue-sensitive opsin. Only the outer segments of blue cones are labeled. (**f**) Retinitis pigmentosa protein 1 (RP1) immunofluorescence is localized to the axoneme of the photoreceptor outer segments. (**g**) Intense immunostaining of sodium/potassium (Na/K) ATPase is observed in photoreceptor inner segments, outer plexiform layer (OPL), and inner nuclear layer (bipolar cells) of the retina. (**h**) Intense immunolabeling of postsynaptic density protein 95 (PSD95) is detected in the upper portion of the OPL of the retina.

2. Materials

2.1. Labeling of Retinal Cryosections for Immunofluorescence Microscopy

2.1.1. Dissection and Fixation of Retina

1. Small curved scissors.

2. Sorensen's phosphate buffer (PB), 0.1 M, pH 7.4.

3. 16% Paraformaldehyde (PFA) (Electron Microscopy Sciences, Fort Washington, PA).

4. 4% PFA in PB, diluted from 16% PFA (see Note 1).

5. Shallow flat-bottom dissecting dishes, preferably polyethylene.

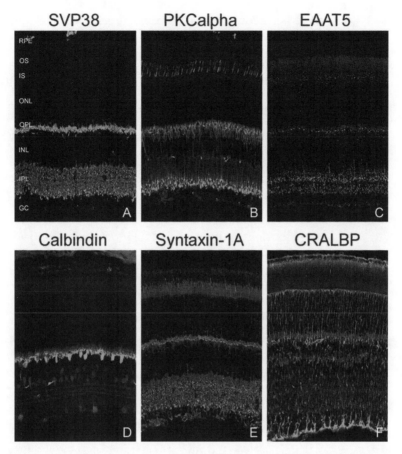

Fig. 4. Immunofluorescence of mouse retinal cryosections labeled with cellular markers for inner retina. (**a**) Intense punctate immunofluorescence of synaptophysin (SVP38) is observed in both the outer and inner plexiform layers (IPLs). (**b**) Section immunostained for the α isoform of protein kinase C (PKCα). Blue cones and rod bipolar cells are labeled. (**c**) Immunolabeling of the excitatory amino acid transporter 5 (EAAT5) is detected in two strata of processes in the IPL, with the OFF-cone bipolar cells in the upper strata and the ON-cone bipolar cells in the lower strata of the layer. (**d**) Calbindin immunofluorescence is prominent in the cell bodies of horizontal cells. (**e**) Syntaxin-1A immunoreactivity is found on amacrine cell processes of the IPL, horizontal cell processes in the outer plexiform layer, and in the inner segment of photoreceptors. (**f**) Cellular retinaldehyde binding protein (CRALBP) labeling is robust in RPE and Müller cells which span throughout the retina vertically.

6. 26 Gauge syringe needle.

7. Medium curved and pointed forceps.

8. Small spring scissors with narrow, sharp tips.

9. Dissecting microscope with illuminator.

2.1.2. Cryo-Protection and Freezing of Retina

1. Sucrose (Fisher Scientific, Ottawa, ON).

2. Sucrose solution (5, 8, 12, 16, 20% w/v) in PB.

3. Embedding molds (Polysciences Inc., Warrington, PA).

4. Polyfreeze Tissue Freezing Medium (Polysciences Inc., Warrington, PA).

5. Liquid nitrogen.

2.1.3. Sectioning of Retina

1. Microscope glass slides, precleaned (Fisher Scientific, Ottawa, ON).
2. Cryostat.
3. Slide boxes for storage (Evergreen Scientific, Los Angeles, LA).

2.1.4. Labeling of Retinal Cryosections

1. Elite PAP pen (Diagnostic BioSystems, Pleasanton, CA).
2. Moisture chamber for slides (Evergreen Scientific, Los Angeles, LA).
3. Sorensen's phosphate buffer, 0.1 M, pH 7.4.
4. Normal goat serum (NGS) (Sigma, St. Louis, MO).
5. Triton X-100 (Sigma, St. Louis, MO).
6. Blocking solution (10% NGS (see Note 2), 0.2% Triton (see Note 3) in PB.
7. Labeling solution (2.5% NGS, 0.1% Triton in PB).
8. Primary antibodies (see Note 4).
9. Secondary antibodies (see Note 5).
10. Mowiol 4-88 mounting media (Polysciences Inc., Warrington, PA).
11. Dihydrochloride DAPI (Invitrogen, Burlington, ON).
12. Microscope cover glass, #1 (Fisher Scientific, Ottawa, ON).
13. Nail polish.

2.2. Labeling of Retinal Whole Mount for Immunofluorescence Microscopy

2.2.1. Dissection and Marking of Retinal Whole Mount

1. Surgical small spring scissors with sharp tips.
2. Medium curved and pointed forceps.
3. Permanent marker.
4. Small curved scissors with blunt tips.
5. Dumont forceps.
6. Small vials (labeled with Left eye or Right eye).
7. 4% PFA in PB.

2.2.2. Separation of Retina from Eyecup

1. Very shallow flat-bottomed dissecting dishes, preferably polyethylene.
2. Dissecting microscope with illuminator.
3. Dumont forceps.
4. No. 11 scalpel blade or 22 gauge syringe needles.
5. Surgical small spring scissors with sharp tips.
6. 4% PFA in PB.
7. No. 3 tapered tip synthetic fiber artist's brush.

2.2.3. Labeling of Retinal Whole Mount

1. Sorensen's phosphate buffer, 0.1 M, pH 7.4.
2. Blocking solution (10% NGS, 0.2% Triton X-100 in PB).

3. Labeling solution (2.5% NGS, 0.1% Triton X-100, 0.01% Sodium Azide in PB).

4. Primary antibodies.

5. Secondary antibodies.

2.2.4. Making Support for Whole-Mounting Retina on Glass Slide

1. Black electrician's or clear tape (two or three layers).

2. Single edged razor blade.

3. No. 11 scalpel blade.

4. Microscope glass slides.

2.2.5. Whole-Mounting Retina on Glass Slide

1. Tapered tip synthetic fiber artist's brush (No. 0, 1, 3).

2. No. 11 scalpel blade.

3. Mowiol 4-88 mounting media (Polysciences Inc., Warrington, PA).

4. Glass coverslips, 24 × 50, No. 1.5.

5. Nail polish.

3. Methods

3.1. Labeling of Retinal Cryosections for Immunofluorescence Microscopy

3.1.1. Dissection of Retina

1. Euthanize mice in compliance with institutional animal care committee protocols and guidelines (see Note 6).

2. Enucleate eyes. In order to prevent tearing of the optic nerve and damaging the retina, apply enough pressure with scissors around the eye so that the eye protrudes out of the socket for easy separation of the eye.

3. Immerse eyes in 4% PFA for 1–12 h (see Note 7) at room temperature.

4. Place the eye under a dissecting microscope. Remove anterior segments (cornea, lens, iris) of the eye by making one small puncture on the whitish ora serrata with a 26 gauge syringe needle while holding the eye in place with forceps.

5. Start making small incisions along the ora serrata with a pair of surgical scissors, and cut all the way around to remove the cornea, thus opening the eyecup.

6. With a pair of forceps securing the eyecup, use another pair of forceps to remove the lens and iris carefully, without disturbing the underlying retina.

3.1.2. Cryo-Protection and Freezing of Retina

1. Cryo-protect eyecups in graded sucrose solutions (5, 8, 12, 16, 20%) (see Note 8), 15 min each at room temperature.

2. In a tissue holder filled with Polyfreeze (see Note 9), position eyecup with its opening facing either left or right in order to obtain tangential (longitudinal) sections of the retina.

3. Once the eyecup is aligned perfectly straight with the side of the holder, dip the tissue holder in liquid nitrogen to freeze the tissue.

4. Eyecups are now ready to be sectioned, or can be wrapped with aluminum foil and stored in an airtight bag at –30°C.

3.1.3. Sectioning of Retina

1. Section eyecup vertically at 10–12 μm on a cryostat set at –26°C.

2. Place 2 or more sections in a group on a glass slide, and place 2 groups with good separation between the groups on a slide; this will allow labeling with two different antibodies on the same slide.

3. Once cut, retinal sections can also be stored at –30°C.

3.1.4. Labeling of Retinal Sections

1. Thaw retinal sections to room temperature.

2. Using a PAP pen, draw around the groups of retinal sections. Let PAP pen marking dry.

3. Rehydrate retinal sections with PB.

4. Incubate sections in blocking solution for 30 min.

5. Dilute primary antibody in labeling solution (see Note 10).

6. Incubate retinal sections with primary antibody (see Note 11) overnight at room temperature in a moisture chamber.

7. Wash sections with PB three times, minimally 15 min each.

8. Incubate retinal sections with appropriate secondary antibody diluted in labeling solution containing DAPI (300 nM) for 1 h at room temperature in a moisture chamber.

9. Wash sections with PB three times, minimum 15 min each.

10. Place a small drop of mounting media on the sections.

11. Cover sections with glass coverslips and secure coverslips by applying nail polish around the coverslip.

12. Labeled retinal sections are ready for viewing by using a conventional light or preferably a confocal scanning microscope with appropriate fluorescent filters and imaging software.

3.2. Labeling of Retinal Whole Mount for Immunofluorescence Microscopy

3.2.1. Dissection and Marking of Retinal Whole Mount

1. Euthanize mice in compliance with institutional animal care committee protocols and guidelines.

2. Carefully cut away the eye lids, using the sharp tipped scissors and forceps, to expose the orbits.

3. Mark the superior point of the eye globe using permanent marker.

4. Using the small curved scissors, insert the tips of scissors into the conjunctiva between the eye and the orbit on the side closest to you.

5. Cut the conjunctiva. Be careful not to cut the sclera of the eye.

6. Using the Dumont forceps, grasp the loose conjunctiva and gently pull the eye slightly forward. Reinsert the scissors tips near the first cut under the eye, cutting the attachment around the eye until the back of the orbit is reached.

7. Carefully cut the remaining conjunctiva around the limbus until the eye comes free.

8. Place the eye in a vial filled with 4% PFA. Incubate for 10–15 min.

3.2.2. Separation of Retina from Eyecup

1. Remove the eye from the vial to the dissection dish under the microscope.

2. Using a No. 11 scalpel blade or 22 gauge needle, pierce the side of the eye just rearward (scleral side) of the limbus. Do not go any deeper than necessary to penetrate the eye wall in order to keep the lens intact.

3. Using the spring scissors and the Dumont forceps, insert one of the scissor blades into the slit just created. First cut up into the cornea. Cut around the eye along the limbus until you return to the beginning. Again cut up over it into the cornea to meet your previous cut from the other direction in order to produce a corneal tab to be used for orientation.

4. After removing the cornea and iris, carefully remove the lens from the inside of the eyecup.

5. Fill the eyecup with a drop of fixative. Fix for ~20–30 min.

6. After an eyecup has been fixed, place it under the microscope so that the interior is visible including the optic nerve head (white dot near the retinal center). Using the small spring scissor or No. 11 blade, make a small cut to the right and left of the marker.

7. Hold onto the sclera with the Dumont forceps while using the 22 gauge needle to separate the retina from the sclera. Gently roll the sclera backward to separate the retina away from the back of the eyecup. If needed, use the spring scissor to cut the sclera; be very careful not to cut the retina.

8. The retina will remain attached to the optic nerve head even when the retina is free from the cup edge. Carefully, using the No. 11 blade, reach into the cup between the loosened retina and the sclera, and sever the optic nerve head from the retina.

9. Fix the retina suspended in 4% PFA for 2–4 h in total.

3.2.3. Labeling of Retinal Whole Mount

1. Rinse retina with PB a few times.

2. Incubate retina with blocking solution for 1 h at room temperature.

3. Label retina with primary antibody diluted in labeling solution containing 0.01% sodium azide for 24 h at 4°C.

4. Wash retina gently with PB 3 times, minimum 20 min each.

5. Label retina with appropriate secondary antibody diluted in labeling solution for 12 h at 4°C.

6. Wash retina gently with PB 3 times, minimum 20 min each.

3.2.4. Making Support for Whole-Mounting Retina on Glass Slide

1. In order to preserve the three-dimensional retina, a support can be made from electrician's tape to prevent the coverslip from flattening the tissue.

2. Cut out a 2–3 in. length of electrician's tape. Apply it carefully to the viewing surface of a glass slide, being careful not to trap air bubbles beneath it.

3. Using a single-edged razor blade, cut the tape off at both ends of the slide by scoring it.

4. Apply a second layer of tape as the first.

5. Using a single-edged razor blade, score through the tape layers near the slide's center to form a diamond shape. Using the point of a No. 11 blade applied to one apex of the diamond, peel the tape up and out, leaving a diamond-shaped area of clear glass to mount the retina within.

3.2.5. Whole-Mounting Retina on Glass Slide

1. Decide the side of the retina that will present the best labeling.

2. Using a No. 3 brush, carefully place a retina on a glass slide, with the desired side up.

3. Using a No. 1 or 0 brush, unfold the retina.

4. Using a No. 11 blade, make small cuts at the retina's edge to allow it to lie flat. For proper orientation, rotate the retina so that the deep cut made during retinal removal is at the 12 o'clock position relative to the glass slide.

5. Place a drop of mounting media on the retina, and a drop on the glass coverslip to be used.

6. Turn the cover glass over and combine the two drops of mounting media as you place the glass coverslip on the slide.

7. Seal the coverslip with nail polish.

8. Examine retinal whole mount with a light or confocal microscope (see Note 12).

4. Notes

1. Alternative fixatives are ice-cold absolute methanol or absolute ethanol. Alcohols do not penetrate as well and consequently do not preserve tissue morphology as well as formaldehyde-based fixatives. Alcohols are primarily used to fix frozen tissue

sections and are more suitable for membrane surface antigens. Another fixative is (4% 1-ethyl-3-(3-dimethylaminopropyl)) carbodiimide, which is used for labeling certain synapse-associated proteins (7).

2. For effective blocking of nonspecific staining from the secondary antibody, choose a serum identical to the host animal of the secondary antibody or from an unrelated species. Addition of 1% bovine albumin serum may also enhance the blocking effect.

3. Percentage of Triton X-100 needed varies depending on the localization and nature of targeted protein. For example, proteins residing in the nucleus require higher percentage of Triton X-100 (0.5% for blocking and 0.3% for labeling of primary and secondary antibody). Triton X-100 is a nonionic detergent that permeabilizes cell membranes, and at high concentration it can destroy tissue morphology.

4. Dilution of primary antibodies should be determined empirically by the investigator with the consideration of manufacturer's recommendation.

5. Secondary antibodies coupled to the Alexa family of dyes (Molecular Probes) give bright, nonfading fluorescent signal that is more superior to that of conventional FITC- or rhodamine-coupled secondary antibodies.

6. The timing of tissue collection may influence the localization of certain proteins. It has been shown that visual signaling proteins such as arrestin (22), recoverin (23), and transducin (24) undergo translocation between the outer and inner segments of the photoreceptors in a light-dependent manner. Therefore it is important to be consistent with the collection time.

7. Length of fixation is dependent on the antibody. The ideal length of fixation would preserve tissue morphology and still retain the antigenicity of the target protein. In general, 15 min to 1 h is sufficient to fix the eyecup properly. However, there are proteins that require longer fixation, such as recoverin (3 h (7)). When punctate staining is expected as in labeling synaptic vesicles and cilia, shorter fixation times should be employed.

8. Some protocols cryo-protect the eyecup in 30% sucrose or higher but in our experience, we find 30% is too viscous and leaves residue in the eyecup during the embedding step. Any residual sucrose in the embedded eyecup can lead to tearing of the tissue during sectioning.

9. Most protocols use OCT instead of Polyfreeze. We find that the use of Polyfreeze minimizes static during sectioning.

10. It is critical to ensure that labeling of primary antibody is not a result of nonspecific labeling or background staining; control experiment should be carried out in parallel. When using

antibodies whose specificity has been tested, it is still good practice to carry out simple labeling controls by omitting the primary antibody; this should reveal whether the secondary antibody is contributing to any nonspecific background staining. If the antibody has yet to be tested, its specificity for the antigen of interest can be proven by the following ways:

(a) Pre-absorb the antibody with the antigen (purified proteins or peptides). The antigen-to-antibody mixture should be made at a working dilution of 10:1 (molar ratio) and be pre-incubated overnight at 4°C. The pre-absorbed antibody can then be incubated with retinal section in place of the primary antibody. The staining intensity produced by the pre-absorbed antibody should be significantly lower compared to that of the primary antibody.

(b) If a knockout mouse model is available for your protein of interest, the retinal sections of the knockout mouse can be labeled with the primary antibody. The absence of labeling would attest to the specificity of the antibody.

11. Labeling of two or even three proteins can be carried out simultaneously by using a combination of primary antibodies generated in different host animals and secondary antibodies conjugated to different fluorophores.

12. Thickness of the mouse retina and the densities of cells vary between central and peripheral retina; in order to achieve consistency, make sure to take photomicrographs from sections of the same region.

Acknowledgments

We thank Dr. Eric Pierce and Dr. John Saari for polyclonal antibodies to RP1 and CRALBP, respectively, and Laurie Molday for helpful discussions on technical details. This work was supported by a grant from the Canadian Institutes for Health Research (CIHR RMF-92101).

References

1. Jeon C-J, Strettoi E, Masland RH (1998) The major cell populations of the mouse retina. J Neurosci 18:8936–8946

2. Applebury ML et al (2000) The murine cone photoreceptor: a single cone type expresses both S and M opsins with retinal spatial patterning. Neuron 27:513–523

3. Curcio CA, Sloan KR, Kalina RE, Hendrickson AE (1990) Human photoreceptor topography. J Comp Neurol 292:497–523

4. Szél Á et al (1992) Unique topographic separation of two spectral classes of cones in the mouse retina. J Comp Neurol 325:327–342

5. Peichl L, González-Soriano J (1994) Morphological types of horizontal cell in rodent retinae: a comparison of rat, mouse, gerbil, and guinea pig. Vis Neurosci 11:501–517

6. Euler T, Wässle H (1995) Immunocytochemical identification of cone bipolar cells in the rat retina. J Comp Neurol 361:461–478

7. Haverkamp S, Wässle H (2000) Immunocytochemical analysis of the mouse retina. J Comp Neurol 424:1–23

8. MacNeil MA, Masland RH (1998) Extreme diversity among amacrine cells: implications for function. Neuron 20:971–982

9. Dräger UC, Olsen JF (1981) Ganglion cell distribution in the retina of the mouse. Invest Ophthalmol Vis Sci 20:285–293

10. Molday RS, MacKenzie D (1983) Monoclonal antibodies to rhodopsin: characterization, cross-reactivity, and application as structural probes. Biochemistry 22:653–660

11. Komaromy AM et al (2008) Targeting gene expression to cones with human cone opsin promoters in recombinant AAV. Gene Ther 15:1049–1055

12. Roberts MR, Hendrickson A, McGuire CR, Reh TA (2005) Retinoid X receptor γ is necessary to establish the S-opsin gradient in cone photoreceptors of the developing mouse retina. Invest Ophthalmol Vis Sci 46:2897–2904

13. Blackmon SM et al (2000) Early loss of synaptic protein PSD-95 from rod terminals of rhodopsin P347L transgenic porcine retina. Brain Res 885:53–61

14. Koulen P, Fletcher EL, Craven SE, Bredt DS, Wässle H (1998) Immunocytochemical localization of the postsynaptic density protein PSD-95 in the mammalian retina. J Neurosci 18:10136–10149

15. Greferath U, Grünert U, Wässle H (1990) Rod bipolar cells in the mammalian retina show protein kinase C like immunoreactivity. J Comp Neurol 301:433–442

16. Wässle H, Peichl L, Airaksinen MS, Meyer M (1998) Calcium-binding proteins in the retina of a calbindin-null mutant mouse. Cell Tissue Res 292:211–218

17. Voigt T (1986) Cholinergic amacrine cells in the rat retina. J Comp Neurol 248:19–35

18. Barnstable CJ, Dräger UC (1984) Thy-1 antigen: a ganglion cell specific marker in rodent retina. Neuroscience 11:847–855

19. Raymond ID, Vila A, Huynh U-CN, Brecha NC (2008) Cyan fluorescent protein expression in ganglion and amacrine cells in a thy1-CFP transgenic mouse retina. Mol Vis 14:1559–1574

20. Dräger UC (1983) Coexistence of neurofilaments and vimentin in a neurone of adult mouse retina. Nature 303:169–172

21. Bunt-Milam AH, Saari JC (1983) Immunocytochemical localization of two retinoid-binding proteins in vertebrate retina. J Cell Biol 97:703–712

22. Nair KS et al (2005) Light-dependent redistribution of arrestin in vertebrate rods is an energy-independent process governed by protein–protein interactions. Neuron 46:555–567

23. Strissel KJ et al (2005) Recoverin undergoes light-dependent intracellular translocation in rod photoreceptors. J Biol Chem 280: 29250–29255

24. Sokolov M et al (2002) Massive light-driven translocation of transducin between the two major compartments of rod cells: a novel mechanism of light adaptation. Neuron 34:95–106

25. Molday LL, Rabin AR, Molday RS (2000) ABCR expression in foveal cone photoreceptors and its role in Stargardt macular dystrophy. Nat Genet 25:257–258

26. Bonilha VL, Finnemann SC, Rodriguez-Boulan E (1999) Ezrin promotes morphogenesis of apical microvilli and basal infoldings in retinal pigment epithelium. J Cell Biol 147: 1533–1547

27. Liu Q, Zuo J, Pierce EA (2004) The retinitis pigmentosa 1 protein is a photoreceptor microtubule-associated protein. J Neurosci 24:6427–6436

28. Hendrickson A, Troilo D, Djajadi H, Possin D, Springer A (2009) Expression of synaptic and phototransduction markers during photoreceptor development in the marmoset monkey Callithrix jacchus. J Comp Neurol 512:218–231

29. Haverkamp S, Ghosh KK, Hirano AA, Wässle H (2003) Immunocytochemical description of five bipolar cell types of the mouse retina. J Comp Neurol 455:463–476

30. Pow DV, Barnett NL (2000) Developmental expression of excitatory amino acid transporter 5: a photoreceptor and bipolar cell glutamate transporter in rat retina. Neurosci Lett 280:21–24

31. Dyer MA, Cepko CL (2001) The p57Kip2 cyclin kinase inhibitor is expressed by a restricted set of amacrine cells in the rodent retina. J Comp Neurol 429:601–614

Chapter 13

A Method of Horizontally Sliced Preparation of the Retina

Ryosuke Enoki and Amane Koizumi

Abstract

Various types of retinal neurons, including amacrine, ganglion, and horizontal cells, expand neurites (dendrites or axons) in horizontal direction and make synaptic or electrical contacts with other cells to integrate the visual information. Many types of ion-channels and receptors are located along these neurites, and these horizontal connections critically contribute to the information processing in the retinal circuits. However, many of previous electrophysiological and immunocytochemical studies employed slice preparations cut by vertical direction in which most of these cells and their neurites were severely damaged and removed. This might lead to the underestimation of active and passive conductance in horizontally expanding neurites, and also missing of morphological information of horizontal structures. Here, we describe an alternative slicing method of horizontally cut preparation of the retina. The slice is made horizontally at the inner layer of the retina using a vibratome slicer after the retina is embedded in the low-temperature melting agarose gel. This horizontal slice preparation enables us to directly access cells in the inner retina by patch-clamp recording, calcium imaging, single RT-PCR, and immunocytochemistry. The method described here would offer an alternative strategy for studying the functions of neurons and neural circuits in the retina.

Key words: Retina, Amacrine cell, Ganglion cell, Horizontal cells, Patch-clamp recording, RT-PCR, Immunocytochemistry, Slice

1. Introduction

Many of previous electrophysiological and immunocytochemical studies on amacrine cells, horizontal cells, and ganglion cells used vertically sliced preparation or dissociated cells. This traditional preparation method enables us to study the many physiological and anatomical characteristics of the light-induced signaling in the retinal circuits. However, the neurites, such as dendrites and axons, of the horizontally expanding cells are severely damaged or even removed in the process of vertical cut or dissociation. A serious concern arises because dendrites and axons are known to have various kinds of active and passive conductance in extensively enriched

Bernhard H.F. Weber and Thomas Langmann (eds.), *Retinal Degeneration: Methods and Protocols*, Methods in Molecular Biology, vol. 935, DOI 10.1007/978-1-62703-080-9_13, © Springer Science+Business Media, LLC 2013

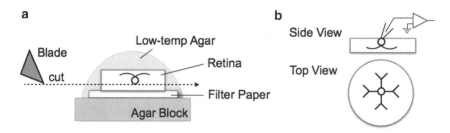

Fig. 1. Schematic procedures for making horizontal slice preparation of the retina. (**a**) The retina was isolated from the eyecup and attached to filter paper, which was flattened on an agar block and covered by low-temperature melting agarose gel. The retina was cut at the level of the inner nuclear layer with a vibratome. (**b**) Side and top view of the horizontal slice. Dendritic arbors of the cells are well preserved.

dendritic morphology (1). The input resistance determined by passive or active conductance of the cells determines the spread of voltage changes in the dendrites and the integration of synaptic inputs, which finally influence the output of signals (2). Also, relative horizontal locations and orientations of cell bodies and dendrites determine characteristics of various types of visual information processing, such as directional selectivity of the moving stimuli (3). Therefore, it was expected to establish an alternative slicing method to preserve horizontal structure of the retina for better understanding of the retinal circuit. In the present chapter, we describe a protocol for alternative slicing method, horizontally sliced preparation of retina (Fig. 1).

There are several important advantages of the horizontal slice preparation. *First*, the morphology of the cells that expand dendrites and axons horizontally, such as amacrine cells and horizontal cells, is well preserved. It has been shown previously that there are over 20 types of amacrine cells in the retina and each subtype of amacrine cells has different functional properties (4). To investigate the functions of these amacrine cells, it is required to preserve their dendritic morphologies. *Second*, in the whole-mount retina, the tight and extensive coverage of Mueller glial cell's endfeets prevents the access of patch pipettes to cells in the inner retina such as amacrine cells and horizontal cells. In contrast, the soma of amacrine cells is exposed to the surface of the horizontal slice preparation (2, 5). *Third*, chemical reagents can easily reach targeted cells and their neurites. Because cell bodies and neurites are located on the surface of the slices, chemical drug application and its removal are fast and easy. *Fourth*, fluorescent ion imaging such as calcium imaging is performable (5). In the traditional vertical slices or the whole-mount retina, excitation light for imaging itself activates photoreceptors. In the horizontal slice preparation, photoreceptors and photopigments are removed so that there is no excitation light-evoked artifact. In addition, the signal-to-noise ratio of imaging is much higher because the background activity of photoreceptors is eliminated. *Finally*, the vertical connection between photoreceptors and ganglion cells is cut, so that light-evoked visual information processing is not intact in the slice. This is the advantage for investigating merely membrane properties and synaptic properties of these cells, although it could not be applied for the study of light-evoked visual information processing.

This unique slice technique is applicable to the retina of any species such as goldfish, mouse, and rabbit. The method of the horizontal slice may offer an alternative way in investigating the function of neurons and neural circuits in the retina.

2. Materials

2.1. Equipment

1. Microwave for dissolving agar solution.
   Hot water bath at 35°C.
2. Vibratome slicer (Leica VT1000S).
3. Membrane filter paper with pore size 0.45 μm (Millipore, HAWP01300).
4. Dissection tools: Forceps, blade, pinch, tweezers.
5. 50 ml Syringe and syringe filter (Millipore, SX0001300).

2.2. Reagents

1. Agar for the block (Sigma, A-1296).
2. Agarose L as low-temperature melting agarose (Wako, 317-01182).
3. Hyaluronidase Type I-S (300 units/mg, Sigma).
4. Cutting solution: 102 mM NaCl, 3.1 mM KCl, 2.0 mM $CaCl_2$, 1.0 mM $MgCl_2$, 23 mM $NaHCO_3$, and 10 mM glucose, maintained at pH 7.8.
5. Ames' solution (Sigma).
6. Instant glue (Alonalpha, Krazy Glu).

3. Methods

1. Prepare a 3% agar with distilled water. Dissolve, microwave, and pour it into a glass dish. Keep the dish in a refrigerator at 4°C (see Note 1).
2. Prepare a 2.5% low-temperature-melting agarose gel with medium. Dissolve using a microwave. Keep it in a water bath at 3°C (see Note 2).
3. Euthanize the animal by anesthesia or decapitation, enucleate an eyeball, and open it as an eyecup. To liquefy the vitreous

humor, the opened eyecup is soaked for 10 min in hyaluronidase in the medium (0.07 mg/ml) if necessary.

4. Cut the agar into a 1 cm × 1.5 cm block for the mouse retina and firmly attach it on a vibratome stage by instant glue. Keep the agar block wet by using cutting solution.

5. Place the blade at 5–10° at the slicer. Gently cut the top surface of the agar block at approximately 50 μm/s speed with a frequency of 50 Hz (see Note 3).

6. Rinse the eyecup with the medium without hyaluronidase. Isolate the retina from a pigment epithelium and place it photoreceptor-side down on a piece of filter paper. To firmly attach the retina to the filter paper, vacuum the retina on the filter paper several times by using a 50 ml syringe (see Note 4).

7. Gently wipe and take out the excess medium on the agar block and carefully place the retina on the filter paper on the agar block. To firmly place the filter paper on the agar block, attach instant glue on the edges of the filter paper (see Note 5).

8. Gently pour the low-temperature-melting agarose gel over the retina. Wait for 1 min and gently pour the cold solution. The agarose gel becomes solidified quickly (see Note 6).

9. Lift the blade position to several hundred microns above the top surface of the agar block and gently cut the top of the solidified agarose gel.

10. Lower down the blade position toward the preparation. Cut the retina at the level of the proximal one-third of the inner nuclear layer for amacrine cells (approximately between 200 and 250 μm above the top surface of the agar block) (see Notes 7 and 8).

11. Notice that the amacrine cells are now face-down position. Carefully pick up the slice of the retina together with the solidified agarose gel by forceps, and place it face-up in a chamber or a dish.

4. Notes

1. The agar block should be prepared in advance and kept in a refrigerator until use.

2. Keep the agarose gel at appropriate temperature. Do not use a hot gel. If it is too hot, it takes a long time to be solidified, and the gel irreversibly destroys the retina.

3. Ensure that the top surface of the agar block is completely smooth and flat. Making several cuts (at least three times) is needed to get a smooth and flat surface.

4. Ensure that the retina is attached to the filter paper completely flat. After placing the retina on the filter paper, cut the excess portion of filter paper surrounding the retina and make a minimal preparation. The excess portion of paper often prevents a blade from going into the appropriate layer of the retina.

5. To avoid unexpectable cracking of the tissue, place the retina as near as possible to the blade on the agar block.

6. When it is too hot, the agarose gel kills the cells.

7. A high-speed blade will damage the retina. Set the speed at approximately 50 μm/s (50 Hz). The appropriate location of the cut depends on the animal species and age.

8. Because the mouse retina is tiny and wavy, it is difficult to obtain a perfect horizontal slice at an appropriate layer. An "oblique" (tilted) slice may be an alternative method to get the relative flat slice of the retina. To do this, put another filter paper in between the retina on the filter paper at the corner and the agar block. Although you cannot expect a perfect horizontal slice, there are always some areas where the soma of amacrine cells is on the surface of the slice.

Acknowledgement

We thank Drs. Richard H. Masland and Akimichi Kaneko for giving us valuable advices and suggestions to establish the procedure of the horizontal slice preparation of the retina.

References

1. Masland RH (2001) The fundamental plan of the retina. Nat Neurosci 4(9):877–886

2. Koizumi A, Jakobs TC, Masland RH (2004) Inward rectifying currents stabilize the membrane potential in dendrites of mouse amacrine cells: patch-clamp recordings and single-cell RT-PCR. Mol Vis 10:328–340

3. Briggman KL, Helmstaedter M, Denk W (2011) Wiring specificity in the direction-selectivity circuit of the retina. Nature 471(7337): 183–188

4. MacNeil MA, Masland RH (1998) Extreme diversity among amacrine cells: implications for function. Neuron 20(5):971–982

5. Azuma T, Enoki R, Iwamuro K, Kaneko A, Koizumi A (2004) Multiple spatiotemporal patterns of dendritic Ca2+ signals in goldfish retinal amacrine cells. Brain Res 1023(1):64–73

Chapter 14

Detection of DNA Fragmentation in Retinal Apoptosis by TUNEL

Francesca Doonan and Thomas G. Cotter

Abstract

Terminal dUTP nick end labeling (TUNEL) is an invaluable technique used in the study of late-stage apoptosis. The technique is based upon detection of fragmented DNA, a well-recognized characteristic of apoptosis, usually with fluorescent markers. Here, we describe the TUNEL technique (1) employing two different detection techniques, fluorescence microscopy and fluorescence-activated cell sorting (2) which can be applied to the analysis of apoptosis in retinal tissues or retinal cell cultures, respectively.

Key words: Retina, TUNEL, Fluorescence microscopy, Flow cytometry, Tissue, Adherent cell

1. Introduction

Apoptosis is a process of programmed cell death occurring in multicellular organisms. It is characterized by cell shrinkage, condensation of chromatin, fragmentation of nuclei, blebbing of plasma membranes, formation of apoptotic bodies, and finally phagocytosis (3). Ideally, for the term apoptosis to be correctly applied, several of these hallmarks should be identified in dying cells. However, DNA fragmentation is considered as an acceptable marker for the diagnosis of apoptosis in vivo since many of the indicators of advanced or late-stage apoptosis are never visualized in tissues, as cells are often engulfed before these indicators are detected (4). A method commonly used to detect DNA fragmentation is terminal dUTP nick end labeling (TUNEL). Exogenously applied terminal transferase labels the terminal ends of nucleic acids with dUTP (1). The newly incorporated dUTP nucleotides are labeled, usually with fluorescent reporter molecules such as fluorescein isothiocyanate (FITC) or rhodamine, to allow visualization. TUNEL staining can be applied to fixed cells followed by fluorescence microscopy or flow cytometry.

Bernhard H.F. Weber and Thomas Langmann (eds.), *Retinal Degeneration: Methods and Protocols*, Methods in Molecular Biology, vol. 935, DOI 10.1007/978-1-62703-080-9_14, © Springer Science+Business Media, LLC 2013

Usually microscopy is the detection method of choice in tissues since it provides spatial and temporal information (5). Furthermore it helps to distinguish individual cells which are likely engaged in an apoptotic death pathway from potentially necrotic tissue characterized by clusters of dying cells. One disadvantage of microscopy is that it can be very user dependent, relying on the classification technique used by each individual to define an apoptotic cell. Fluorescence-activated cell sorting (FACS), a specialized type of flow cytometry, is more useful in cultures of retinal cells providing accurate, rapid quantification of TUNEL-positive cells in a given population and lacking the person-to-person bias of microscopy (6). Therefore the choice of detection method will often depend on which of these factors is more important and whether the researcher is working with retinal tissue or retinal cell lines. As a final point, if it is crucial for the researcher to definitively assign apoptosis as the particular type of cell death taking place, examining nuclear/cellular morphology in tandem with TUNEL analysis is quickly and easily achieved (see Note 1).

2. Materials

Store all reagents at –20°C unless otherwise stated. Prepare the TUNEL reaction mix just prior to use.

2.1. Tissue/Cell Preparation

1. Neutral buffered formalin.
2. Phosphate-buffered saline (PBS), pH 7.4.
3. Triton® X-100.
4. Sucrose, 30% in dH_2O, store at 4°C.
5. Cryochrome.
6. Super-frost plus slides.

2.2. TUNEL Staining

1. Terminal Deoxynucleotidyl Transferase (TdT).
2. Recombinant (30 U/µl) TdT reaction buffer: 500 mM cacodylate buffer (pH 6.8), 5 mM $CoCl_2$, and 0.5 mM DTT.
3. Fluorescein-12-2′-deoxy-uridine-5′-triphosphate (Fluorescein-12-dUTP) (1 nmol/µl) (see Notes 2 and 3).
4. Hoechst 33342 to counterstain: Stock solution 1 mg/ml in PBS, store at 4°C.

2.3. Microscopy

Mowiol mounting medium:

1. Add 2.4 g Mowiol 4-88 and 6 g glycerol to a 50 ml beaker.
2. Add 6 ml of dH_2O and stir for several hours at room temperature.

3. Add 12 ml 0.2 M Tris–HCl (pH 8.5) and incubate at ±53°C until the Mowiol has dissolved.

4. Clarify by centrifugation of the solution at $500 \times g$ for 20 min.

5. Carefully remove the supernatant and store aliquots at –20°C. These aliquots remain stable for 12 months, once thawed aliquots are stable for 1 month at 4°C.

---

3. Methods

3.1. TUNEL Staining of Retinal Sections for Microscopy

1. Fix whole eyes by immersion in 2 volumes of neutral buffered formalin overnight at 4°C (see Note 4). Immersion of fixed tissues, especially those kept in fixative for an extended time, i.e., greater than a week, before the TUNEL assay is carried out can affect in situ end labeling (7).

2. Cryoprotect whole eyes by immersion in 2 volumes of 30% sucrose for 5–24 h at 4°C.

3. Cut 7 μm sections and mount on super-frost plus slides.

4. Allow the slides to air-dry for 5 min at room temperature (RT). Freeze at –20°C for later use or proceed with staining procedure.

5. To remove residual cryochrome, wash the slides in 1× PBS for 5 min on a rocking platform.

6. Place the slides in a slide staining tray and when they are dry, draw around the section with a hydrophobic pen.

7. Permeabilize sections with 0.1% Triton® X-100/1XPBS, 50 μl per slide for 2 min at RT.

8. Wash the slides in 1× PBS, 3 washes 5 min each (see Note 5).

9. Make up the TUNEL solution as follows for 1 ml of reaction (50 μl per slide) (see Notes 6 and 7): 200 μl TdT Buffer (5×), 10 μl TdT Enzyme (30 U/μl), 3 μl Fluorescein–dUTP (1 nmol/μl), 1 μl Hoechst (1 mg/ml), and 786 μl dH$_2$O.

10. Pipette 50 μl of reaction mix onto each slide; position some damp tissue in the bottom of the staining tray to maintain humidity and place in a 37°C incubator for 1 h (see Note 8).

11. Wash the slides in the dark (black polyoxymethylene-poly-acetal plastic containers are recommended) in 1× PBS, 3 washes 5 min each.

12. Carefully dry the slides without touching the section.

13. Pipette 7 μl Mowiol mounting media onto a coverslip (20×20) and gently place the coverslip over the section. Using a forceps

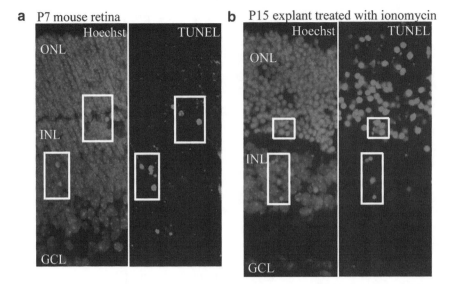

Fig. 1. Detection of terminal dUTP nick end labeling (TUNEL) by microscopy. (**a**) Cells undergoing apoptosis during retinal development were detected using the TUNEL technique. TUNEL-positive cells are visible in the INL and ONL of the retina at postnatal day (P) 7. (**b**) P15 retinal explants were treated with 5 μM ionomycin for 24 h, inducing apoptosis primarily in the ONL. In both cases sections were counterstained with Hoechst dye and the areas highlighted in the box indicate dying cells exhibiting condensed chromatin, a morphological indicator of apoptosis (*INL* inner nuclear layer, *ONL* outer nuclear layer).

push firmly around but not on the section to remove air bubbles.

14. Dry overnight at RT or for 1 h at 37°C before viewing under a fluorescence microscope (Fig. 1).

3.2. TUNEL Staining of Adherent Retinal Cell Cultures for FACS

1. Collect the medium from each well (assuming 6-well plates are used—see Note 9) into separate 25 ml tubes to retain any cell apoptotic cells that have lifted from the plate.

2. Harvest the remaining cells by gentle scraping or with 200 μl Trypsin for 1–2 min and add to the medium in the 25 ml tubes. The trypsin reaction will be stopped by adding the cells to the medium as long as it contains serum.

3. Centrifuge the cells at 1,100 rpm ($200 \times g$) for 5 min.

4. Decant the supernatant and wash the cells in 1 ml of 1× PBS. Transfer to a 1.5 ml Eppendorf tube (see Note 10).

5. Centrifuge the cells at 1,100 rpm ($200 \times g$) for 5 min.

6. Fix the cells with neutral buffered formalin on ice for 20 min.

7. Centrifuge the cells at 1,100 rpm ($200 \times g$) for 5 min.

8. Decant the supernatant and wash the cells in 1 ml of 1× PBS.

9. Centrifuge the cells at 1,100 rpm ($200 \times g$) for 5 min.

10. Decant the supernatant and permeabilize the cells for 2 min on ice in 0.1% Triton® X-100/1× PBS.

11. Centrifuge the cells at 1,100 rpm ($200 \times g$) for 5 min.

12. Decant the supernatant and wash the cells in 1 ml of 1× PBS.

13. Centrifuge the cells at 1,100 rpm (200×*g*) for 5 min and decant the supernatant.

14. Make up the TUNEL reaction mix as in step 9 above and resuspend the cell pellet in 50 µl of TUNEL reaction per sample.

15. Incubate for 1 h at 37°C with resuspension every 30 min (see Note 11).

16. Centrifuge the cells at 1,100 rpm (200×*g*) for 5 min and decant the supernatant (see Note 12).

17. Wash the cells in 1 ml of 1× PBS.

18. Centrifuge the cells at 1,100 rpm (200×*g*) for 5 min and resuspend in 300 µl of 1× PBS.

19. Read the samples on the FACS, keeping them in the dark prior to analysis.

20. Record the data as dot plots with forward scatter (FSC) on the *x*-axis and FL-1 on the *y*-axis (Fig. 2).

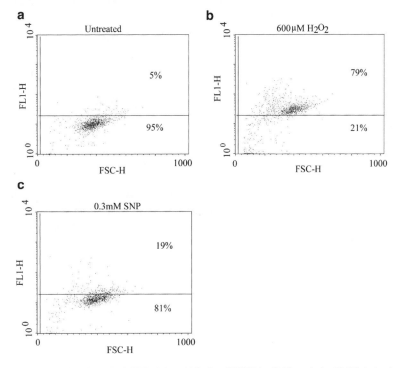

Fig. 2. Detection of terminal dUTP nick end labeling (TUNEL) by FACS analysis. 661 W derived photoreceptor cells which had been allowed to adhere overnight were (**a**) untreated, (**b**) treated with 600 µM H_2O_2, (**c**) treated with 0.3 mM sodium nitroprusside (SNP) for 24 h. After TUNEL staining cells were analyzed by flow cytometry. Increased fluorescence in FL1 indicating TUNEL labeling and therefore apoptosis was indicated by an upward shift in the cell population. The FL1 channel measures fluorescence from 515 to 545 nm and forward scatter (FSC) is a measure of cell volume. CellQuest Pro software was used to calculate the percentage of cells above and below the line.

4. Notes

1. One potential disadvantage of this assay is that TUNEL-positive cells can also be observed in cells undergoing necrosis (8). Therefore this method alone does not definitively establish apoptosis. As mentioned above it is desirable to identify at least one other characteristic of apoptosis to be sure that this is the mode of cell death. One way to address this problem is to co-stain retinal sections with Hoechst dye alongside TUNEL and then analyze nuclear morphology (Fig. 1). Nuclei of cells undergoing apoptosis appear rounded due to condensation of chromatin (9) and can therefore be distinguished from necrotic cells which do not exhibit condensed chromatin (10). To confirm apoptosis in cultured retinal cells, look for cell shrinkage and rounding under the light microscope prior to FACS analysis (11).

2. If greater sensitivity is required Br-dUTP can be used as it is more readily incorporated into DNA strand breaks than larger ligands such as fluorescein. TUNEL-positive cells are then identified by a fluorescently labeled anti-BrdU monoclonal antibody.

3. If the user does not have access to a fluorescence microscope a colorimetric staining protocol can be used. A biotinylated nucleotide is incorporated instead of a fluorescently labeled one. Streptavidin–HRP is added which reacts with the biotinylated nucleotides and the HRP enzymes of the streptavidin complex catalyze the chromogen reaction to form a colored complex, brown in the case of diaminobenzidine which can be viewed under a light microscope.

4. TUNEL-positive cells stain particularly well in formalin-fixed tissue compared to other fixatives. Formaldehyde prevents the loss of the fragmented DNA by cross-linking the low-molecular-weight DNA fragments to other cell constituents. Omission of this step decreases the incorporation of dUTP.

5. For a positive control treat cells or tissue sections with 10 U/ml of DNaseI for 10 min at RT. Wash these slides separately as residual DNaseI activity may contribute to false positives.

6. Keep the TdT enzyme out of the freezer for the minimum amount of time it takes to add it to the reaction mix.

7. The suppliers of TdT (Promega) recommend using the enzyme at a concentration of 1/50 μl/slide. We have optimized this further and use only 0.5/50 μl/slide. Once the TUNEL mix has been applied keep the slides/samples in the dark for all steps thereafter.

8. To obtain minimal background, do not let the sections dry out at any point after the TUNEL reaction has been applied; ensure

that the expiry date of the FITC-dUTP has not passed and use Mowiol aliquots for a maximum of 1 month.

9. Due to loss of cells during the many washing steps it is advisable to pool three 6-well plates or use a small flask for each sample so that there are enough cells to read on the FACS at the end of the experiment.

10. Take care when decanting the supernatant, as the cell pellet can be quite small and loosely attached.

11. A 1-h incubation time with the TUNEL mix is sufficient for 661 W cells but some cultured cells require a longer incubation. If using a longer incubation time pay particular attention to the untreated samples to ensure that the length of the incubation in TdT buffer does not start to affect the integrity of the cells.

12. The cells do not pellet easily after the TUNEL staining step. Confirm the presence of a pellet before decanting the supernatant. If there is no visible pellet spin the samples again. If there is still no visible pellet increase the rpm.

References

1. Gavrieli Y, Sherman Y, Ben-Sasson SA (1992) Identification of programmed cell death in situ via specific labeling of nuclear DNA fragmentation. J Cell Biol 119:493–501

2. Tanke HJ, van der Keur M (1993) Selection of defined cell types by flow-cytometric cell sorting. Trends Biotechnol 11:55–62

3. Kerr JF, Wyllie AH, Currie AR (1972) Apoptosis: a basic biological phenomenon with wide-ranging implications in tissue kinetics. Br J Cancer 26:239–257

4. Kroemer G, Galluzzi L, Vandenabeele P et al (2009) Classification of cell death: recommendations of the nomenclature committee on cell death 2009. Cell Death Differ 16:3–11

5. Doonan F, Donovan M, Gomez-Vicente V et al (2007) Bim expression indicates the pathway to retinal cell death in development and degeneration. J Neurosci 27:10887–10894

6. Miller TJ, Schneider RJ, Miller JA et al (2006) Photoreceptor cell apoptosis induced by the 2-nitroimidazole radiosensitizer, ci-1010, is mediated by p53-linked activation of caspase-3. Neurotoxicology 27:44–59

7. Lucassen PJ, Chung WC, Vermeulen JP et al (1995) Microwave-enhanced in situ end-labeling of fragmented DNA: parametric studies in relation to postmortem delay and fixation of rat and human brain. J Histochem Cytochem 43:1163–1171

8. Grasl-Kraupp B, Ruttkay-Nedecky B, Koudelka H et al (1995) In situ detection of fragmented DNA (tunel assay) fails to discriminate among apoptosis, necrosis, and autolytic cell death: a cautionary note. Hepatology 21:1465–1468

9. Reme CE, Grimm C, Hafezi F et al (2000) Apoptosis in the retina: the silent death of vision. News Physiol Sci 15:120–124

10. Trichonas G, Murakami Y, Thanos A et al (2010) Receptor interacting protein kinases mediate retinal detachment-induced photoreceptor necrosis and compensate for inhibition of apoptosis. Proc Natl Acad Sci U S A 107: 21695–21700

11. Ebert S, Schoeberl T, Walczak Y et al (2008) Chondroitin sulfate disaccharide stimulates microglia to adopt a novel regulatory phenotype. J Leukoc Biol 84:736–740

Chapter 15

High-Throughput RNA In Situ Hybridization in Mouse Retina

Seth Blackshaw

Abstract

The introduction of large-scale gene expression profiling studies has greatly increased the need to rapidly obtain high-quality cellular expression patterns of genes found to exhibit differential expression. The use of large-scale nonradioactive RNA in situ hybridization makes this possible, and greatly increases the general usefulness of this data. Here, we describe protocols for parallel analysis of up to 50 different gene-specific probes in mouse retinal sections.

Key words: RNA, Gene expression, Cellular resolution, Hybridization, Digoxigenin, Riboprobe, Chromogenic, Retina, Photoreceptor, Development

1. Introduction

RNA in situ hybridization (1, 2) can be used to characterize the cellular expression pattern of any RNA species. By designing antisense probes that can undergo complementary base pairing with a target sequence of interest, one can readily design a probe that can strongly and selectively bind to virtually any target RNA, whether or not it codes for protein. The high stability of RNA–RNA hybrids means that hybridization conditions can be made especially stringent, thus resulting in both low background signal and high sensitivity. Complementary RNA (cRNA) probes are typically generated from linear DNA templates, using recombinant viral RNA polymerases to directly incorporate modified bases that contain a label of choice to allow detection of probe–target hybrids. Radioactive nucleotide triphosphates can be used to allow for direct detection of bound probe. Alternatively, chemically modified bases can be used, allowing indirect probe detection using immunodetection. Critical improvements came with the use of bases conjugated to the highly antigenic small molecule digoxigenin for probe labeling,

Bernhard H.F. Weber and Thomas Langmann (eds.), *Retinal Degeneration: Methods and Protocols*, Methods in Molecular Biology, vol. 935, DOI 10.1007/978-1-62703-080-9_15, © Springer Science+Business Media, LLC 2013

which allowed the use of highly specific alkaline phosphatase-conjugated antibodies for immunohistochemistry (2, 3). These modifications improved the specificity and sensitivity of the protocol to the point where it could be used to analyze many different probes in parallel. One of the most spectacular uses of this approach has been the effort of the Allen Brain Atlas consortium to map the expression of all annotated mouse genes in the adult brain (4).

In the retina, large-scale in situ hybridization has been instrumental in analyzing the results of SAGE (5, 6) and microarray (7, 8) data obtained by profiling different developmental stages, or mutant animals exhibiting developmental defects or retinal degeneration. While global expression profiling of this sort generates vast amounts of data, it is very hard to interpret meaningfully unless one also knows the cellular expression pattern of any differentially expressed genes. Even in cases where isolated cell subtypes or even individual cells are profiled (9, 10), it is important to use a different experimental approach to confirm the validity of any results obtained. The regular structure of the retina enables the major cell types that express a given gene to be identified on the basis of their laminar position, making this data particularly useful. Since up to 50 different cRNA probes can be run in parallel by a single investigator, with results obtained within 3–5 days, it is now feasible to rapidly sort through all of the most potentially interesting hits obtained in such experiments.

2. Materials

2.1. RNAse-Free Solutions

1. DEPC-treated water: Add DEPC to 0.1% final concentration in MilliQ ddH$_2$O. Shake solution to mix, and leave overnight at room temperature. Inactivate DEPC by autoclaving (15–25 min at 15 psi) prior to use (see Note 1).

2. DEPC-treated PBS, SSC, EDTA, LiCl: Prepare these as described above for DEPC-treated water. Do not treat any buffer containing amines (e.g., triethanolamine, Tris, etc.) with DEPC (see Note 2).

2.2. Probe Preparation

1. 10× RNA polymerase buffer (Roche).

2. 10× DIG NTP mix (Roche).

3. RNAse-free ddH$_2$O (not DEPC treated).

4. RNAse inhibitor (Roche).

5. RNA polymerase (T7, T3, or Sp6).

6. RNAse-free DNAse to degrade probe.

7. RNAse-free 1.5 ml Eppendorf tubes or RNAse-free 96-well plates.

8. DEPC-treated 3 M NaOAC.

9. RNAse-free 100% EtOH.

10. 70% EtOH prepared with DEPC ddH$_2$O.

2.3. Tissue Pretreatment, Probe Hybridization, and Washes

1. 4% Paraformaldehyde (PFA): 45 ml ddH$_2$O, 4 g PFA.

   To prepare, heat to 60–70°C, add 1 drop 10 N NaOH, stir to dissolve. Once PFA has fully dissolved, add 5 ml 10× PBS, pH 7.5. Sterile filter and store on ice. Use PFA solution on the day of preparation. Alternatively, stocks of 20% PFA in water (dissolve as above) can be prepared ahead of time. These can be thawed, and brought to 4% in 1× PBS prior to use.

2. Hybridization buffer (50 ml volume): 25 ml 100% ultrapure formamide, 12.5 ml 20× SSC, pH 6.0, 5 ml 50× Denhardt's solution, 250 μg/ml final yeast tRNA in DEPC water (store resuspended aliquots at –80°C), 500 μg/ml final salmon sperm DNA, DEPC ddH$_2$O (to 50 ml).

3. 20× SSC, pH 6.0 (1 l): Add 175.9 g NaCl and 88.2 g Na$_3$(C$_3$H$_5$O(COO)·2H$_2$O) to 800 ml of ddH$_2$O. Adjust pH to 6.0 with concentrated HCl. Adjust volume to 1,000 ml final.

4. 50× Denhardt's solution (1 l): 900 ml ddH$_2$O, 5 g Ficoll 400, 5 g polyvinylpyrolidone, 5 g BSA (Fraction V), adjust volume to 1,000 ml with ddH$_2$O. Filter through a 0.2 μm filter. Store in aliquots at –20°C.

5. Protease K solution: Dissolve at 0.5 mg/ml in DEPC-treated water. Freeze in aliquots and store at –20°C. Do not reuse aliquots.

6. RNAse buffer: 0.5 M NaCl, 10 mM Tris pH 7.5, 5 mM EDTA.

7. B1 buffer: 0.1 M Tris pH 7.5, 0.15 M NaCl.

8. B2 buffer: B1 + 5% heat-inactivated normal sheep serum (HISS).

   Place serum in a water bath at 56°C, 30 min to heat inactivate. Store HISS at –20°C in aliquots.

9. B3 buffer: 0.1 M Tris–Cl pH 9.5, 0.1 M NaCl, 50 mM MgCl$_2$.

   Filter through a 0.45 μm filter (see Note 3).

10. B4 buffer: 3.375 μl/ml NBT (100 mg/ml in 70% dimethyl-formamide), 3.5 μl/ml BCIP (50 mg/ml in ddH$_2$O), 0.24 mg/ml levamisole in B3 buffer.

11. Gelvatol mounting media: 21 g PVA, 42 ml, 52 ml, 0.2 M Tris, pH 8.5, 3–5 crystals of NaN$_3$, ddH$_2$O.

    Preparation of Gelvatol: Add PVA to glycerol followed by ddH$_2$O. Add 3–5 crystals of NaN$_3$. Stir with low heat for a few hours or until reagents dissolved. Clarify the mixture by centrifugation at $5,000 \times g$ for 15 min. Aliquot and store at 4°C. See Note 4 for details on Gelvatol preparation.

12. 3 M NaOH.

13. 1% SDS in ddH$_2$O.

14. Tissue-Tek plastic slide boxes and slide holders (Fisher).

15. Siliconized 24×60 mm coverslips.
    To prepare, load coverslips onto 24-slot Tissue-Tek slide holder. In a fume hood, dip twice into 3% Sigmacote (Sigma) in chloroform (dip 2×), then dip twice into 100% EtOH. Air-dry coverslips in hood. Prepare several hours in advance to allow sufficient time for drying.

3. Methods

Carry out all procedures at room temperature unless otherwise specified.

3.1. Probe Preparation for Linearized Templates (See Note 5)

1. Prepare plasmid DNA using Qiagen miniprep kit or equivalent. Digest 5–10 µg of template DNA to completion using restriction enzyme of choice. Confirm completeness of digestion using gel electrophoresis.

2. Following digestion, add 0.5 µg protease K to the enzyme digestion buffer and incubate at 37°C for 15 min.

3. Increase volume to 200 µl with DEPC-treated TE.

4. Extract once with 200 µl TE-buffered phenol, and then once with 200 µl chloroform.

5. Precipitate with 600 µl volumes of EtOH and 20 µl DEPC-treated 3 M NaOAc.

6. Spin for 15 min at maximum speed to collect pellet, and then wash twice in 200 µl 70% EtOH prepared with DEPC-treated water.

7. Air-dry the pellet and resuspend at 1 µg/µl in TE.

3.2. Alternative Protocol: Probe Preparation for PCR-Generated Templates

1. Amplify the probe template using primers that include the promoter sequence for the RNA polymerase used for probe generation. Primers commonly used for this include M13 forward and reverse, and primers targeting the T7, T3, and Sp6 RNA polymerase promoter sequences (see Note 6). Use approximately 0.1 ng of plasmid template, running 25–30 cycles of amplification.

2. Confirm that a correctly sized band is amplified using agarose gel electrophoresis.

3. Purify amplified DNA using a Qiagen spin column, eluting in TE.

4. Following purification of template DNA, synthesize probe by mixing the following components in the order indicated. Use RNAse-free aerosol tips for all procedures: 2 μl 10× RNA polymerase buffer, 2 μl 10× DIG NTP mix, RNAse-free ddH$_2$O (to 17 μl final), 1 μl RNAse inhibitor, and 1 μl RNA polymerase (T7, T3, or Sp6) to 19 μl final volume. Generate a master mix using these specifications when screening multiple probes. Finally, add 0.5–1 μg of template in 1 μl TE. This reaction can be performed in RNAse-free Eppendorf tubes or in 96-well RNAse-free PCR plates.

5. Incubate for 60 min at 37°C.

6. Add 2 μl RNAse-free DNAse. Incubate for 15 min at 37°C to degrade probe template.

7. Run denaturing gel with RNA size marker to check probe yield and integrity.

8. If probe yield and integrity are satisfactory, add 2.5 μl 4 M DEPC-treated LiCl and 75 μl 100% EtOH to precipitate. Vortex at maximum speed for 5 s. If probe synthesis is performed in 96-well plate format, transfer the product to RNAse-free Eppendorf tubes prior to precipitation.

9. Store at –80°C for at least 2 h. Precipitate by centrifuging at maximum speed.

10. Wash twice in 200 μl 70% EtOH prepared with DEPC-treated water. Air-dry the pellet and resuspend at 1 μg/μl in TE. The probe can be stored in EtOH indefinitely, or in TE for at least 2 years at –80°C.

3.3. Preparation of Fresh-Frozen Tissue Sections (See Note 7)

1. Remove eyes and embed directly in O.C.T. compound (VWR) in Peel-A-Way disposable plastic mold (Polysciences) and snap freeze on dry ice. Store block at –80°C prior to sectioning.

2. Allow block to warm to cutting temperature for a minimum of 20 min.

3. Cut 15–20 μm sections using a cryostat or freezing microtome onto Superfrost Plus slides (VWR, 48311-703) (see Note 8).

4. Air-dry sections for at least 20 min. Slides can be dried for several hours if necessary. Do not allow to dry overnight, however. Use dried slides immediately for in situ hybridization analysis or store at –70°C in sealed slide box (can store for 1–2 years without appreciable loss of signal). If using stored sections for analysis, allow them to equilibrate to room temperature in a closed slide box.

3.4. Alternative Protocol: Preparation of Immersion Fixed Sections

1. Remove cornea, lens, and sclera from dissected eyes to create eyecup preparation. Fix tissue by overnight immersion at 4°C in 4% PFA in 1× PBS.

2. Transfer to 30% sucrose in 1× PBS for 24 h at 4°C.

3. Mount in O.C.T. compound and section as described for Method 1.

4. Air-dry for at least 20 min. Slides can be dried overnight if needed. Use immediately or freeze at −20°C as described above.

3.5. Pretreatment of Sections

1. Before beginning: Remove all RNAse contamination from slide racks and chambers by rinsing with 0.3 M NaOH, rinsing with MilliQ water, treating with RNAseZap or 1% SDS in MilliQ water, and then rinsing once again with MilliQ water. Wipe clean with Kimwipes (see Note 9). Use DEPC-treated solutions for all treatments prior to hybridization (see Note 10).

2. Fix in fresh 4% PFA in 1× PBS for 10 min.

3. Wash 3× with PBS, 5 min each (see Note 11).

4. If tissue was fixed in 4% PFA before embedding, treat with 2 μg Protease K in PBS for 10 min, followed by 2× 5-min washes in PBS, a 5-min refix in 4% PFA/PBS (see Note 12), and 2× 5-min PBS washes.

5. Incubate for 10 min in a mixture of 270 ml DEPC-treated water/30 ml 1 M triethanolamine, pH 8.0/0.75 ml acetic anhydride. Mix solution in an RNAse-free glass bottle and mix well by shaking after addition of acetic anhydride (see Note 13).

6. Wash 3× 5 min with PBS.

3.6. Riboprobe Hybridization

MilliQ water is adequate for this and all subsequent steps.

1. Place slides in a chamber constructed from a 245×245 mm BD Falcon* Square BioDish XL (Fisher, 02-667-21) square Petri dish on a raised platform constructed from two 2 ml polystyrene pipettes taped to the surface of the chamber with waterproof tape. Alternatively, these can be bonded directly to the surface of the dish using chloroform (see Note 14).

2. Place 500–1,000 μl of hybridization buffer on slide. Cover sections completely (see Note 15).

3. Leave in humidified chamber (keep moist with strips of gel blot paper soaked in 5× SSC) for at least 90 min.

4. Prepare siliconized 24×60 mm coverslips several hours in advance to allow sufficient time for drying.

5. Pour off prehybridization solution and blot off edges by direct touching to bench paper. To reduce costs, prehybridization solution can be saved, stored at −20°C, and reused 3–4 additional times. Add 75–100 μl hybridization solution containing

       200–300 ng/ml DIG RNA which has been heated at 80°C for 5 min, vortexed for 5 s, and then snap-chilled on ice. Add probe along bottom, long edge of the slide.

6. Clean coverslips using blown compressed air or manual tapping if visible dust is present.

7. Coverslip slides by slowly lowering down a siliconized coverslip. Place long edge, in contact with probe, down first and lower the rest slowly using fingers or a bent needle. Go slowly, to avoid trapping of air bubbles. Once on the slide, raise and lower the coverslip a couple of times to mix the probe with the prehybridization solution that remains on the slide (see Note 16).

8. Place slides horizontally in a humidified chamber (use 20 slide capacity microslide boxes) (VWR). If possible, place slides with different probes in separate boxes. However, if running many probes in one experiment, place abundant probes at the bottom. Make sure that long edge of slides is not in contact with the back of the box, as this can promote capillary transfer of the hybridization buffer away from the slide. Insert at least four blank slides (pushed all the way to the back of the box) to avoid this problem (see Note 17). Place a couple of Kimwipes (VWR) soaked in 5–10 ml 50% formamide/5× SSC in the bottom of the box to ensure that slides do not dry out.

9. Seal with waterproof tape (incubate at 65–72°C overnight) (see Note 18).

3.7. Washes, Antibody Binding, and Signal Detection

1. Place slides in rack, submerged in 5× SSC to remove coverslips. If coverslips are slow in falling off, the solution temperature can be increased to 65–70°C. Carefully remove slides from solution with forceps, grasping the frosted end. Coverslips should fall off into the solution when slides are lifted up (see Note 19).

2. Transfer slides with forceps into metal racks.

3. Incubate in 0.2× SSC at 65°C for 1 h in a water bath. After 30 min, jostle the slides a bit to remove bubbles that may have accumulated on the slides. Slides can be washed longer if needed, but not longer than 3 h total (sections will often fall off the slide if heated longer) (see Note 20).

4. Wash with RNAse buffer for 5 min at 37°C.

5. Wash in RNAse buffer containing 10 μg/ml RNAse A for 30 min at 37°C (see Note 21).

6. Wash in RNAse buffer for 5 min at room temperature.

7. Wash 2× for 30 min in 0.2× SSC, 65°C.

8. Wash in 0.2× SSC for 5 min.

9. Wash in B1 for 5 min.

10. Place 1 ml buffer B2 on horizontal slides for 1 h (see Note 22).

11. Place 0.5 ml anti-DIG Ab (1:5,000 in buffer B2) on each slide. Incubate in humidified chamber at 4°C overnight (see Note 23).

12. Wash with buffer B1 3× for 5 min.

13. Wash with buffer B3 for 5 min, keeping slides horizontal in humidified chamber (use the same prehyb chamber), puddle on buffer B4. Keep in the dark (reaction is photosensitive) at RT (cover chamber with foil). Check color after 15 min, 1 h, and then again after 3 h and 6 h using a low-power microscope (see Note 24). Can leave reaction for up to 3 days at either room temperature or 4°C, and for even longer if background is low.

3.8. Coverslipping and Mounting

1. Rinse slides in TE.

2. Rinse slides in ddH$_2$O.

3. Mount in 4 drops Gelvatol per slide, using 24×60 mm coverslips. Leave overnight before examining. Once dry, wash away excess Gelvatol with tap water, and then air-dry (see Note 25).

4. Notes

1. DEPC is highly toxic. Use caution when preparing solutions, and do not breathe vapor. Autoclaving will fully inactivate 0.1% DEPC, and the faint smell detectable after autoclaving reflects residual ethanol contamination.

2. DEPC reacts with amine, hydroxyl, and thiol groups of proteins, thus inactivating RNAse, as well as any other protein with which it comes into contact. As a result, it is highly toxic and should be handled with great care.

3. The filter unit used to prepare B3 can be wrapped with parafilm and reused.

4. The viscosity of the Gelvatol requires optimization for each batch prepared. When making the solution, add PVA in step 4 until the solution is clear and is slightly less viscous than molasses. Then refrigerate the beaker of Gelvatol overnight at 4°C (after step 5 and before step 6), and check it the next morning to be sure that the viscosity is that of molasses. If it is, continue on to step 6. If it is too viscous, add a little more glycerol to lower the viscosity and then go on to step 6. If it is not viscous enough, add more PVA with heat and refrigerate for a few more hours, again checking the viscosity before going on to step 6. Continue until viscosity is optimal. Gelvatol can be stored at 4°C indefinitely, or at room temperature for 1 month.

5. DNA templates used for cRNA probe synthesis should be between 300 and 2,000 bp in length, with 700–1,000 bp being optimal. Probe sequences should lack any repeat sequences longer than 40 bp, and should not show more than 90% identity over any continuous stretch of 150 bp or more, or cross-reactivity will result. Probe templates must be cloned into vectors (such as pBluescript) in which the insert is flanked by T7, T3, or Sp6 RNA polymerase promoters, so as to allow generation of labeled cRNAs. Many 3′ directed ESTs, such as those from the BMAP project or other large-scale cDNA sequencing efforts, work very well as ISH probes, and can be easily ordered from companies such as Thermo-Fisher. Alternatively, PCR amplification followed by cloning into an appropriate vector (such as the TOPO-TA vector) can be used if repeat-free ESTs are not already available as probe templates. Only cloned sequences should be used as templates for probe generation. While PCR can be used to simultaneously amplify template sequences from complex target preparations (e.g., reverse-transcribed cDNA), this introduces a strong possibility of contamination. Once a clone containing the probe sequence has been obtained, a linearized template must be generated in order to conduct run-off transcription for cRNA synthesis. All experiments should include both a positive and a negative control sample. Positive control probes should robustly recognize target mRNAs in retina, but not be so abundant that contamination of other slides is a real risk. Good negative control probes should target transcripts that are not detectably expressed in retina (such as albumin, cardiac albumin, GFP, etc.). Use of sense control probes is not usually recommended, as a sizeable minority of mammalian genes have associated antisense transcripts (11).

6. When using PCR primers that target an RNA polymerase promoter sequence (i.e., T3, T7, or Sp6), it is important to include 2–3 bases of 5′ overhang outside the primer sequence. This substantially improves the efficiency of cRNA synthesis.

7. Fixed tissue generally produces weaker signal intensity than fresh-frozen, though use produces superior morphology and better overall signal–noise ratio. Fresh-frozen tissue is often easier to section consistently than fixed tissue, and is particularly useful for analyzing embryonic samples.

8. It is advantageous to fill as much as the slide as possible with sectioned samples (although make sure that O.C.T. from other sections does not overlap your tissue). The more sections present on a slide, the greater the likelihood of obtaining high-quality data in a given experiment. It is also the best way to directly compare results from different samples, since placing them on the same slide effectively eliminates slide-to-slide variation in signal intensity and probe spreading.

9. RNAses are very resistant to inactivation, so pretreatment is designed to simply denature and remove any proteins that might come into contact with the slides. In this step, this is accomplished by treatment with detergent and a strong base.

10. Avoiding RNAse contamination during the first day of the procedure is critical. RNAses can come from human and animal skin and hair, or very often as contamination from other experimental procedures, particularly plasmid DNA preparation. The danger is greater to the probe than to the sample, as target RNA sequences in fixed tissue are much less accessible to RNAses than are cRNAs in solution. Do everything possible to avoid these sources of contamination. Wear a clean lab coat to cover arms, tie back long hair, and avoid working in lab areas where animals are sacrificed. Use aerosol tips for all solutions that require pipetting. Put down fresh bench paper before beginning the procedure, and change gloves whenever the possibility of contamination arises. We have often used a fume hood to conduct all the steps up until the prehybridization step, which both protects your sample from airborne debris and removes any PFA vapors from the work area.

11. Dunk sections several times during each wash to ensure good mixing.

12. This refixation is important to maintain tissue integrity following the protease K treatment.

13. Acetic anhydride modifies positively charged amine groups in proteins and lipids, greatly reducing nonspecific binding by the negatively charged cRNA probe. However, acetic anhydride hydrolyzes rapidly in aqueous solution, and it is extremely important that the solution be applied immediately to the slides once mixed.

14. It is important that slides rest above the surface of the box so as to avoid capillary transfer of solution away from the sections.

15. Do not allow the tissue to dry out at this or any other successive stage. This will result in a loss of signal in the affected area. Chill prehybridization solution on ice prior to applying to reduce surface tension and ensure an even spread. Solution used for prehybridization can be reused 3–4 times. Pour into 50 ml conical tubes prior to adding probe and store at −80°C (reused solution should not be mixed with probe and used for hybridization).

16. Probe must be well mixed to ensure even signal intensity across the slide.

17. It is critically important to change gloves between probes. Failure to do so will result in cross-contamination.

18. 70–72°C is an optimal hybridization temperature for perfect match probes that are longer than 300 bases. 65°C is better for

shorter probes or an imperfect match (i.e., rat probe used on mouse tissue).

19. Do not use any force or pressure to remove the coverslip. Doing so will result in damage to the tissue.

20. In this and every subsequent step, preheat solutions in a water bath prior to washing.

21. The RNAse treatment degrades the single-stranded cRNA probe while leaving double-stranded RNA–RNA hybrids intact. This results in a considerable reduction in background signal. However, it requires great caution, as the RNAse used in this step can contaminate materials used prior to the hybridization step. Every effort should be made to prevent this. Make sure that slide boxes and racks used for RNAse treatment are treated with 0.3 M NaOH and RNAseZap after use. Change gloves after handling slides during this step.

22. To ensure even spread of solution across the slide and to reduce the amount of serum used, chill B2 solution on ice prior to application.

23. For abundant RNA a 1-h incubation is sufficient, but overnight incubation greatly enhances the signal and reduces color reaction time.

24. Optimizing the ratio of target to background signal is crucial for obtaining high-quality data using this procedure. To this end, it is essential to vigilantly track the progress of the color reaction so as to assess when it should be terminated. The most efficient way to do this is to directly view the slides in their chamber against a white background using a dissecting microscope such as a Leica Stemi 2000-C or an Olympus BH-2 at roughly 10× magnification. Stop the reaction before any obvious background is visible, but slightly past the point at which the color exposure appears optimal to the eye, as the cellular signal intensity will look weaker at the 200× magnification usually used for photographing retinal sections.

25. Gelvatol automatically seals the slide once it dries, which reduces labor substantially when running large number of slides. One can also use Aquamount (Fisher, 14-390-5) or an equivalent water-based solution to mount the slides, but they must then be sealed with clear nail polish to prevent drying during long-term storage.

References

1. Jamrich M, Mahon KA, Gavis ER, Gall JG (1984) Histone RNA in amphibian oocytes visualized by in situ hybridization to methacrylate-embedded tissue sections. EMBO J 3:1939–1943

2. Schaeren-Wiemers N, Gerfin-Moser A (1993) A single protocol to detect transcripts of various types and expression levels in neural tissue and cultured cells: in situ hybridization

using digoxigenin-labelled cRNA probes. Histochemistry 100:431–440

3. Young WS 3rd (1989) Simultaneous use of digoxigenin- and radiolabeled oligodeoxyribonucleotide probes for hybridization histochemistry. Neuropeptides 13:271–275

4. Lein ES, Hawrylycz MJ, Ao N, Ayres M, Bensinger A, Bernard A, Boe AF, Boguski MS, Brockway KS, Byrnes EJ et al (2007) Genome-wide atlas of gene expression in the adult mouse brain. Nature 445:168–176

5. Blackshaw S, Fraioli RE, Furukawa T, Cepko CL (2001) Comprehensive analysis of photoreceptor gene expression and the identification of candidate retinal disease genes. Cell 107:579–589

6. Blackshaw S, Harpavat S, Trimarchi JM, Cai L, Huang H, Kuo WP, Weber G, Lee K, Fraioli RE, Cho SH et al (2004) Genomic analysis of mouse retinal development. PLoS Biol 2:E247

7. Corbo JC, Myers CA, Lawrence KA, Jadhav AP, Cepko CL (2007) A typology of photoreceptor gene expression patterns in the mouse. Proc Natl Acad Sci U S A 104:12069–12074

8. Punzo C, Cepko CL (2007) Cellular responses to photoreceptor death in the rd1 mouse model of retinal degeneration. Invest Ophthalmol Vis Sci 48:849–857

9. Trimarchi JM, Stadler MB, Cepko CL (2008) Individual retinal progenitor cells display extensive heterogeneity of gene expression. PLoS One 3:e1588

10. Trimarchi JM, Stadler MB, Roska B, Billings N, Sun B, Bartch B, Cepko CL (2007) Molecular heterogeneity of developing retinal ganglion and amacrine cells revealed through single cell gene expression profiling. J Comp Neurol 502:1047–1065

11. Katayama S, Tomaru Y, Kasukawa T, Waki K, Nakanishi M, Nakamura M, Nishida H, Yap CC, Suzuki M, Kawai J et al (2005) Antisense transcription in the mammalian transcriptome. Science 309:1564–1566

Chapter 16

Assessment of Mitochondrial Damage in Retinal Cells and Tissues Using Quantitative Polymerase Chain Reaction for Mitochondrial DNA Damage and Extracellular Flux Assay for Mitochondrial Respiration Activity

Stuart G. Jarrett*, Bärbel Rohrer*, Nathan R. Perron, Craig Beeson, and Michael E. Boulton

Abstract

Mitochondrial dysfunction and genomic instability are associated with a number of retinal pathologies including age-related macular degeneration, diabetic retinopathy, and glaucoma. Consequences of mitochondrial dysfunction within cells include elevation of the rate of ROS production due to damage of electron transport chain proteins, mitochondrial DNA (mtDNA) damage, and loss of metabolic capacity. Here we introduce the quantitative polymerase chain reaction assay (QPCR) and extracellular flux assay (XF) as powerful techniques to study mitochondrial behavior. The QPCR technique is a gene-specific assay developed to analyze the DNA damage repair response in mitochondrial and nuclear genomes. QPCR has proved particularly valuable for the measurement of oxidative-induced mtDNA damage and kinetics of mtDNA repair. To assess the functional consequence of mitochondrial oxidative damage, real-time changes in cellular bioenergetics of cell monolayers can be measured with a Seahorse Biosciences XF24 analyzer. The advantages and limitations of these procedures will be discussed and detailed methodologies provided with particular emphasis on retinal oxidative stress.

Key words: Mitochondria, Retinal pigment epithelium, Photoreceptor cell, Oxidative stress, Quantitative polymerase chain reaction, Extracellular flux assay

1. Introduction

Mitochondria are critical organelles for cell function and survival with principal functions including provision of chemical energy through ATP production, modulation of cellular metabolism, and regulation of cell death (1). Since mitochondria are vital components

---

*Authors Stuart G. Jarrett and Bärbel Rohrer contributed equally to this work.

Bernhard H.F. Weber and Thomas Langmann (eds.), *Retinal Degeneration: Methods and Protocols*, Methods in Molecular Biology, vol. 935, DOI 10.1007/978-1-62703-080-9_16, © Springer Science+Business Media, LLC 2013

in cellular metabolism and function, it is not surprising that dysfunction of this organelle impacts severely on tissue homeostasis. A major theory of aging and disease is that oxidative damage can result in mitochondrial dysfunction and ultimately tissue malfunction. Damage to the mitochondrial DNA appears to have more relevance to mitochondrial impairment due to the fact that it encodes components of the electron transport chain (ETC) and thus controls the entire cells' metabolic capacity. Numerous retinal pathologies are associated with oxidative stress, mitochondrial DNA (mtDNA) damage, and changes in mitochondrial metabolic capacity, in part, due to the retina's highly oxidizing microenvironment (2–5). Chronic mitochondrial dysfunction is associated with a number of age-related degenerative diseases including age-related macular degeneration (AMD), diabetic retinopathy, and glaucoma (6). In this article, we describe two powerful techniques that will help readers design experiments to aid in the investigation of mitochondrial genomic injury and metabolic alterations in the pathogenesis of retinal degenerations.

1.1. Analysis of Mitochondrial DNA Damage and Repair: Quantitative Polymerase Chain Reaction Assay

Over the past decade the Quantitative polymerase chain reaction (QPCR) assay technique has been utilized to analyze genomic injury in multiple species and cell types (2, 5, 7–15). The QPCR assay has the ability to detect multiple classes of DNA damage and include oxidative stress-generated mtDNA damage (blue light, decarbomoyl mitomycin, menadione, hydrogen peroxide (H_2O_2)) (2, 15, 16), methylation (methyl methanesulfonate) (2, 15–17), helical distorting adducts (UV) (17), DNA cross-links (cisplatin), and double-strand breaks (etoposide) (2, 15, 17). The QPCR assay works on the simple premise that DNA damages (i.e., strand breaks, base modifications, bulky adducts, cross-links (cisplatin), and apurinic sites) are all capable of blocking the progression of a DNA polymerase (18). Therefore, only the DNA templates that do not contain blocking lesions will be amplified. As a result, the amount of PCR product is inversely proportional to the amount of template DNA damage. The major strength of the QPCR assay is that it is based on genome-specific primers, thus negating the necessity to isolate mitochondria prior to analysis, a procedure which is associated with extensive artifactual mtDNA damage (19). Furthermore, the genome-specific primers allow a direct comparison between the mtDNA and nuclear DNA (nDNA) damage response simultaneously (20). Defects in DNA repair pathways have been implicated in retinal aging and degeneration; thus this assay has the unique potential to provide a greater understanding of the contribution of mtDNA repair in retinal cell dysfunction (2). In addition, a particular gene or region of interest can be specifically investigated via the use of specific primer sets, i.e., transcribed vs. non-transcribed genes (7). Another major benefit of QPCR is the detection of a wide array of endogenously and exogenously induced

DNA damage (18). Finally, only very low amounts of input DNA (~10–100 ng) are required, making this assay suitable for limited or small-scale samples, e.g., RPE isolated from either human and mouse donors (5). A limitation of QPCR, however, is that it is unable to distinguish between the different types of DNA lesions generated due to the nondiscriminatory nature of QPCR (however, this property may be advantageous depending on the experimental outcomes required). Further, QPCR only provides relative quantification of DNA damage and not an absolute level, as all lesion measurements are expressed using a control sample that is defined as "undamaged," even though the extent of endogenously generated DNA lesions is unknown.

1.2. Measurement of Mitochondrial Respiration Activity: Extracellular Flux Assay

Although genetic and environmental factors contribute to retinal degenerative disease, the underlying etiology common to many retinal diseases arises from the extremely high energy demand of the retina and surrounding microenvironment. Significant energy is required in the retina, particularly in the outer retina. The retina consumes ATP in both the presence and absence of light. In the dark-adapted photoreceptors, the main energy consumption is driven by ion pumps to maintain homeostasis and synaptic transmitter release; light-adapted photoreceptors require energy for phototransduction and light adaptation (21). The RPE on the other hand requires energy for maintaining ion homeostasis of the subretinal space, which rapidly changes in response to light, in addition to its other functions that include epithelial transport of molecules; re-isomerization of the chromophore 11-*cis*-retinal; daily removal of photoreceptor outer segments by phagocytosis; and production and secretion of molecules (22). The production of ATP in the outer retina is primarily dependent upon glucose and oxygen (23). However, since the outer-retina environment is highly nutrient- and oxygen-rich, together with the presence of light and high levels of poly-unsaturated fatty acids, the high metabolic demands may cause persistent mitochondrial damage in the retina. Since ATP utilization and these biochemical processes are intimately linked, changes in energy metabolism are among the earliest and most informative markers of cellular stress and evidence of mtDNA damage.

Traditionally, metabolic fluxes associated with energy metabolism have been determined by time-dependent accumulation of radionuclide-labeled metabolites. For example, accumulation of ^3HOH water from 3-^{3}H-D-glucose is a measure of glycolytic flux through glyceraldehyde-phosphate dehydrogenase (GAPDH). These radiometric assays are highly specific but are also labor intensive and require substantial quantities of tissue or cells. Recent work shows that measurement of metabolite fluxes like O_2, lactate, and total acid can estimate intracellular fluxes with accuracies comparable to radiometric assays (24, 25). The advantages of extracellular flux assays include higher throughput, reduced sample size, and substantially improved kinetic resolution. These extracellular flux assays recapitulate the classical methods used to study isolated mitochondria with the added advantage of using whole cells or tissues that retain intact cellular processes and signaling.

Until recently, methods for measuring energy metabolism by extracellular flux analysis relied on Clark electrode chambers or the Cytosensor® microphysiometer. The Clark electrode is an electrode that measures oxygen on a catalytic platinum surface, measuring electron flow in response to oxidative phosphorylation. While the readouts are highly reproducible, the measurements require large amounts of tissue or cells suspended in solution that needs to be stirred constantly, and only one sample can be examined at a time. The Cytosensor® microphysiometer on the other hand is a device that measures extracellular acidification (rate of acid efflux) for four samples in parallel. It uses an ~10 μl sensor perfusion chamber to provide sensitive rate measurements for a small number of cells (e.g., 10^4–10^5 per chamber). During a rate measurement, flow is momentarily stopped to measure specific changes of extracellular pH as the cells respire within the small volume. After such measurements, flow is restored to prevent oxygen depletion and accumulation of metabolic wastes.

More recently, a multiwell plate-based assay platform was developed, the Seahorse Biosciences Extracellular Flux (XF) Analyzer, that uses fluorescent optode detectors to combine measurements of oxygen consumption rates (OCR) and extracellular acid release (ECAR) from cells plated in multiwell plates. The instruments are available in 24- and 96-well plate-based formats, using the same basic technology (26). The three technologies have been developed to either address basic physiological questions or to assess oxygen consumption in large tissue (Clark electrode); for basic drug screening in cell-based assays before the advent of higher throughput instruments (Cytosensor® microphysiometer); or for high-throughput screening and combined oxygen and extracellular acid release (XF analyzer).

2. Materials

All solutions are prepared using ultrapure water (prepared by purifying deionized water to attain a sensitivity of 18 MΩ cm at 25°C) and cell culture and molecular biology grade reagents.

2.1. QPCR Assay

2.1.1. Cell Culture and Induction of DNA Damage

1. RPE growth media: Ham's F10 medium (Invitrogen) (500 ml) supplemented with 10% heat inactivated fetal calf serum (Invitrogen) (40 ml). The serum is heat-inactivated by incubation at 65°C for 2 h. Growth media is supplemented with 100 μl/ml streptomycin, 100 μl/ml kanamycin, and 60 μl/ml

penicillin (Invitrogen). All media are filtered (0.2 μm) and stored at 4°C and warmed to 37°C for 30 min before the start of a QPCR experiment.

2. RPE cell lines (transformed and primary cultures; see Subheading 3.1.1) are maintained using standard cell culture procedures. For routine cell expansion, RPE cells are grown until ~80% confluence is achieved followed by a 1:3 split. For QPCR analysis, RPE are grown to confluence followed by withdrawal of serum-*containing* Ham's F10 media and replacement with serum-*free* Ham's F10 media for 24 h before the DNA damage treatment. This step promotes cellular quiescence and mimics the in vivo RPE microenvironment (15).

3. Hydrogen peroxide (H_2O_2) is diluted in Hams's F10 media without the addition of fetal calf serum and other supplements. H_2O_2 is prepared in the dark to prevent degradation using sterile tubes covered in aluminum foil. In addition, H_2O_2 is stored at 4°C until the day of the experiment and added to prewarmed serum-free Ham's F10 media to give the desired molarity to generate detectable DNA damage. To initiate RPE mtDNA damage final H_2O_2 concentrations of 100–500 μM are recommended. Please note that if long-term studies are to be performed, H_2O_2 should be filtered with 0.2 μm filters to ensure sterility.

2.1.2. DNA Isolation and Quantification

1. DNA isolation is performed using a DNeasy Blood and Tissue kit (Qiagen). This kit contains buffers that enable optimal DNA binding conditions, removal of contaminants, and pure DNA elution. All reagents should be handled with gloves to avoid the introduction of contaminants that can cause degradation of template DNA (see Note 1). The isolation procedure is designed for rapid DNA purification that does not require phenol/chloroform extraction or alcohol precipitation, thus limiting artifactual DNA oxidation. DNA is quantified using Quant-iT Picogreen dsDNA kit (Molecular Probes), containing PicoGreen dissolved in DMSO, 20× TE (200 mM Tris–HCl, 20 mM EDTA, pH 7.5) and Lambda DNA standard (100 μg/ml in TE). The fluorescence is measured using a microplate reader and standard fluorescein wavelengths (excitation ~480 nm, emission ~520 nm) (see Note 2). All reagents required and detailed protocols are supplied by the manufacturers of the kits.

2.1.3. QPCR Analysis

For QPCR analysis the GeneAmp XL PCR Kit (Applied Biosystems) is used and contains all reagents (except primers) to carry out QPCR. The kit contains rTth DNA polymerase XL (400 U), 3.3× XL PCR buffer, Mg(OAc)$_2$ (25 mM), dNTPs (10 mM).

2.2. Extracellular Flux Assay

2.2.1. Cell Culture and Induction of Oxidative Stress

1. The 661W cell line described here was generously provided by Dr. Muayyad Al-Ubaidi (University of Oklahoma). Cells are grown and expanded in Dulbecco's modified Eagle's medium (DMEM) supplemented with 10% fetal bovine serum (FBS). They are allowed to grow to 90% confluence before harvesting and replating for use in experiments. Alternatively, RPE cells can be cultured as discussed earlier in Subheading 2.1.2.

2. For XF experiments, cells are plated on 24-well custom plates designed for use in the XF24 (20,000 cells/well) and grown to ~90% confluence in DMEM + 5% FBS (48 h).

3. Treatment with the phosphodiesterase inhibitor, IBMX, induces cell death in 661W cells mediated by calpain and caspase-3. IBMX treatment results in the rapid increase in intracellular calcium, the generation of reactive oxygen species (ROS), and the activation of oxidative stress enzymes (22). Cell death involves mitochondrial damage as documented by Bid cleavage, mitochondrial depolarization, and cytochrome *c* release (27). IBMX is made as a 100 mM stock solution in DMSO plus 20% pluronic F-127 (w/v) and added to cells at 300–600 μM to initiate oxidative stress; corresponding DMSO plus 20% pluronic F-127 concentrations are added as controls.

3. Methods

3.1. QPCR Analysis

3.1.1. Oxidative Stress Exposure and Mitochondrial DNA Damage and Repair

1. To analyze the mtDNA damage response, we have routinely used primary human RPE isolated from human eyes obtained from donors up till the age of 70 years and processed within 48 h following death. All human eyes *must be* obtained from a registered eye bank or alternative authorized source and researchers *must* have the appropriate institutional approval for their use in laboratory research. A spontaneously transformed RPE cell line, derived from a 19-year-old male donor (ARPE-19, American Type Culture Collection; Accession No. CRC-23021), has also been used extensively in QPCR studies (4). All cultures are maintained at 37°C in a humidified incubator at 5% CO_2/95% during DNA damage and repair experiments. In addition, it is vital to carry out the three procedures of the QPCR protocol, i.e., (1) oxidative stress exposure; (2) DNA isolation and quantification; and (3) QPCR, in a separate area of the laboratory to avoid cross-contamination during the QPCR process.

2. RPE cells are cultured in Ham's F10 medium supplemented with heat-inactivated fetal calf serum (10%), 100 μl/ml streptomycin, 100 μl/ml kanamycin, and 60 μl/ml penicillin and allowed to grow to form a confluent monolayer. Cells are

maintained in serum-free Ham's F10 growth media for 24 h before treatment with the DNA-damaging agent.

3. Oxidative stress should be initiated with H_2O_2 diluted in serum-free Hams's F10 media to give a final concentration of 250 μM for 1 h. The concentration of H_2O_2 and length of exposure, however, depend on the oxidative sensitivity of the particular cell type and need to be optimized (see Note 3).

4. After the DNA damage exposure, H_2O_2 is aspirated and the cells washed twice with sterile PBS. For DNA damage studies, genomic DNA should be extracted at this point (see Subheading 3.1.2). For DNA repair assessment, serum-free medium is to be added with the cultures maintained at 37°C and allowed to recover for various time points. We suggest a starting point for RPE DNA repair analysis of 0.5, 1, 3, 6, and 12 h repair time-points. It is important to always include control cultures in the QPCR that are mock treated.

3.1.2. DNA Isolation and Quantification

All procedures involving isolated DNA should be carried out on ice and all reagents maintained at 4°C throughout the experimental protocol unless otherwise specified (see Note 4).

1. At the appropriate repair time point, serum-free Ham's F10 media should be aspirated and the cells washed twice with PBS followed by trypsinization (0.05% trypsin–EDTA, Invitrogen) to detach the cells. The cell pellet obtained by centrifugation at $500 \times g$ for 5 min is used for DNA isolation according to the instructions provided by the manufacturer of the DNeasy Blood and Tissue kit (see Subheading 2.1.2). DNA purity should be confirmed prior to QPCR, determined by the A_{260}/A_{280} ratio. Only continue with QPCR if the ratios are between 1.7 and 1.9, confirming high purity. It is important to note to use less than 2×10^6 cells per DNA isolation to allow optimal nucleic acid yields.

2. The Quant-iT PicoGreen dsDNA quantification method is used to determine the amount of DNA in each sample as described in the manufacturer's protocol with minor modifications. Ten microliters of the sample DNA stock is reconstituted with TE buffer (10 mM Tris–HCl, 1 mM EDTA, pH 7.5) and further diluted to give 1:10, 1:50, and 1:100 aliquots. In addition, a standard curve (using Lambda DNA) is generated using a 2 μg/ml stock solution to give final DNA concentrations of 1, 0.5, 0.25, 0.125, 0.0625, 0.031, and 0 μg/ml in TE buffer. DNA is analyzed using a fluorescence plate reader (excitation 480 nm/emission 520 nm). The isolation procedure using 1×10^6 ARPE-19 cells should give ~15 μg DNA dissolved in 100 μl of TE buffer.

3. At this point, the isolated DNA should be stored in separate aliquots at –80°C for long-term storage. It is recommended, however, that fresh DNA that has not been frozen is used for QPCR to limit any effect of nucleic acid degradation in the QPCR analysis

3.1.3. QPCR Analysis

1. For QPCR, the GeneAmp XL PCR kit has been successfully utilized by multiple laboratories (Applied Biosystems). The kit contains all the components required to amplify large DNA fragments (>20 kb) including the rTth DNA polymerase XL (2 U/μl), 3.3 XL PCR buffer (containing potassium acetate, glycerol, and DMSO), Mg (OAc)$_2$ (25 mM), and dNTPs (10 mM).

2. It is important to use a large PCR reaction volume of at least 100 μl which facilitates the amplification of >10 kb DNA fragments. Table 1 shows a standard protocol used to amplify a >10 kb DNA fragment. X refers to a variable volume depending on the quantity of DNA to be used in QPCR. Please note that each specific set of primers will involve optimization of QPCR conditions (see Notes 5–14 and Table 1).

3. PCR fragments are amplified using the following thermocycling profile: The PCR is initiated with a hot-start with the addition of the 1 U of XL r*Tth* polymerase when samples have reached a temperature of 75°C. This is followed by an initial denaturation for 1 min at 94°C, cycles of denaturation at 94°C for 30 s, and primer extension at X°C for 12 min for a total of X cycles. After the PCR cycles have been completed, a final extension at 72°C for 10 min is performed. Please note that the annealing

Table 1
QPCR components and concentrations

Component	Volume (μl)	Final concentration
Sterile water	X	–
XL PCR buffer	31	1×
dNTP mix (10 mM)	8	800 μM
Primer 1 (10 μM)	1	0.1 μM
Primer 2 (10 μM)	1	0.1 μM
Mg(OAc)$_2$ (25 mM)	4	1 mM
rTth DNA polymerase	1	2 U
DNA	X	15–100 ng
Total volume	100	

temperatures and cycle numbers will need to be optimized for each set of primers used in this assay (see Notes 5–8).

4. It is necessary to normalize QPCR results for endogenous damage and copy number to make sure that changes in amplification levels are due to DNA damage. Normalization is performed by amplifying a small mitochondrial DNA fragment (~100–800 bp). It is also beneficial to compare the amplification of a short nuclear DNA fragment between samples to verify identical starting amounts between samples. Primers for the generation of short products have been presented previously (2) (see Notes 9–14).

5. After the completion of QPCR, the extent of PCR product amplified can be determined via two methods, either agarose gel electrophoresis or Picogreen analysis. For agarose gel electrophoresis, 18 μl of reaction sample is mixed with 6× loading dye (0.4% orange G, 0.03% bromophenol blue, 0.03% xylene cyanol FF, 15% Ficoll® 400, 10 mM Tris–HCl (pH 7.5), and 50 mM EDTA (pH 8.0); Promega) and DNA fragments resolved on a 0.7% agarose gel (Invitrogen) dissolved in Tris–borate–EDTA (45 mM Tris–borate, 1 mM EDTA, pH 8.0) with ethidium bromide added to the gel (final concentration 0.5 μg/ml; Sigma). The intensity of the PCR product bands can be quantified with Scion Image analysis software (Scion Corp). For Picogreen analysis, product DNA is analyzed using a fluorescence plate reader (excitation 480 nm/emission 520 nm) as described previously (see Subheading 3.1.2).

6. The QPCR assay measures the average lesion frequency and a detailed data analysis protocol has been previously described in detail (2). Briefly, the resulting DNA amplification values are converted to relative lesion frequency by assuming a random distribution of damage. The lesion frequency (λ) is calculated as the amount of amplification of damaged DNA samples (A_d) relative to the amplification of control (A_0) (no damage).

3.2. XF Analysis

3.2.1. The Seahorse Biosciences Extracellular Flux Analyzer

The XF analyzer uses two light sources, to excite hydrogel optodes deposited on the plunger heads of the sensor plates. One optode is a pH-sensitive fluorophore and the second contains an oxygen-sensitive, fluorescent metal complex. The plungers normally reside about 5 mm above the cells within about 1 ml of buffer. During a rate measurement, the plungers descend to ~300 μm above the surface of the plates to entrap ~7 μl of buffer immediately overlying with limited diffusion to create a "virtual chamber."

As the plunger entraps cells in a limited diffusion region, analyte concentrations in each well are measured over a period of ~1 min. The initial changes of concentrations, such as the decrease of O_2, are calculated to give a rate. After rate measurements, the plungers return to their original position and vibrate to mix the buffer and re-equilibrate the formerly entrapped region with the bulk medium. Also above each well of the Seahorse plate are cylindrical reagent reservoirs, which can be used to eject reagents into the wells. Thus, each well can be injected with four different reagents during an experiment. Rate measurements can be made every few minutes without significant depression of oxygen tension or acidification of the medium. In this way, the Extracellular Flux Analyzer achieves sensitivities comparable to those of the microphysiometer without the need for cumbersome perfusion microfluidics.

3.2.2. OCR and ECAR Measurements

1. OCR and ECAR measurements of 661W cells are performed using a Seahorse Bioscience XF24 instrument (Seahorse Bioscience, Billerica, MD). O_2 leak through the plastic sides and bottom of the plate is accounted for using the Akos algorithm in the XF24 software package.

2. Cells are plated (see Subheading 2.2.1 and Note 15). Prior to running the experiment, the growth medium is removed and the cells are washed with PBS containing Ca^{2+}/Mg^{2+} (pH 7.4), which is then aspirated and replaced with 700 µl of RS buffer.

3. The buffer used for testing is a reduced serum (RS) buffer. The RS buffer contains $CaCl_2$ (1.8 mM), $MgCl_2$ (0.6 mM), KH_2PO_4 (0.5 mM), KCl (5.33 mM), Na_2HPO_4 (0.5 mM), NaCl (130 mM), glucose (5.6 mM), glutamax, minimum essential medium (MEM) amino acids solution, MEM nonessential amino acids, MEM vitamin solution, penicillin/streptomycin, 1% bovine serum albumin (BSA, factor V fatty acid free), 1% FBS, and insulin (100 nM). All components except FBS and insulin are combined prior to filter sterilization. Following addition of FBS and insulin (usually 24–48 h pre-experiment), the RS buffer is warmed to 37°C and the pH is adjusted to 7.4.

4. A typical experiment to evaluate the cellular metabolic capacity and mitochondrial coupling includes testing ECAR and OCR in the presence of the following agents: a protonophore that depolarizes the inner mitochondrial membrane potential (FCCP), and a mitochondrial inhibitor of cytrochrome c oxidase (sodium azide) or complex I (rotenone) or ATP-synthase (oligomycin).

5. The template for testing is set up as follows. Measurements will be performed every 5 min, repeating metabolic measurements 3–4 times per condition for averaging purposes. The 5-min cycle includes a 2-min mix period, 1-min wait, and a 2-min measuring time. After measurements of baseline activity, FCCP is injected, rates are measured, and finally rotenone (a Complex I inhibitor) is injected followed by a final measuring of the rates (see Notes 16–18).

3.2.3. Interpretation of Fluxes

Extracellular O_2, pH, and lactate fluxes provide estimates of glucose utilization in cells and tissues that are comparable to those obtained with radiometric assays (24, 25). When glucose is the primary metabolic substrate, O_2 flux is a good estimate of glucose oxidation, whereas lactate flux is a good measure of the Embden–Meyerhof pathway flux, which is particularly useful for the study of cancer cell metabolism (e.g., the Warburg effect) (see Note 19).

3.3. Results

3.3.1. Example of QPCR Data

As an illustration of QPCR, we present data from an experiment, simultaneously analyzing mitochondrial and nuclear DNA repair capacities in RPE cells following oxidative stress. Cells were exposed to H_2O_2 (250 µM) and allowed to repair for 1, 3, 6, and 12 h (see Subheading 3.1), DNA isolated and quantified (see Subheading 3.2), and QPCR performed (see Subheading 3.3). As shown in Fig. 1a, b, both the nDNA and mtDNA showed equal susceptibility to H_2O_2-induced DNA damage by sustaining ~1.1–1.3 lesions/10 kb. However, mtDNA showed a reduced capacity to repair H_2O_2-induced lesions compared to nDNA up to 3 h post H_2O_2 exposure ($P < 0.05$).

3.3.2. Example of XF Data

A representative example in Fig. 2 shows the effects of a typical experiment, analyzing baseline, and effects of FCCP and rotenone on both OCR (Fig. 2a, closed symbols) and ECAR (Fig. 2a, open symbols).

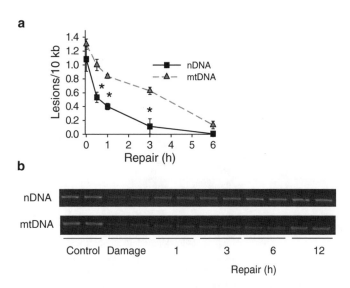

Fig. 1. A comparison of nDNA and mtDNA damage and repair in a primary human RPE cell culture following H_2O_2 exposure. Cells were treated with 250 µM H_2O_2 for 1 h and allowed to recover for 1, 3, 6, and 12 h. The cells were harvested, the DNA was extracted, and QPCR was performed. DNA damage was quantified by comparing the relative efficiency of amplification of large fragments of DNA (16.2 kb for the mtDNA and 10.4 kb for the *hprt* gene) and normalizing this to the amplification of smaller 100 bp fragment, which have a statistically negligible likelihood of containing damaged bases (1). (a) The nDNA and mtDNA lesion repair after H_2O_2-induced oxidative stress. (b) Agarose gels (0.7%) derived from QPCR analysis of nDNA and mtDNA amplification. Significantly different number of lesions per 10 kb between nDNA and mtDNA: *$P < 0.05$. The data are expressed as the means ± SEM from three separate experiments and were performed in duplicate.

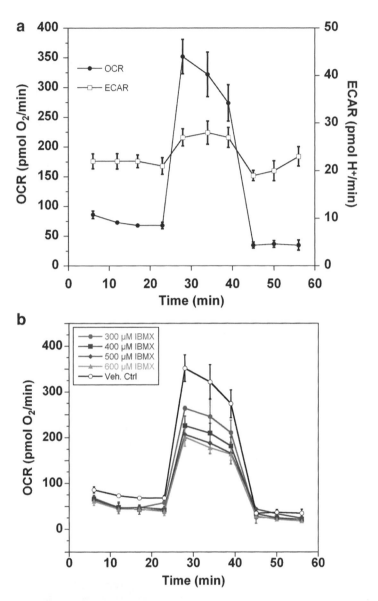

Fig. 2. Mitochondrial respiration and glycolytic capacity of 661W cells. (**a**) Typical O_2 consumption rates (OCR) and extracellular acidification rates (ECAR) of 661W cells as measured with an XF24 Seahorse Biosciences instrument are shown. After measuring four basal rates, the cells are sequentially treated with FCCP (1 μM) and rotenone (500 nM). (**b**) OCR rates in response to increasing doses of IBMX are shown. While basal respiration rates are slightly reduced after 24 h of IBMX treatment, a significant dose-dependent decrease is measured in the FCCP uncoupled rates. The average rates (mean ± SEM for $n = 3–4$ wells) are plotted.

As indicated in Subheadings 2 and 3, treatment with FCCP (1 μM) collapses the proton gradient across the inner mitochondrial membrane. In response, the mitochondria increase their flux through the ETC in order to restore the proton gradient. In the presence of sufficient substrates for production of NADH (e.g., pyruvate or palmitic acid) this increase in OCR represents the maximal respiratory capacity of the mitochondria (24, 25). In 661 W cells, the maximal FCCP-uncoupled OCR response ranges from 1.5- to 3.5-fold higher than the basal OCR (Fig. 2a). Rotenone (500 nM), which is a complex I inhibitor, causes an immediate decrease in OCR. The response that can be blocked by rotenone corresponds to the fraction of measured respiration that is entirely mitochondrial. Here, rotenone decreased OCR by 90% (Fig. 2a), indicating that other oxygen-dependent processes (peroxisome, NAD(P)H-oxidases, etc.) only contribute ~10% to the overall oxygen consumption of these cells. When analyzing the ECAR responses, it is observed that FCCP causes a rapid increase in ECAR (Fig. 2a, open symbols). This increase in ECAR is due to a shift towards glycolysis and increased lactic acid extrusion—or the Pasteur effect as has previously been described by Winkler and colleagues using retinal cells (2003).

Second, we provide representative data for the mitochondrial oxygen consumption of 661W cells as they are exposed to IBMX for 24 h (Fig. 2b). Previous work in our lab has shown that IBMX damages 661W cells via a mitochondrial oxidative dysfunction (see above). IBMX at all four concentrations (300–600 µM) causes a small decrease in basal respiration rates. But, when the mitochondria are uncoupled (FCCP treatment), the untreated cells show an almost fourfold increase in respiration (i.e., their capacity is about fourfold of their basal) (open symbols); in contrast, the cells that had been treated with different concentrations of IBMX for 24 h show up to a 50% loss in metabolic capacity as measured from the FCCP responses (closed symbols).

4. Notes

1. To limit the chance of DNA contamination during the QPCR process, it is vital to set up all the reaction mixes for this part of the protocol in a separate area in the laboratory that has not been used for DNA isolation or PCR product analysis. In addition, it is important to use dedicated pipettes for each stage of the protocol, i.e., DNA preparation, reaction mixing/PCR, and DNA fragment analysis.

2. To ensure that the DNA sample readings are in the detectable range of the microplate reader, the gain settings should be adjusted to the DNA sample containing the highest DNA concentration to yield a fluorescence intensity near, but below, the fluorometer's maximum. In addition, to prevent photobleaching, the time taken for fluorescence measurement should be constant for all samples.

3. The QPCR assay has the ability to detect multiple classes of DNA damage. However, to investigate oxidative stress, H_2O_2 is an excellent model compound that can be used as a starting point for mtDNA damage studies. We and others have determined a cell type- and donor-specific sensitivity to H_2O_2 exposure. Thereby, the appropriate H_2O_2 dose used in a particular study must be determined from a dose–response curve.

4. It is critical to isolate high-molecular-weight, high-quality DNA suitable for PCR amplification. In order to prevent any artifactual damage during (e.g., strand breaks and oxidative damage) the DNA isolation procedure we use the DNeasy Blood and Tissue Kit (Qiagen). Harsh methods of DNA isolation using phenol and chloroform should be avoided.

5. The hot start procedure is highly recommended for QPCR, as it improves the procedure by reducing any initial mis-priming and primer oligomerization by-reactions.

6. The optimum amount of DNA polymerase enzyme to use will depend on the DNA fragment length and source of template DNA. For most samples 2 U of rTth DNA polymerase should suffice; however, if fragments >20 kb are amplified 4 U of rTth DNA polymerase should be used (one unit of rTth DNA polymerase is defined as the amount that will incorporate 10 nmol of dNTPs into acid-insoluble material per 30 min in a 10-min incubation at 74°C).

7. The optimum annealing temperature can be determined empirically by analyzing 2–3°C increments until maximum product yield is reached. The rTth polymerase has the greatest activity between 60 and 70°C. Thereby, it is recommended that primers designed are suitable for this temperature range. In addition, two-temperature rather than three-temperature cycling should be used if the QPCR is employing annealing temperatures over 60°C.

8. Special care must be taken to ensure that the QPCR cycle conditions are quantitative, thus ensuring that any reduction in DNA fragment amplification is due to DNA damage. Thereby, cycle test analyses must be performed to determine quantitative QPCR conditions, e.g., 23, 26, 29, 31, 33, and 36. The DNA fragment of interest should be amplified within the exponential range of QPCR.

9. The optimal primer concentrations for QPCR will need to be determined as concentrations that are too low will result in suboptimal levels of PCR product, whereas concentrations that are too high will result in the amplification of nontarget sequences. It will be necessary to test primer concentrations in the range of 20–100 pmol/run in 5 pmol/run increments.

10. Primers for the generation of small and long fragments (10–21 kb) are described in detail for human, mice, rat, yeast, melanogaster, adenovirus, killifish, and zebrafish (1, 16).

11. The optimal magnesium concentration for each set of QPCR primers should be determined. The amplification of the DNA fragment should be analyzed using magnesium concentrations ranging from 0.8 to 1.5 mM in 0.1 mM increments.

12. It is recommended that a 50% undamaged template (containing half the DNA content, but equal reaction volume) always be included in QPCR. This is an internal control and thus gives a 50% reduction of the DNA product amplification. If a 50% reduction in PCR product is not observed then the reaction cannot be considered as quantitative in nature.

13. It is important that no nonspecific amplification products are observed following QPCR. If they are observed, QPCR conditions need to be re-optimized (see Notes 5–11).

14. It is useful to always include a positive control in QPCR. A model DNA-damaging agent that generates bulky helical distorting adducts is UVC. This geno-toxic agent is a well-established substrate for QPCR (2). However, if access to UVC is not available, compounds such as etoposide (Sigma) are also excellent positive controls for DNA damage detection as they generate polymerase stalling double-strand breaks (12).

15. It is critical to establish an optimal plating density for the XF plates prior to running experiments. Typical seeding densities are 10–20,000 cells/well and these are typically grown over 24–48 h. We recommend then testing the cells on the XF instrument measuring four basal rates followed by injection of 0.5 μM FCCP and measuring an additional four rates. An ideal plating density will give robust basal and FCCP-uncoupled rates. If the cells are too dense, the basal rates might be low and the uncoupled rate will often be unstable.

16. For most cells an ~5-min XF cycle time is adequate with 2 min for measurement, 1-min mix, and 2-min wait but these times might need to be adjusted to accommodate cells that have unusually high rates (lower measure times, longer mixing times) or unusually low rates (longer measure times).

17. The medium used here is DMEM modified to use low phosphate (1 mM) to accommodate ECAR changes. The manufacturer also provides a low buffer DMEM but many other buffers can be used as long as they do not contain bicarbonate, as there is no CO_2 atmosphere control in the instrument. Other media will typically have higher buffer capacity that will lower sensitivity of the ECAR measurements but the final calculation of proton production rates is unchanged as this takes into account the buffer capacity.

18. Pharmacological agents used to perturb bioenergetic metabolism, such as the ATPsynthase inhibitor oligomycin, uncouplers such as FCCP, and ETC inhibitors such as rotenone should be titrated with new cell lines to determine the concentration that gives maximum effect without killing the cells outright. Although the instrument enables four different injections per well, the effect of one drug on the response to a subsequent drug treatment should be separately evaluated.

19. Normalization of data is often done via cell number, protein content, or to the basal OCR and ECAR rates. Alternatively, each well can be gently washed, lysed with detergent, and analyzed for protein content with a BCA assay. Care should be taken in doing so as after treatments, and the plunging of the sensor, some cells are prone to lifting up easily during the wash step. The use of sulforhodamine B staining of cells directly in the wells and then measuring of absorbance exhibit artifacts and are not reliable. Fixing the cells with paraformaldehyde and then staining with a nuclear dye, such as DAPI, enable very reliable cell counts via automated imaging.

Acknowledgment

This work was supported by NIH grants EY019688 and EY021626 (M.E.B.) and a Foundation Fighting Blindness Wynn-Gund Translational Research Acceleration grant (B.R.).

References

1. Scheffler IE (2001) A century of mitochondrial research: achievements and perspectives. Mitochondrion 1:3–31

2. Ayala-Torres S, Chen Y, Svoboda T, Rosenblatt J, Van Houten B (2000) Analysis of gene-specific DNA damage and repair using quantitative polymerase chain reaction. Methods 22:135–147

3. Jarrett SG, Lin H, Godley BF, Boulton ME (2008) Mitochondrial DNA damage and its potential role in retinal degeneration. Prog Retin Eye Res 27:596–607

4. Liang FQ, Godley BF (2003) Oxidative stress-induced mitochondrial DNA damage in human retinal pigment epithelial cells: a possible mechanism for RPE aging and age-related macular degeneration. Exp Eye Res 76:397–403

5. Lin H, Xu H, Liang FQ, Liang H, Gupta P, Havey AN, Boulton ME, Godley BF (2011) Mitochondrial DNA damage and repair in RPE associated with aging and age-related macular degeneration. Invest Ophthalmol Vis Sci 52:3521–3529

6. Carelli V, Ross-Cisneros FN, Sadun AA (2004) Mitochondrial dysfunction as a cause of optic neuropathies. Prog Retin Eye Res 23:53–89

7. Ballinger SW, Van Houten B, Jin GF, Conklin CA, Godley BF (1999) Hydrogen peroxide causes significant mitochondrial DNA damage in human RPE cells. Exp Eye Res 68:765–772

8. Kalinowski DP, Illenye S, Van Houten B (1992) Analysis of DNA damage and repair in murine leukemia L1210 cells using a quantitative polymerase chain reaction assay. Nucleic Acids Res 20:3485–3494

9. Liang FQ, Alssadi R, Morehead P, Awasthi YC, Godley BF (2005) Enhanced expression of glutathione-S-transferase A1-1 protects against oxidative stress in human retinal pigment epithelial cells. Exp Eye Res 80:113–119

10. Liang FQ, Green L, Wang C, Alssadi R, Godley BF (2004) Melatonin protects human retinal pigment epithelial (RPE) cells against oxidative stress. Exp Eye Res 78:1069–1075

11. Santos JH, Meyer JN, Mandavilli BS, Van Houten B (2006) Quantitative PCR-based measurement of nuclear and mitochondrial DNA damage and repair in mammalian cells. Methods Mol Biol 314:183–199

12. Stuart GR, Santos JH, Strand MK, Van Houten B, Copeland WC (2006) Mitochondrial and nuclear DNA defects in Saccharomyces cerevisiae with mutations in DNA polymerase gamma associated with progressive external ophthalmoplegia. Hum Mol Genet 15:363–374

13. Van Houten B, Cheng S, Chen Y (2000) Measuring gene-specific nucleotide excision repair in human cells using quantitative amplification of long targets from nanogram quantities of DNA. Mutat Res 460:81–94

14. Van Houten B, Gamper H, Sancar A, Hearst JE (1987) DNase I footprint of ABC excinuclease. J Biol Chem 262:13180–13187

15. Yakes FM, Van Houten B (1997) Mitochondrial DNA damage is more extensive and persists longer than nuclear DNA damage in human cells following oxidative stress. Proc Natl Acad Sci U S A 94:514–519

16. Godley BF, Shamsi FA, Liang FQ, Jarrett SG, Davies S, Boulton M (2005) Blue light induces mitochondrial DNA damage and free radical production in epithelial cells. J Biol Chem 280:21061–21066

17. Yang M, Jarrett SG, Craven R, Kaetzel DM (2009) YNK1, the yeast homolog of human metastasis suppressor NM23, is required for repair of UV radiation- and etoposide-induced DNA damage. Mutat Res 660:74–78

18. Miller H, Grollman AP (1997) Kinetics of DNA polymerase I (Klenow fragment exo-)

activity on damaged DNA templates: effect of proximal and distal template damage on DNA synthesis. Biochemistry 36:15336–15342

19. Lim KS, Jeyaseelan K, Whiteman M, Jenner A, Halliwell B (2005) Oxidative damage in mitochondrial DNA is not extensive. Ann N Y Acad Sci 1042:210–220

20. Jarrett SG, Boulton ME (2005) Antioxidant up-regulation and increased nuclear DNA protection play key roles in adaptation to oxidative stress in epithelial cells. Free Radic Biol Med 38:1382–1391

21. Okawa H, Sampath AP, Laughlin SB, Fain GL (2008) ATP consumption by mammalian rod photoreceptors in darkness and in light. Curr Biol 18:1917–1921

22. Strauss O (2005) The retinal pigment epithelium in visual function. Physiol Rev 85:845–881

23. Ames A 3rd, Li YY, Heher EC, Kimble CR (1992) Energy metabolism of rabbit retina as related to function: high cost of Na+ transport. J Neurosci 12:840–853

24. Eklund SE, Taylor D, Kozlov E, Prokop A, Cliffel DE (2004) A microphysiometer for simultaneous measurement of changes in extracellular glucose, lactate, oxygen, and acidification rate. Anal Chem 76:519–527

25. Wiley C, Beeson C (2002) Continuous measurement of glucose utilization in heart myoblasts. Anal Biochem 304:139–146

26. Ferrick DA, Neilson A, Beeson C (2008) Advances in measuring cellular bioenergetics using extracellular flux. Drug Discov Today 13:268–274

27. Sharma AK, Rohrer B (2007) Sustained elevation of intracellular cGMP causes oxidative stress triggering calpain-mediated apoptosis in photoreceptor degeneration. Curr Eye Res 32:259–269

Chapter 17

Analysis of Photoreceptor Rod Outer Segment Phagocytosis by RPE Cells In Situ

Saumil Sethna and Silvia C. Finnemann

Abstract

Counting rhodopsin-positive phagosomes residing in the retinal pigment epithelium (RPE) in the eye at different times of day allows a quantitative assessment of engulfment and digestion phases of diurnal RPE phagocytosis, which efficiently clears shed photoreceptor outer segment fragments (POS) from the neural retina. Comparing such activities among age- and background-matched experimental wild-type and mutant mice or rats serves to identify roles for specific proteins in the phagocytic process. Here, we describe experimental procedures for mouse eye harvest, embedding, sectioning, immunofluorescence labeling of rod POS phagosomes in RPE cells in sagittal eye sections, imaging of POS phagosomes in the RPE by laser scanning confocal microscopy, and POS quantification.

Key words: Mouse eye, Retina, Retinal pigment epithelium, Diurnal photoreceptor outer segment phagocytosis, Rhodopsin-positive phagosome quantification, Immunofluorescence microscopy, Paraffin sectioning

1. Introduction

Prompt and complete clearance by phagocytosis of shed photoreceptor outer segment fragments (POS) by the underlying retinal pigment epithelium (RPE) is essential for life-long visual function (1, 2). In mammals, rod POS shedding and RPE phagocytosis are regulated and coordinated by the circadian rhythm such that they occur in a daily peak at light onset (3). Quantification of POS phagosome load of the RPE in eyes derived from experimental animals sacrificed at precise times before and after light onset therefore allows analysis of kinetics and capacity of POS phagocytosis of RPE cells in situ. Quantification of POS numbers per length of RPE in sagittal sections of fixed, paraffin-embedded eyecups has proven to be a reliable method to assess RPE phagosome load in individual eyes. Comparing POS load of the RPE in wild-type mice with POS

Bernhard H.F. Weber and Thomas Langmann (eds.), *Retinal Degeneration: Methods and Protocols*, Methods in Molecular Biology, vol. 935, DOI 10.1007/978-1-62703-080-9_17, © Springer Science+Business Media, LLC 2013

load of RPE in age-matched mutant mice of the same genetic background is an efficient method to identify components and pathways relevant to POS uptake or digestion.

Transmission electron microcopy can identify engulfed POS in the RPE based on their morphological appearance (4, 5). This method is powerful but cost- and labor-intensive. Light microscopy can demonstrate POS in the RPE in frozen or paraffin eyecup sections stained with histological dyes (6). This method is fast and economical but it is only appropriate for eyes derived from albino animals because RPE melanosomes may obscure phagosomes. Here, we describe the use of immunofluorescence laser scanning confocal microscopy to rapidly and unambiguously identify POS phagosomes in RPE in cross sections of paraffin-embedded mouse or rat eyes (7). We further discuss methodology to reliably quantify POS phagosome load per length of retina.

2. Materials

Prepare all solutions using double-distilled water (ddH$_2$O) or a similar quality water and analytical grade reagents. Prepare and store all reagents at room temperature unless indicated otherwise.

2.1. Materials for Enucleation, Fixation, and Lens Removal of Mouse Eyes

1. Mice maintained in a strict 12-h dark/light cycle—at least four animals for each time point (see Note 1).

2. Curved forceps, No.11 blade, sharp edged forceps, microdissection scissors.

3. Davidson's fixative (for 100 mL): Mix in this order: 33.5 mL H$_2$O, 33 mL 95% ethanol, 22 mL formaldehyde 37%, 11.5 mL glacial acetic acid (see Note 2).

2.2. Materials and Equipment for Eyecup Processing and Paraffin Embedding

Make ethanol dilutions using 95% ethanol and ddH$_2$O. Use 2 L plastic cylinders to make alcohol dilutions.

1. Automatic Tissue Processer (e.g., Leica TP1020).

2. Plastic processing cassettes and fitting metal molds.

3. 50% Ethanol.

4. 85% Ethanol.

5. 95% Ethanol.

6. 100% Ethanol (200 proof).

7. Histoclear II (Electron Microscopy Sciences).

8. Paraffin (e.g., Peel-A-Way® Micro-Cut Paraffin (Polysciences, Warrington, PA)).

9. Paraffin Embedding Center (e.g., Thermofisher Histostar).

2.3. Materials and Equipment for Paraffin Sectioning, Deparaffinization, RPE Pigment Bleaching, and Immunofluorescence Staining

1. Water bath set to 50°C, incubator set to 45°C, and hot plate set to 62°C.

2. Microtome (e.g., Thermofisher HM325) with low profile microtome blades (e. g. Accu-Edge, Sakura Finetek, Torrance, CA).

3. Superfrost® Plus slides and slide staining jars with slide rack (e.g., EasyDip Slide Staining System, Simport Plastics).

4. Histoclear II, 100% ethanol, 95% ethanol, 70% ethanol, prepared as in Subheading 2.2.

5. PBS: Make a 5× PBS stock: Dissolve 40 g NaCl, 1 g KCl, 1 g KH_2PO_4, 10.8 g Na_2HPO_4 in 500 mL dH_2O. Adjust pH to 7.2 and fill to 1 L with ddH_2O. Dilute fivefold with ddH_2O to make a 1× PBS working solution.

6. Pigment bleaching solution: Weigh 1 g sodium borohydrate and dissolve in 100 mL ddH_2O, prepare fresh daily.

7. Pap pen, kimwipes, slide staining chamber.

8. 1% Bovine serum albumin in PBS: Add 1 mL 30% BSA stock to 29 mL PBS. Store at 4°C, bring to room temperature before use.

9. Mouse anti-rhodopsin antibody (see Note 3).

10. AlexaFluor488-conjugated donkey anti-mouse IgG.

11. DAPI nuclei staining solution: 10 µg/mL 4′,6-diamidino-2-phenylindole DAPI in PBS.

12. Cover glasses (24 mm × 50 mm size).

13. Vectashield (Vector Laboratories, Burlingame, CA).

14. Nail polish.

2.4. Equipment and Software for POS Phagosome Imaging and Counting

1. Laser scanning confocal microscope.

2. Image J Software (NIH—http://rsb.info.nih.gov/ij/download.html).

3. Methods

Carry out all procedures at room temperature unless otherwise specified.

3.1. Enucleation, Fixation, and Lens Removal of Mouse Eyes

1. For each mouse to be sacrificed, prepare two 2 mL flat-bottom microtubes with 1.5 mL each Davidson's fixative. Assign numbers or codes to mice and label tubes accordingly. Record genotype, precise time of sacrifice, and other relevant information.

2. At selected times of day (e.g., 1 h before, 30 min and 8 h after light onset), sacrifice mice using a CO_2 chamber or other suitable and approved method (see Notes 4 and 5).

3. Promptly following sacrifice, enucleate eyes using a curved forceps and place into separate tubes filled with fixative. Make sure that eyes are completely immersed in fixative (see Note 6).

4. Leave eyes at room temperature for 30 min to 12 h before storing fixed eyes at 4°C for at least another 12 h.

5. 24–48 h after sacrifice, dissect cornea and lens from fixed eyes one at a time: Carefully transfer eye into 3 cm tissue culture dish filled with fixative. Under a dissecting microscope, use a sharp-edged forceps to hold the eye in place via the optic nerve, and with the other hand use a No.11 blade to create a 3–5 mm incision in the cornea. Use microdissection scissors to enlarge the incision by cutting in the shape of a cross, ultimately generating an opening in the cornea that is large enough to allow the lens to float out of the eyeball (see Note 7). Place the eyecup back in its tube with fixative for at least 30 min or until all eyes are processed.

3.2. Tissue Processing and Paraffin Embedding

1. Place each eyecup into a separate plastic cassette labeled clearly with pencil and close with plastic lid (see Note 8).

2. Incubate eyecups with solutions in a tissue processor with vacuum using the following protocol:
   (a) 50% Ethanol—1 h.
   (b) 50% Ethanol—1.30 h.
   (c) 85% Ethanol—1.30 h.
   (d) 2×95% Ethanol—1.30 h each.
   (e) 2×100% Ethanol—1.30 h each.
   (f) 2×Histoclear II—1.30 h each.
   (g) 2×Paraffin—2 h each.

3. Remove plastic cassettes from the tissue processor container and place them in the designated preheated area of the Tissue Embedding Center.

4. Embed each eyecup individually as follows. Pour just enough liquid paraffin to cover the bottom of a preheated metal mold (see Note 9). Move mold to cold area of processor. As paraffin hardens, use sharp-tipped forceps to place the eyecup in the center of the mold. Handle the eyecup using the optic nerve only. The eyecup should be placed such that the optic nerve is parallel to the bottom of the mold. Move the mold to the heated area, and wait for the hardened paraffin in the mold to melt slightly before adding more liquid paraffin until the mold is filled completely. Move the mold to the cold area and immediately remove any bubbles that may be trapped in or around the eyecup using the forceps. Place the numbered plastic cassette on top of the metal mold before the paraffin solidifies. Add more paraffin until the plastic cassette is filled completely. Place the entire assembly in the cooling area. Once the paraffin

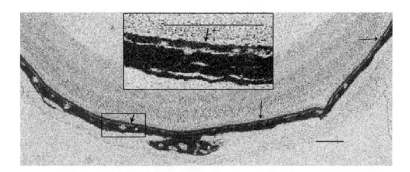

Fig. 1. Bright field image of a 7-μm thick section of a paraffin embedded eyecup of a 2-month-old mouse at the correct orientation. *Arrows* indicate the apical side of the thin, pigmented RPE layer. Note the uniform thickness and appearance of the RPE layer throughout the section. *Inset* shows a magnified image showing the RPE cell layer residing on Bruch's membrane, which is visible as a clear line. Note that most pigment granules localize to the apical aspect of RPE cells. *Scale bars* are 100 μm.

has hardened completely, remove the paraffin block containing the embedded eye along with the plastic mold and store at room temperature.

3.3. Paraffin Sectioning, Deparaffinization, Pigment Removal, and Immunofluorescence Staining

1. Bring water bath temperature to 50°C. Label eight slides with the coded number for each eyecup to be sectioned and consecutive slide numbers.

2. With a razor blade remove excess paraffin surrounding the eyecup, such that a ~1 cm × 1 cm cube is left around the eyecup. Securely mount one paraffin block with eyecup embedded with plastic cassette attached to the microtome. Set section thickness to 25 μm and cut the block until excess paraffin is trimmed. Once the sectioning reaches eyecup tissue reduce section thickness to 7 μm and cut sections as a ribbon and transfer ribbons consisting of 3–4 sections onto the water surface with a paintbrush (No. 6 or smaller) (see Note 10). Collect ribbons on labeled slides. Check under a light microscope for proper alignment after completing two slides (see Note 11). If tissue orientation is correct (Fig. 1), continue sectioning to generate ribbons of 5–7 sections, completing eight slides per eyecup. If not, adjust orientation of tissue block on the microtome, cut one slide, and check again. Repeat checking until orientation is correct, and then cut eight slides.

3. Dry slides at 45°C for 1 h.

4. For phagosome count, use slides numbered 1, 4, and 7.

5. Heat slides on a hot plate set to 62°C for 30 min immediately before tissue deparaffinization.

6. Deparaffinize slides by sequential incubation in slide staining boxes in the following: Histoclear II, 3 × 3 min, 100% ethanol 3 × 1 min, 95% ethanol 2 × 1 min, 70% ethanol 1 × 1 min, ddH$_2$O 1 × 1 min, and PBS 1 × 1 min.

7. Let PBS run off slides, dry areas far away from tissue with Kimwipe, and mark tissue fields to be stained with Pap pen. Transfer slides to humidified chamber and cover sections with PBS. Keep tissue sections covered with solutions at all times for the rest of the procedure. Change solutions by carefully aspirating one solution, immediately replacing it with the next.

8. To remove RPE pigment, incubate in fresh 1% sodium borohydrate solution for 2 min. Rinse with PBS 4×1 min (see Note 12).

9. To block the sections, incubate with 1% BSA in PBS for 20 min (see Note 13).

10. Incubate sections in opsin monoclonal antibody in PBS overnight at 4°C (see Note 14).

11. Wash with PBS 2×5 min and with 1% BSA–PBS 1×5 min.

12. Incubate sections in freshly diluted secondary antibody AlexaFluor488-conjugated donkey anti-mouse IgG (1:250 in PBS) for 2 h.

13. Wash with PBS 2×5 min.

14. Counterstain with DAPI nuclear stain for 30 min. Wash with PBS for 5 min.

15. Mount in Vectashield, cover with cover glass, aspirate excess Vectashield, and seal with nail polish. Store slides in the dark at room temperature for up to 1 week or at 4°C for up to 1 month.

3.4. Microscopy and Quantification of POS Phagosomes

1. Set up a sequential scan with first scan acquisition parameters excitation being at 488 nm, emission at 490–540 nm, and second scan parameters excitation being at 405 nm, emission at 410–480 nm (see Note 15). Use a 40× objective and set zoom such that about half of the length of RPE in a section is visible in the field. Image the central 50% of each eye section.

2. For the 488 scan, increase gain, offset, and laser power until RPE phagosomes are clearly distinguishable. This setting will result in overexposing the opsin signal of the intact outer segment area. Adjust 403 nm scan setting similarly such that RPE nuclei are visible. For each field, acquire an *x–y* image stack of exactly 5 μm height with 0.25 μm distance between individual *x–y* scans (see Note 16). Acquire at least two 5 μm-stacks per slide, for a total for at least six stacks per sample. Once stacks are acquired, add 100 μm scale bars and save maximal projections of channel overlays (see Fig. 2 for example of maximal projection of opsin stain only). Export maximal projections as "tiff" format files.

3. For measuring the length of RPE surveyed in each scan, use Image J software. Open the image, click on "line" tool, and draw a line exactly over the scale bar. Under the "Analyze" menu, click on "set scale." Change "known distance" to 100 and "unit of length" to "μm." Click "OK."

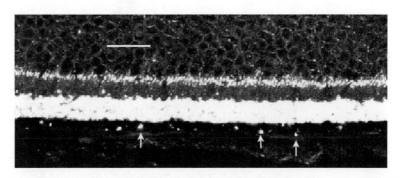

Fig. 2. Maximum projection of a 5-μm stack of *x–y* images acquired at 0.25-μm interval of a paraffin section of an eyecup of a 2-month-old mouse stained with monoclonal opsin antibody clone B6-30 (8). The overexposed, white tissue area is the rod outer segment layer of the mouse retina, while the *arrows* indicate individual POS phagosomes in the RPE. *Scale bar* is 20 μm.

4. Draw another line covering at least 100 μm, just above the RPE layer from which phagosomes will be counted. Under the analyze menu, click on "Measure." The software will give out readout in μm. If there is no continuous area of 100 μm of intact RPE to count, measure and count two smaller stretches totaling at least 100 μm. Count phagosomes under the line and transfer values to an excel file along with the length measurement. Divide phagosome count by length and multiply by 100 to obtain phagosome count per 100 μm length of RPE. Count phagosomes of all images acquired for a total for six times per mouse eyecup sample. Average the six values to obtain the mean number of POS phagosomes residing in 100 μm RPE for that eyecup. Repeat for all eyecup samples.

5. For each sample type (identical age, genotype, and time collected) analyze at least one eye each of four different mice. Calculate average ± SD to obtain average phagosome count for each sample.

4. Notes

1. All animal procedures need to be reviewed and approved by authorities as appropriate. The procedure requires postmortem tissue harvest.

2. Davidson's fixative maintains structural integrity of the retina very well and is hence the preferred fixative for this procedure. Use gloves while preparing and handling Davidson's fixative. White, fine precipitate may form after mixing or with time. This does not inactivate the solution. Remove precipitate by paper filtration before using.

3. A number of rhodopsin monoclonal antibodies are commercially available and many can be used to label early POS phagosomes that still contain intact opsin protein. However, depending on the epitope recognized, antibodies may differ in their recognition of partially digested opsin that is present in phagosomes at later time points. Choice of the appropriate opsin antibody therefore depends on the scientific objective of the experiment.

4. It is imperative to maintain the dark/light cycle precisely for at least 3 weeks before the experiment to ensure that mice are entrained to a specific rhythm. RPE phagocytosis is regulated by the circadian rhythm and influenced by the light cycle in mice and other higher vertebrates. If the light cycle is not maintained precisely, results will be ambiguous. Aspects to consider include access of personnel to animal rooms at dark times, which may cause light on/off at inappropriate times, and changes associated with daylight savings time.

5. If testing mice at time points before light onset, place the required mice in a cage and into an open cardboard box near the door of the animal room the night before the experiment. The day of the experiment, enter the animal room in the dark and place a black photography cloth over the box before moving the box to where euthanization and tissue harvest take place. Sacrifice the mice and remove eyes in the dark under dim red light provided by a darkroom red lamp and/or a red flashlight.

6. Keep the optic nerve intact. Handle the eye grasping only the optic nerve to prevent distorting and damaging the retina. The optic nerve will also be useful to orient the eye during embedding.

7. Make a large enough incision such that the lens floats out. Do not squeeze the eye to remove the lens; this may damage the retina. Trim off any excess connective tissue and muscles on the outside of the eyeball.

8. Write clearly and with a pencil as subsequent alcohol treatments will not have an effect on pencil but will remove permanent markers and ball pen writing.

9. Make sure that there is no paraffin in the mold from previous use. If there is any paraffin, use a Kimwipe to clean it off.

10. If the blade is no longer sharp, sections bunch up or wrinkle, which should be avoided. If the mounted blade fails to cut sections properly, move it sideways to use a different blade area or, eventually, replace blade. Use the paintbrush to smooth out minor wrinkles before placing section ribbons in water bath. Smooth out wrinkles further there if needed, but beware of sections sticking to bristles.

11. Check the tissue for proper orientation where specifically RPE cells are cut perpendicular to Bruch's membrane. The RPE should be visible as a pigmented layer of uniform thickness where pigment is oriented mostly toward the outer segments while the

basal aspect of the RPE faces Bruch's membrane, which should appear as a thin, clear, shiny line (Fig. 1). Incorrect orientation of the section will result in incorrect POS phagosome counts. If needed, adjust the orientation of the paraffin tissue block and repeat checking the orientation until it is correct and a uniform RPE layer can be seen under light microscope.

12. Omitting this step will increase the immunofluorescence staining. However, pigment interference may make phagosome counts unreliable.

13. 5% Normal donkey or goat serum in PBS can be substituted for blocking.

14. Some primary antibodies will yield stronger staining if they are incubated in the presence of 0.1% Triton X-100.

15. The exact acquisition parameters will differ depending on the instrumentation and quality of immunofluorescence staining. It is imperative to only compare samples obtained following identical experimental procedures.

16. Laser scanning confocal microscopy and collapsing image stacks representing a precise tissue volume are imperative. Acquiring POS phagosome signals from an x–y image stack of precise thickness that is identical for all samples is necessary to ensure that sample counts represent load of phagosomes in the same tissue volume. Individual x–y scans or images obtained by epifluorescence (wide-field) microscopy cannot yield such normalized phagosome counts that represent POS phagosome load in the same volume of RPE.

Acknowledgment

This work was supported by NIH grant EY013295.

References

1. Mullen RJ, LaVail MM (1976) Inherited retinal dystrophy: primary defect in pigment epithelium determined with experimental rat chimeras. Science 192:799–801

2. Nandrot EF, Kim Y, Brodie SE, Huang X, Sheppard D, Finnemann SC (2004) Loss of synchronized retinal phagocytosis and age-related blindness in mice lacking αvβ5 integrin. J Exp Med 200:1539–1545

3. LaVail MM (1976) Rod outer segment disk shedding in rat retina: relationship to cyclic lighting. Science 194:1071–1074

4. Young RW, Bok D (1969) Participation of the retinal pigment epithelium in the rod outer segment renewal process. J Cell Biol 42:392–403

5. Bosch E, Horwitz J, Bok D (1993) Phagocytosis of outer segments by retinal pigment epithelium: phagosome-lysosome interaction. J Histochem Cytochem 41:253–263

6. Gibbs D, Kitamoto J, Williams DS (2003) Abnormal phagocytosis by retinal pigmented epithelium that lacks myosin VIIa, the Usher syndrome 1B protein. Proc Natl Acad Sci U S A 100:6481–6486

7. Nandrot EF, Anand M, Almeida D, Atabai K, Sheppard D, Finnemann SC (2007) Essential role for MFG-E8 as ligand for αvβ5 integrin in diurnal retinal phagocytosis. Proc Natl Acad Sci U S A 104:12005–12010

8. Adamus G, Zam ZS, Arendt A, Palczewski K, McDowell JH, Hargrave PA (1991) Anti-rhodopsin monoclonal antibodies of defined specificity: characterization and application. Vision Res 31:17–31

Part V

Tissue Culture and Cell Models

Chapter 18

Ca²⁺ Microfluorimetry in Retinal Müller Glial Cells

Antje Wurm, Thomas Pannicke, and Andreas Reichenbach

Abstract

Calcium acts as a prominent second messenger in virtually every cell type and modulates a plethora of cell functions. Thus, Ca²⁺ microfluorimetry became a valuable tool to assess information about mechanisms involved in the regulation of the intracellular calcium level in research on living tissues. Here we offer insight into distinct approaches to detect changes in calcium levels specifically in Müller cells, the principal macroglial cells of the retina.

Key words: Calcium imaging, Müller glial cells, Neuro-glial signal exchanges, Retinal slice, Retinal wholemount, Cell isolation

1. Introduction

Second messengers are important components of signal transduction cascades. They play a decisive role in transducing the signal of extracellular primary messengers (e.g., hormones, neurotransmitters) into an intracellular response. Typical second messengers are small organic molecules (e.g., cyclic nucleotides) and calcium ions. Under normal conditions there is a large difference between intracellular (about 100 nM) and extracellular calcium concentrations (low millimolar range) (1). Therefore, increases in the intracellular calcium concentration can serve as a valuable signal of cellular activation. A calcium increase can be mediated on one hand by an influx of calcium ions from the external medium through plasma membrane channels, such as voltage-dependent calcium channels in electrically excitable cells. On the other hand, calcium can be released from intracellular stores (e.g., the endoplasmic reticulum).

Bernhard H.F. Weber and Thomas Langmann (eds.), *Retinal Degeneration: Methods and Protocols*, Methods in Molecular Biology, vol. 935, DOI 10.1007/978-1-62703-080-9_18, © Springer Science+Business Media, LLC 2013

This intracellular release is mediated by intracellular calcium channels. These channels can be activated by calcium ions themselves or by other messengers (such as inositol 1,4,5-triphosphate, IP_3) acting on ryanodine receptors or on IP_3 receptors, respectively (2). Alterations of the intracellular calcium concentration then regulate a wide variety of cellular functions (3). Regarding the brain these functions include exocytosis (particularly neurotransmitter release), synaptic plasticity, activation of transcription factors, or sprouting of neurites. Calcium overload by any dysregulation can cause neuronal cell death (1). To regulate the intracellular calcium concentration, cells express not only calcium channels but also a variety of calcium-controlling components, the so-called calcium signaling toolkit (2), among these components are calcium pumps and exchangers as well as calcium-binding proteins (3). The versatility of calcium signaling is the precondition for its universal role in regulating a variety of cellular processes (4). Moreover, the significance of calcium-regulated processes has turned them into an object of research in many fields of life sciences. Therefore, methods of investigation of calcium-signaling processes are of broad interest and widely in use.

In this chapter, we will describe the method of calcium microfluorimetry also known as calcium imaging (5). By loading cells with dyes that change their spectral properties in the absence or presence of calcium, it is possible to record the intracellular calcium concentration (or at least, alterations of intracellular calcium concentration) in living cells. One major advantage of the calcium imaging method is a high temporal and spatial resolution of the measurements of calcium signals within the cell. This is of extreme importance for understanding cell physiology because the spatiotemporal pattern of calcium signaling determines a wealth of cellular processes. To give only one example, the correct function of synaptic transmission in neurons depends on the increase of the calcium concentration within a few microseconds in a minute cellular domain, the presynaptic ending.

Within the field of neurobiology, physiological research was focused on the neurons for a long time. Since the 1980s it turned out that also the second element of the nervous tissue, the glial cells, may play an active functional role. The focus of research in our lab is on the retinal Müller glial cell which will therefore serve as the object in the following description of the calcium imaging method. Calcium channels in Müller cells were described for the first time by Newman (6). Ten years later, calcium waves were recorded in isolated Müller cells from the tiger salamander (7). Since then, the importance of calcium signaling in Müller cells for retinal function has been elucidated in a large number of articles, many of them based on the calcium imaging technique.

2. Materials

A number of factors determine the methodical details in calcium imaging experiments. Here we concentrate on investigation of the retina and the Müller cells in particular. Howsoever, the protocols might be modified and adapted to work with other tissues and cell types.

2.1. Microsurgical Instruments/Materials for Tissue Preparation

1. Two pairs of fine forceps (i.e., Dumont #5 Forceps, Fine Science Tools GmbH (FST), Heidelberg, Germany).

2. Adequately sized scissors, i.e., spring scissors (8 mm blades, sharp, from FST) for small eyes from mouse or standard scissors (11 mm blades, sharp, from FST) for bigger eyes such as from rat or guinea pig.

3. Curved self-closing forceps.

4. Nitrocellulose filter: pore width, 0.45 μm; diameter, 50 mm; Schleicher & Schuell Microscience; Dassel, Germany.

2.2. Calcium-Sensitive Dye

Fluo-4/AM is the calcium indicator most commonly used to detect changes of the intracellular calcium concentration in Müller cells. A more sensitive, but easily saturated alternative is Oregon Green® 488 BAPTA-1. For more detailed information about the choice of the appropriate calcium-sensitive dye see Note 1.

2.3. Solutions

1. Oxygenated extracellular solution (ECS): 110 mM NaCl, 3 mM KCl, 1 mM $MgCl_2$, 1 mM Na_2HPO_4, 10 mM HEPES, 2 mM $CaCl_2$, 10 mM glucose, 25 mM $NaHCO_3$. It is possible to generate a fivefold concentrated stock solution which contains all the before mentioned substances except glucose and $NaHCO_3$. This can be stored at 4°C for maximally 1 month until usage. At the day of the experiment the working concentration is adjusted by dilution with deionized water (electrical conductivity of 18 MΩ cm at 25°C) and addition of glucose. Subsequently, adjust the pH to 7.4 with Tris-(hydroxymethyl)-aminomethane hydrochloride (Tris) and only thereafter add $NaHCO_3$ (see Note 2). Finally, bubble the solution with carbogen (95% O_2, 5% CO_2) for at least 30 min.

2. ECS without oxygenation: 138 mM NaCl, 3 mM KCl, 1 mM $MgCl_2$, 10 mM HEPES, 2 mM $CaCl_2$, 10 mM glucose. A stock solution can be prepared and used as described for the oxygenated ECS. At the day of the experiment the working concentration is adjusted by dilution with deionized water (electrical conductivity of 18 MΩ cm at 25°C) and addition of glucose. Subsequently, adjust the pH to 7.4 with Tris.

3. Staining solution: Dissolve the calcium-sensitive dye in 2% Pluronic F-127 in dimethylsulfoxide and then further dilute in

ECS (with or without oxygenation depending on the tissue preparation) to the final working concentration (see Note 3).

4. ECS containing 50 μM adenosine-5′-triphosphate (ATP, Sigma Aldrich, Deisenhofen, Germany) (see Note 4).

5. Calcium- and magnesium-free phosphate-buffered saline (PBS), pH 7.4 (Biochrom, Berlin, Germany).

2.4. Technical Prerequisites for Imaging

1. First, it should be checked whether the setup at the microscope allows convenient imaging of the fluorescence signal with the chosen calcium-sensitive dye. This includes appropriate means to excite the dye as well as to filter and to detect the signal at a sufficient spatial and temporal resolution to address your experimental question.

2. Recording chamber depending on the tissue preparation you chose (Fig. 1).

3. Perfusion system: (1) The simplest solution is a gravity-fed perfusion system consisting of several reservoirs that are connected with tubes to one common main tube (see Note 5). Plug opening/closing of the respective tube enables a fast exchange of different test solutions. The velocity of the perfusion can be modulated by hose clamps and should be adapted to the volume of the respective measuring chamber. (2) The perfusion system might also be driven by a pump system. The principal is the same—it should be possible to initiate application of test substances by rapid substitution of the chamber volume. Assure removal of excess of fluid, i.e., by drainage with a vacuum pump-based system.

4. Suitable software that enables the online imaging of calcium responses (in our case—Zeiss LSM Image Examiner Version 3.2.0.70 or the Till Vision software, both adapted to the respective setup) and subsequent evaluation of the gathered data (by programs such as SigmaPlot 2000, SPSS, Inc., Illinois, USA or Prism, Graphpad Software, San Diego, CA).

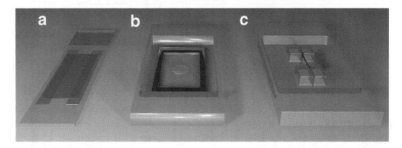

Fig. 1. Schematic drawings of recording chambers for measurements on Müller cells in different tissue preparations. (**a**) A chamber for measurements on isolated Müller cells is shown. (**b**) To image Müller cells in the retinal wholemounts, the tissue should be kept in place by a grid with nylon strings. (**c**) Retinal slice preparations need to be fixed on a nitrocellulose filter (*black stripe*), to orient them properly in the measuring chamber.

3. Methods

All experimental procedures are carried out at room temperature unless otherwise stated.

3.1. Preparation of Vital Retina

1. Cautiously enucleate eyes immediately after the animal was sacrificed avoid rupture of the eye ball.

2. Use a scalpel to make a small incision approximately 1 mm from the corneal-scleral junction.

3. Get hold of the cornea with a pair of fine forceps and insert a spring scissor to do a circumferential cut to remove the cornea at the plane of the ora serrata (Fig. 2a) (see Note 6).

4. After the eye has been opened, the lens can easily be taken out from the eye cup (see Note 7).

5. Transfer the opened eye cup into a petri dish filled with ECS.

6. Gently pull out the vitreous body with fine forceps (see Note 8).

7. Use curved self-closing forceps to gently scratch the retina out of the eye cup. To this end, fix the eye cup by grabbing the sclera (without touching the retina) with forceps. Subsequently place the curved self-closing forceps underneath the retina and scratch it out (thereby cutting the optic nerve as the last tight contact of the retina with the residual eye structures) (Fig. 2b).

3.2. Dye Loading of Müller Cells

Please note that all detailed descriptions and notes in the following sections refer to experiments done with the calcium indicator mentioned therein. Application of alternative dyes is possible, but differences in loading properties and response pattern are probable and should be tested comprehensively.

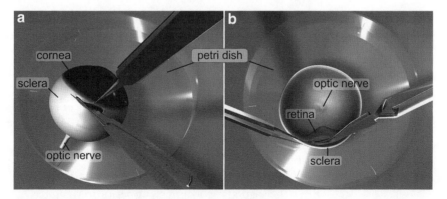

Fig. 2. Key steps during the preparation process to obtain an isolated vital retina. (**a**) Schematic drawing depicting the location of the circumferential cut to remove the cornea and to open the eye cup. (**b**) Orientation of the forceps to gently scratch the retina out of the eye cup after the lens and vitreous have been removed.

3.2.1. Staining of Isolated Müller Cells

1. After the retinal tissue has been removed from the eye cup (see Subheading 3.1), transfer it into an adequate volume of PBS containing papain (2 mg/ml, Roche, crystal suspension of 100 mg in 10 ml).

2. Incubate for 30 min at 37°C to digest components of the extracellular matrix.

3. Freshly prepare the fluo-4/AM (Molecular Probes) staining solution from the stock by diluting it into ECS (*without oxygenation*) to a concentration of 1 μM.

4. Carefully wash the tissue five times in PBS by removing the supernatant. Avoid that tissue is sucked into the pipette tip, as this would result into damaging of the cells.

5. Incubate the retinal pieces in 500 μl PBS containing DNase (200 U/ml, Sigma, D-5025) at room temperature for 2 min. This is important to avoid clumping of the cells by sticky DNA set free from cell debris.

6. Discard the supernatant and replace it with staining solution. Only thereafter, dissociate the cells by gently sucking the retinal tissue up and down with a pipette for 2–3 times (use blue 1 ml pipette tips) (see Note 9).

7. Transfer the cell suspension into the recording chamber (Fig. 1a) (approximately 150 μl, if you use 24 × 32 mm glass slides) (see Note 10). Allow the cells to settle and to load with the dye for at least 15 min at 37°C in the dark.

3.2.2. Staining of Retinal Wholemount Preparations

1. Always prepare stock solutions of fluo-4/AM (180 μM, Molecular Probes, Leiden, Netherlands) or x-rhod-1/AM (1.2 mM) in 2% Pluronic F-127 in dimethylsulfoxide directly at the day of the planned experiment and protect them from light during the whole course of the experiment. Dilute them to the final concentration of 40 and 1.2 μM, respectively, in oxygenated ECS. Vortex thoroughly for 10 s to assure efficient dispersion of the stock solution.

2. Cut the freshly isolated retinal wholemount into pieces (approximately 2 × 2 mm) and transfer them into the staining solution (see Note 11). Incubate at room temperature in the dark for 30–45 min (see Note 12).

3. To image calcium responses in Müller cell endfeet in the retinal wholemount preparation, place the retina into the recording chamber with the photoreceptors down (see Note 13). To avoid drifting of the sample during active perfusion, the tissue should be kept in place by a grid with nylon strings (Fig. 1b).

4. Place the loaded recording chamber onto the microscope stage and adjust the perfusion to a velocity of 1.5 ml/min to wash out excess dye with oxygenated ECS.

<table>
<tr><td>

3.2.3. Staining of Retinal Slices

</td><td>

1. Prepare the staining solution by diluting fluo-4/AM (40 μM) in oxygenated ECS as described in Subheading 2.3.

2. Cut freshly isolated retina into halves.

3. Use forceps to pin down the tissue onto a nitrocellulose filter. To assure firm attachment of the tissue, put the filter—with the retina on top—onto a paper towel and let excess fluid be sucked by the towel. Place the retina/filter back into a petri dish filled with staining solution.

4. Incubate for 30–45 min at room temperature in the dark.

5. To obtain even retinal slices cut the filter with the attached retina by hand with a common razor blade.

6. Only cut one slice at once and immediately transfer it into the measuring chamber (Fig. 1c) filled with ECS (see Note 14).

7. The velocity of the perfusion should be adjusted to 3 ml/min to assure rapid exchange of the chamber volume. Wash out excess dye with oxygenated ECS.

</td></tr>
</table>

3.3. Imaging of Calcium Signals in Müller Cells

Changes of intracellular calcium levels in Müller cells occur in the context of information processing in the retina during light stimulation (8, 9). Alternatively, the intracellular calcium concentration can be directly modified by administration of substances that act as agonists on calcium channels or on G_{q11}-coupled receptors. Adenosine-5′-triphosphate (ATP) certainly is the most comprehensively studied agonist eliciting calcium responses in Müller cells (10–12). In the following sections, several experimental designs are briefly introduced as examples of how calcium responses in Müller cells can be studied.

3.3.1. Detection of Calcium Responses in Isolated Müller Cells from Rat Retina with Fluo-4/AM

1. Prepare solutions and isolate Müller cells as described in Subheadings 2.3 and 3.2.3.

2. After dye loading, place the recording chamber onto the microscope and start the perfusion (1.5 ml/min) with ECS (*without oxygenation*) to wash out excess dye.

3. Use an Achroplan 63×/0.9 long distance water immersion objective (Zeiss) and focus on single Müller cells (Fig. 3a) (see Note 15) without residual photoreceptors attached, and as few as possible neurons located in their vicinity. This ensures that indirect activation effects, due to agonist induced substance release from neurons, are kept as small as possible (see Note 16).

4. Use the experimental setup described in Subheading 3.3.3.

5. Record one picture every second with a spatial resolution of 512×512 pixels over the whole time course of the experiment.

6. As described for imaging on retinal slices (Subheading 3.3.2), record the calcium levels of the cells for several minutes to

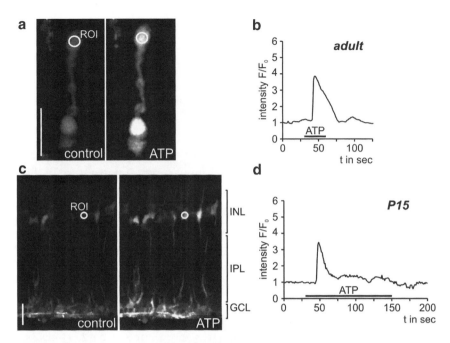

Fig. 3. Calcium imaging on Müller cells in different tissue preparations from rat retina. (**a**) Exemplary image of an isolated Müller cell from a adult rat loaded with fluo-4/AM before and during stimulation with ATP (50 μM). The *circle* marks the area, also called region of interest (ROI), wherein the fluorescence intensity of fluo-4/AM was measured for further data analysis as described in Subheading 3.4. The resulting trace is shown in (**b**). (**c**) A retinal slice from a P15 animal where the typical morphology of Müller cells (endfeet in the ganglion cell layer (GCL), inner stem process spanning the inner plexiform layer (IPL) and a soma in the inner nuclear layer (INL)) is visualized by loading the cells with fluo-4/AM. Single cells show an enhanced fluo-4/AM-signal during ATP application indicating an intracellular calcium increase. A representative trace for a measurement on a Müller cell soma is shown in (**d**). *Scale bars*, 20 μm.

gather reference values before you apply the test substance (i.e., 50 μM ATP, Fig. 3b) by fast exchange of the perfusate.

7. Wash out the test substance for several minutes to test the recovery of the intracellular calcium level in the absence of the stimulus.

3.3.2. Calcium Responses in Müller Cells in Retinal Wholemount Preparations from Guinea Pig During Full-Field Light Stimulation

1. For this experiment x-rhod-1/AM is suitable, as it has been shown that it highly selectively stain Müller cells in the guinea pig retina, while other dyes such as fura-2/AM, though preferentially labeling Müller cells, also stain retinal neurons (9).

2. The setup to image x-rhod-1/AM fluorescence includes the following components: an upright microscope (Axioskop, Zeiss, Jena, Germany) equipped with a 40×/0.75 water immersion objective (Zeiss), Till-Photonics imaging system including a conventional mercury arc lamp, a monochromator (Polychrom IV) to selectively allow light of the desired wavelength to pass for excitation, a dichroic mirror (590 nm, Omega Optical), an emission filter (600 nm, Omega Optical), an Imago-VGA camera (PCO, Kehlheim, Germany) to detect the emitted light, and Till Vision software for data processing.

3. Prepare solutions and retinal wholemounts as described in Subheadings 2.3 and 3.2.1 with one major amendment: All tissue preparation steps need to be accomplished under dim light conditions (i.e., low intensity deep red light). Before each single measurement the tissue should be allowed to dark-adapt for at least 15 min after the desired focus plane was set (i.e., onto Müller cell somata in the inner nuclear layer).

4. Stimulate the tissue and excite x-rhod-1/AM with a 200 ms light pulse (590 nm), record one picture every second over a time course of 10 min.

5. Depending on the test substance, preincubation, if necessary, might be performed during the dark adaptation step, otherwise the substance can be acutely administered during light stimulation by fast exchange of the perfusate.

3.3.3. Response Induction by Activation of Purinergic Receptors with Adenosine-5′-Triphosphate in Retinal Slice Preparations from Rat Retina

1. Prepare solutions and retinal slices as described in Subheadings 2.3 and 3.2.2.

2. The setup includes the following components: Confocal laser scanning microscope LSM 510 Meta (Zeiss, Oberkochen, Germany) equipped with an argon laser (488 nm), a main dichroic beam splitter (488 nm), a long pass emission filter (505 nm), and the LSM 510 META software.

3. Place the measuring chamber loaded with a retinal slice in ECS onto the microscope stage and connect it with the perfusion system to wash the slice for at least 10 min in oxygenated ECS.

4. Use a 63×/0.9 long distance water immersion objective (Zeiss) and adjust the focus plane such as that Müller cells can clearly be identified in the slice (Fig. 3c) (see Note 17).

5. Use the "time series" function to scan a picture every second with a spatial resolution of 512×512 pixels, over the whole time course of the experiment (see Note 18).

6. After all settings are fixed, start the measurement and image the tissue in oxygenated ECS (but still in the absence of any test substance) for several minutes, to obtain data about baseline calcium levels in the cells.

7. Thereafter, wash in ATP (50 μM) for 60 s.

8. Wash out ATP for at several minutes to test the reversibility of the response (Fig. 3d).

3.4. Data Analysis

1. Define an area (also called region of interest, ROI, Fig. 3a, c) from which changes in the intensity pattern of the fluorescence of the calcium-sensitive dye should be quantified (i.e., a single Müller cell soma or endfoot).

2. Export numerical raw data into a suitable statistics program (i.e., SigmaPlot 2000, SPSS, Inc., Illinois, USA).

3. Define the baseline fluorescence F_0 of the calcium-sensitive dye in the unexcited cell by calculation of the mean value measured before onset of the stimulation.

4. Divide each single value measured during the experiment by the baseline intensity, according to F/F_0.

5. To minimize the unwarranted effects of unequal dye-loading (which may occur in different individual experiments) it is highly recommended to normalize the absolute numbers (see Note 19).

4. Notes

1. Due to proceeding development of calcium-sensitive dyes to improve their usability in terms of specific cell loading, maintenance within the cell, sensitivity, signal intensity, and fluorescence pattern, the decision which of the numerous possibilities will optimally meet the needs of one's research interest might be challenging. So, how to choose the right calcium-sensitive dye? Since there is already lots of comprehensive literature referring this issue (i.e., see information material from Molecular Probes (13)), we advert to only few general points you should consider:

   (a) What kind of technical devices you have access to (light source to excite the dye, specific filters, sensitive detection system)?

   (b) Do you expect the calcium response to be large scale or only localized and rather small? Especially if you expect only minor calcium changes to occur, you should consider the application of a ratiometric calcium-sensitive dye such as fura-2/AM, which shows a spectral shift in excitation or emission upon binding of calcium ions. As an example, fura-2/AM is excited successively at two distinct wavelengths (340 and 380 nm). The emission (~550 nm) in response to intracellular calcium increases is enhanced at one wavelength, while it decreases at the other. Formation of an emission intensity ratio from both excitation wavelengths yields data about changes in calcium levels independent from dye loading, photobleaching, or unequal thickness of the cells. Additionally, you efficiently eradicate any unspecific noise signals. Additionally, if you need to assess data about calcium concentrations in absolute numbers, you have to choose ratiometric dyes since they allow the application of calibration protocols and, thus, allow to estimate absolute calcium concentrations (14–17).

   However, please note that the protocols described in the following sections primarily refer to the use of non-ratiometric dyes. Like the most commonly used dye fluo-4, these dyes are optimized for fast cell-loading and high emission intensity which makes them optimal for more qualitative measurements and fast screening for calcium responses; however the calcium responses can hardly be quantified with this method.

Beyond the ratiometric properties of a dye, its K_D value is of importance and may vary remarkably between different probes. Again, it depends on whether you need to detect small alterations of the calcium level and saturation of the probe is of less importance (preferably chose dyes with a low K_D value), or you decide to apply a dye which allows detection of a broad range of calcium concentrations, but is rather insensitive to small calcium changes.

(c) Do you intend to co-stain the cells with other vital dyes which might interfere with the signal from the calcium-sensitive dye? To date there exists a huge palette of calcium-sensitive dyes which strongly differ in their excitation/emission spectra. If you plan to identify a specific cell population via co-labeling with an additional vital dye, you should consequently choose a calcium indicator with a nonoverlapping excitation/emission pattern. In our experience, Müller cells tend to take up virtually every dye. In contrast, there are remarkable cell type-specific differences in how the dye is incorperated into retinal neurons.

2. Resolution of $NaHCO_3$ causes a successive increase of pH which is only balanced by sufficient bubbling with carbogen.

3. Co-application of Pluronic F-127 helps to prevent unwanted compartmentalization of the dye into distinct subcellular structures, and thereby assures an even distribution of the dye all over the cytoplasm.

4. Always prepare the ATP-containing solution freshly as ATP is prone to enzymatic hydrolysis and rapidly becomes degraded to adenosine-5′-diphosphate and other derivatives.

5. It is important to keep the common tube section of the perfusion system as short as possible, since its fluid content adds to the chamber volume which has to be exchanged to successfully apply test substances after the initial control measurements.

6. Note that it is important to cut not directly at the junction between cornea and sclera, but approximately 1 mm towards the scleral tissue. This assures a neat separation of the lens including lens fibers from the retina. Otherwise often the retina may stay attached to the lens, and subsequent separation by pulling with forceps causes an undesirable stretching of the tissue which might lead to a partial dysfunction of the normal Müller cell physiology (18).

7. Especially in rat eyes, it is possible to slowly extricate the lens from the eye cup (still laying on the work space and not yet in ECS) such as that the vitreous body stays attached to it. This eradicates the subsequent step of removal of the vitreous by pulling it out with fine forceps, which is much more complicated.

8. Complete removal of the vitreous body is essential for successful dye loading of Müller cells. However, depending on the species, it might be difficult to assure complete extraction. In mice, we strongly recommend to include an intermediate digestion step of the vitreous as follows. After eye opening and lens extraction, the eye cup is transferred into ECS containing 2 mg/ml Collagenase/Dispase (Roche). Incubate for 10–15 min at room temperature. After three short washing steps with ECS, proceed as described in Step 7 of Subheading 3.1.

9. Dissociation of the cells with the pipette is a crucial step and should be done with care. The tissue falls into pieces and this process should be observed under the microscope, because the number of dissociated cells may vary between experiments. Normally, after a first dissociation procedure a lot of destroyed cells (often photoreceptors) are visible, whereas the Müller cells are still hidden in the larger pieces. After additional sucking of the retina, more and more Müller cells (partly with adhering photoreceptors) appear. Microscopic control helps to optimize the procedure, because too many dissociation steps do severely stress the cells. Cell swelling indicates such stress.

10. Chambers for measurements on isolated Müller cells can easily be self-made. Just cut 5 mm stripes from a 24×50 mm sized coverslip with a diamond knife, and glue it onto an object slide as space holders. Place a 24×32 mm sized coverslip on top such as that the cell suspension can be pipetted underneath.

11. Use a large-pore (2 mm in diameter) plastic or even better glass Pasteur pipette (retinal tissue sometimes tends to stick to plastic) to transfer retinal pieces. This avoids additional tissue damage due to grabbing it with forceps.

12. The time for optimal tissue loading depends on the dye and the species used. We approved an incubation time of 45 min for fluo-4/AM to be sufficient for retinal wholemounts of mouse, rat, guinea pig, rabbit, pig, and cynomolgus monkey (*Macaca fascicularis*) and 90 min for x-rhod-1/AM in guinea pig.

13. Generally it is rather simple to identify the orientation of the retinal tissue. As it lines the eye bulb, it tends to coil up even when removed from the eye cup such that the photoreceptors are lying outside and the ganglion cell layer faces the interior. The easiest way to flat-mount the retina is to get hold of one edge of the tissue. Afterwards remove almost the complete ECS from the chamber (e.g., with a plastic Pasteur pipette)

and unfold the retinal tissue by gently smoothening it with a second pair of forceps. The advantage of a low fluid level in the chamber is that the retina does not continuously curl up again, as it would do if the chamber was completely filled with ECS. Place a nylon grid on top of the retina and only thereafter refill the chamber with ECS.

14. Always cut the slice directly before the measurement and image the freshly cut surface. This assures that predominantly Müller cells are stained and, hence, can easily be identified in the slice.

15. Müller cells are easily identified owing to their distinct morphology, including their prominent, thick stem processes and a "rough" surface texture. In contrast, retinal neurons display a "smooth" superficial structure and very fine axonal and dendritic structures. Of course, a partial shortening of the cells, or even a rupture of one stem process (most often the outer stem process gets lost together with the attached photoreceptors) may occur as a consequence of the isolation procedure. To our experience this does not significantly comprise the Müller cell physiology (in respect to electrophysiology, volume regulation, or calcium responses). However, if the cells appear extremely swollen and have lost their elongated morphology, you should consider to adjust the conditions of cell isolation (such as to lower the enzyme concentration or to accomplish less trituration steps).

16. To design your experiment, consider that some agonists (aside from their effect on Müller cells) might also trigger transmitter release from neurons. On the other hand, these same substances might elicit calcium responses in the Müller cells proper, via alternative receptors. Thus, it is recommended to block the respective receptors on Müller cells (which would respond to the substance released from the neurons) to avoid indirect effects and unmask the direct action of the original agonist on Müller cells.

17. To allow neat imaging of Müller cells it is absolutely mandatory to cut the tissue exactly in the plane parallel to their processes. Otherwise it is almost impossible to trace individual cells from endfoot to soma.

18. Of course, the choice of image resolution, scan speed, and interval to acquire pictures depends on your research interest and on the characteristics of the calcium response you want to measure (duration, amplitude, and intended spatial resolution). These parameters thus should be adjusted to your needs. In principal, you lose spatial resolution with faster picture acquisition, but you gain an increased temporal resolution and vice versa.

19. Note that normalization of the data does not exclude changes in the fluorescence intensity of the dye due to cell volume

alterations (and the resulting dilution or accumulation of the calcium-sensitive dye) in response to the applied stimulus. Such "side effects" can only unequivocally be delineated from the actual changes in the calcium levels by the use of ratiometric dyes such as fura-2/AM.

Acknowledgments

This work was supported by the Deutsche Forschungsgesellschaft (SPP 1172: T.P., A.R.; FOR748: A.W., A.R.; GRK 1097: A.R.; PA 615/2-1). The authors are indebted to Jens Grosche (effigos AG, www.effigos.de) for professional assistance with the illustrations.

References

1. Zündorf G, Reiser G (2011) Calcium dysregulation and homeostasis of neural calcium in the molecular mechanisms of neurodegenerative diseases provide multiple targets for neuroprotection. Antioxid Redox Signal 14:1275–1288

2. Berridge MJ, Bootman MD, Roderick HL (2003) Calcium signalling: dynamics, homeostasis and remodelling. Nat Rev Mol Cell Biol 4:517–529

3. Clapham DE (2007) Calcium signaling. Cell 131:1047–1058

4. Berridge MJ, Lipp P, Bootman MD (2000) The versatility and universality of calcium signalling. Nat Rev Mol Cell Biol 1:11–21

5. Tsien RY (1988) Fluorescence measurement and photochemical manipulation of cytosolic free calcium. Trends Neurosci 11:419–424

6. Newman EA (1985) Voltage-dependent calcium and potassium channels in retinal glial cells. Nature 317:809–811

7. Keirstead SA, Miller RF (1995) Calcium waves in dissociated retinal glial (Müller) cells are evoked by release of calcium from intracellular stores. Glia 14:14–22

8. Newman EA (2005) Calcium increases in retinal glial cells evoked by light-induced neuronal activity. J Neurosci 25:5502–5510

9. Rillich K, Gentsch J, Reichenbach A, Bringmann A, Weick M (2009) Light stimulation evokes two different calcium responses in Müller glial cells of the guinea pig retina. Eur J Neurosci 29:1165–1176

10. Newman EA (2001) Propagation of intercellular calcium waves in retinal astrocytes and Müller cells. J Neurosci 21:2215–2223

11. Uckermann O, Uhlmann S, Weick M, Pannicke T, Francke M, Reichenbach A, Wiedemann P, Bringmann A (2003) Upregulation of purinergic P2Y receptor-mediated calcium responses in glial cells during experimental detachment of the rabbit retina. Neurosci Lett 338:131–134

12. Wurm A, Erdmann I, Bringmann A, Reichenbach A, Pannicke T (2009) Expression and function of P2Y receptors on Müller cells of the postnatal rat retina. Glia 57:1680–1690

13. Takahashi A, Camacho P, Lechleiter JD, Herman B (1999) Measurement of intracellular calcium. Physiol Rev 79:1089–1125

14. Baylor SM, Hollingworth S (1988) Fura-2 calcium transients in frog skeletal muscle fibres. J Physiol 403:151–192

15. Roe MW, Lemasters JJ, Herman B (1990) Assessment of Fura-2 for measurements of cytosolic free calcium. Cell Calcium 11:63–73

16. William DA, Fay FS (1990) Intracellular calibration of the fluorescent calcium indicator Fura-2. Cell Calcium 11:75–83

17. Barreto-Chang OL, Dolmetsch RE (2009) Calcium imaging of cortical neurons using Fura-2 AM. J Vis Exp Pii:1067

18. Lindqvist N, Liu Q, Zajadacz J, Franze K, Reichenbach A (2010) Retinal glial (Müller) cells: sensing and responding to tissue stretch. Invest Ophthalmol Vis Sci 51:1683–1690

Chapter 19

Functional Analysis of Retinal Microglia and Their Effects on Progenitors

Debra A. Carter, Balini Balasubramaniam, and Andrew D. Dick

Abstract

The identification of stem/progenitor cells within the retinal neural environment has opened up the possibility of therapy via cellular replacement and/or reprogramming of resident cell populations (1–4). Within the neuro-retinal niche, following injury or in disease states (including inflammation and degeneration), cellular responses affect tissue homeostasis, reduce cell density, disrupt tissue architecture, and produce scar formation. Microglia (resident retinal immune cell tissue macrophage) are key to the maintenance of retinal homeostasis and are implicated in responses that may influence the control and behavior of retinal progenitors (5, 6). Factors to consider in the generation of a transplantable cell resource with good migratory and integrative capacity include their yield, purity, and functional viability. Utilizing human postmortem retina, we have created a research platform to isolate, culture, and characterize adult retinal microglia as well as analyze their effect on retinal progenitors. Here, we describe techniques using magnetic labeled bead cell separation to isolate pure populations of retinal CD133+ precursor cells and CD11b+ microglia from primary adult retinal cell suspensions (RCSs), enabling flow cytometric cell phenotypic and qPCR genotypic analysis, as well as functional analysis by real-time ratiometric calcium imaging.

Key words: Primary retinal cells, CD133, CD11b, Magnetic labeled cell separation, Flow cytometry, RNA isolation, qPCR, Calcium imaging

1. Introduction

To achieve a greater understanding of retinal microglia and their effects on retinal precursor cells, assessment of pure cell populations are required to elucidate the microenvironmental signals associated with inflammation, injury, and/or proliferation. Within the adult human retina we have demonstrated a successful purification protocol (to 95%) for adult retinal precursor cells, via magnetic separation from primary retinal cell suspensions (RCSs), using a stem cell marker CD133 (7). Purified retinal CD133+ cultures, examined in the presence of specified growth factors and

Bernhard H.F. Weber and Thomas Langmann (eds.), *Retinal Degeneration: Methods and Protocols*, Methods in Molecular Biology, vol. 935, DOI 10.1007/978-1-62703-080-9_19, © Springer Science+Business Media, LLC 2013

cytokines (including FGF2 and LIF) demonstrated proliferative capacity by BrdU incorporation and positive phenotypic expression of Ki67 and cyclin D (8). Differentiation potential of established neurospheres from retinal precursor cell suspension cultures (in the absence of LIF) was confirmed by positive flow cytometric as well as immunocytochemical expression profiles of retinal cell lineage markers (8, 9). Altered gene expression profiles observed in CD133⁺ cells under varied culture conditions included upregulation of genes associated with cell proliferation and cell cycling (Ki67 and Cyclin D1) in addition to other stem cell markers including Nestin, CD135, Pax-6, and Notch (Affymetrix, data deposited in NCBI's Gene Expression Omnibus GSE14733) (8). Utilizing the myeloid-derived macrophage marker CD11b, expressed by human microglia and a modified magnetic cell separation technique, we have isolated a sufficient yield of primary retinal microglia (60%) to enable phenotyping (via flow cytometry), genotyping (by qPCR), and functional studies (using ratiometric calcium imaging) (9). Purified retinal cell isolates of CD133⁺ progenitor cells and CD11b⁺ microglia generated using magnetic separation of primary RCS has allowed further analysis of the effect of retinal microglia on retinal progenitor cell proliferation and differentiation. Here, we demonstrate methods we have developed and modified to isolate CD133⁺ and CD11b⁺ cells from primary human retinal explants, as well as perform flow cytometric phenotyping, and ratiometric functional analysis of purified cell populations.

2. Materials

2.1. Reagents and Supplies

1. Dissociation enzyme solution: 50 ml of MEM, 2.5 ml Trypsin (0.5%)—EDTA (0.2%), 1 ml Collagenase III (10 mg/ml), and 1 ml DNAase I_{IV} (1 mg/ml). Aliquot into working volumes and store at –80°C for up to 3 months.

2. Trypsin Deactivation Wash Buffer: On the day of cell isolation, add 1 ml of fetal bovine serum (FBS) to 9 ml of DMEM/RPMI to make a 10% solution. Keep incubated at 35°C until needed.

3. Isolation buffer: To 100 ml of phosphate-buffered saline add 2 mM of EDTA. Allow the EDTA to dissolve completely using a beaker stirrer. Adjust the pH to 7.2 and then add 0.5 g of bovine serum albumin (BSA) and mix to dissolve using a beaker stirrer. Recheck pH of solution to ensure a pH of 7.2 is achieved. Store at 4–8°C until needed. Make up fresh each week.

4. Retinal microglia culture media: To 100 ml of RPMI-glutamax, add 5 ml FBS, 1 ml sodium pyruvate, 1 ml nonessential amino acids (NEAA), 1 ml of Glucose, 10 ng/ml macrophage colony

stimulating factor (M-CSF). Store at 4–8°C until needed. Make up fresh each week.

5. Progenitor cell media: To 100 ml of DMEM-glutamax add 1 ml of Neural 2 Supplement (N2), 5 ng/ml of basic fibroblast growth factor (bFGF), 10 ng/ml of epidermal growth factor (EGF). Store at 4–8°C until needed. Make up fresh each week.

6. Retinal Microglia Culture Conditions for Calcium Imaging Studies: CD11b + MG cells are cultured post-magnetic sorting on uncoated 13 mm diameter glass coverslips (aliquot approx 100 µl/well) within a 24-well plate at a standard density from initial sort (approximately 0.11×10^6 per 2 globes). Microglia are cultured in 1 ml of RPMI (GIBCO-Invitrogen Ltd, Paisley, UK) supplemented with 5% FCS, 1% PSA (Sigma-Aldrich, Missouri, USA), and 10 ng/ml recombinant human (rhu) M-CSF (R&D Systems, Abingdon, UK) per well.

7. Fura-2AM and HEPES constituents for calcium ratiometric imaging: To enable measurements of intracellular Ca^{2+} concentration $((Ca^{2+})_i)$, preload the cells with 2 µM (2 µl/1 ml) of Fura-2 acetoxymethylester (Fura-2AM, Molecular Probes), 25 µl of 20% DMSO, and 0.02% (25 µl of 10%) Pluoronic F-127 (Molecular Probes). Allow to stand for 30 min in culture media at 37°C, prior to mounting the glass coverslip loaded cells into the low volume perfusion chamber. To facilitate calcium imaging, the cells are maintained under continuous perfusion in an extracellular solution containing 135 mM NaCl, 5 mM KCl, 1 mM $MgCl_2$, 2 mM $CaCl_2$, 30 mM d-glucose, 10 mM HEPES–NaOH, with a pH of 7.3 and 310 mOsm osmolarity.

8. Tools and settings for radiometric calcium imaging: Fura-2AM loaded CD11b+ microglia cells on glass coverslips are mounted onto a low-volume chamber (Warner, RC21) and maintained under continuous perfusion using a peristaltic pump at a rate of ~1 ml/min. The perfused chamber is then placed on an inverted microscope (Nikon, TE2000) connected to a charge coupled device (CCD) camera (Hamamatsu, ORCA 12AG, Japan) with capacity to capture emitted fluorescence light. The time-lapse ratiometric calcium images acquired are recorded on a personal computer (PC) using "Velocity 5" software (Improvision, UK) that permits further qualitative and quantitative data analysis of individual cell profiles. All images are performed using the 40× fluorescence objective and recorded in time-lapse every 5 s as the Fura-2AM loaded microglia are exposed to 200 ms duration pulses of 340 nm wavelength UV light, immediately followed by an identical exposure period of 380 nm wavelength light (from a Xenon light source). Calcium mobilization within microglia cells is reflected as Fura-2AM is excited at wavelengths of 340 nm (calcium bound) and 380 nm (calcium unbound).

3. Methods

3.1. Extraction of Ocular Tissue from Donor/Dissection of Neurosensory Retina

Dissection of eye globes (acquired for example from an Eye Bank following their removal and storage of the corneas for transplant, with ethical and research permission) is performed within 24 h postmortem as outlined below.

1. Using sharp sterile scissors, cut around the iris and remove from the eyecup. The lens should be removed easily at the same time as the iris (see Note 1).

2. Using one pair of rounded forceps and one pair of straight sharp pointed forceps (sterile), firstly take hold of the vitreous using the rounded forceps (see Note 2).

3. Begin to lift the vitreous out of the eyecup by pulling gently. When the edge of the retina is recognized, use the sharp pointed forceps to detach the retina from the vitreous. Keeping hold of the vitreous gently pull from the eyecup allowing the retina to slide off and remain in the eye cup (see Note 3).

4. Using the rounded forceps cut the retina at the optic nerve and remove the neurosensory retina from the eyecup.

5. Place the retinal tissue in a Petri dish and wash with warm media to remove any retinal pigment epithelial cells that may remain attached.

6. Transfer the washed whole retinal explant into a clean Petri dish, now you are ready to generate adult human RCS.

3.2. Formation of Primary Retinal Cell Suspension

1. Using forceps and a curved blade, the dissected retina is cut up into very small pieces.

2. Pipette pre-warmed dissociation enzyme mix into the Petri dish and collect both fluid and retinal pieces into a 15 ml centrifuge tube.

3. Place centrifuge tube into a tube rotator inside an incubator heated to 35°. Incubate while spinning for 20 min (see Note 4).

4. Centrifuge retinal enzyme mix for 5 min at $337 \times g$, following which remove supernatant.

5. Flick cell pellet into suspension and add 2 ml of Trypsin deactivator washing buffer to the tube (see Note 4).

6. Transfer retinal suspension into a 7 ml Bijou.

7. Using a 19 gauge (G) needle and sterile syringe, pass the retinal suspension through the needle three times. Repeat process using 21G needle (see Note 5).

8. Add a further 2 ml of Trypsin deactivation wash buffer to the 7 ml Bijou. Now pass the cell suspension through a 0.4 μm

sieve into the remaining 6 ml of Trypsin deactivation wash buffer. This will remove any retinal tissue that has not been digested properly (see Note 6).

9. Centrifuge the cell suspension for 5 min at 1,500 rpm, then remove supernatant.

10. Flick cell pellet into suspension, you are now ready to isolate specific cell types from your cell suspension.

3.3. Magnetic Cell Separation of CD11b⁺MG/CD133⁺ Progenitors from Retinal Cell Suspension

The cell separation protocol outlined below may be used to isolate either retinal progenitor cells using the CD133 Micro Beads or retinal microglia cells using the CD11b Micro Beads.

1. Add 1 ml of isolation buffer to the cell suspension, then pass through a 0.4 μm sieve to promote single cells and remove any cell aggregates (see Note 7). Determine cell number.

2. Firstly isolate CD11b microglia cells (see Note 8). CD11b Micro Beads (Miltenyi Biotec) are used for the positive selection of microglia cells from cell suspensions. For 10^7 cells/ml of RCS (achieved using a pair of globes) add 100 μl of CD11b micro beads. If cell numbers are higher, scale up accordingly. Mix well and then incubate at 2–8°C for 30 min (see Note 9).

3. Wash the cells by adding up to 10 ml of isolation buffer for 5 min at 1,500 rpm. Remove the supernatant completely leaving only the cell pellet. Flick the cell pellet into suspension and add 3 ml of isolation buffer and mix well using a pipette.

4. Set up an MACS column in an MACS separator by placing a 30 ml sterile tube underneath to catch the flow through cells. To prepare the column pass 1 ml of isolation buffer through the column to rinse before adding the cell suspension.

5. Place a 0.4 μm sieve on top of the MACS column, then pass the 3 ml of cell suspension through the sieve and onto the column. Cells within the buffer will drip slowly through the column. Labeled cells will stay within the column and unlabeled cells pass through the column and into the collection tube (see Note 10).

6. When the whole volume of cell suspension has passed through the column, remove and place in a new sterile 15 ml tube. Collect the unlabelled cells in a separate clean tube to use later for CD133 progenitor cell removal.

7. Add 3 ml of isolation buffer to the top of the column and using the plunger supplied push with force the liquid through the column into the new sterile 15 ml tube. Labeled cells will be flushed from the column into the tube. To improve purity pass the labeled cells through a new column and repeat the process to collect the CD11b cells. Finally wash cells by adding up to 10 ml of isolation buffer into the 15 ml tube and

centrifuging for 5 min at 1,500 rpm. Determine cell numbers then seed into 3 ml of microglia media within a 25 ml tissue culture flask. Microglia will adhere to the plastic within 3–5 days and can be maintained in culture long term if media is changed at least every 5 days (see Note 11).

8. For the unlabeled cells, transfer into a new 15 ml tube and add up to 10 ml of isolation buffer, then centrifuge for 5 min at 1,500 rpm. Resuspend the cell pellet in 1 ml of isolation buffer and then pass through a 0.4 μm sieve to generate single cells while removing any cell aggregates. Determine cell number.

9. Add 200 μl of Fragment Crystallizable Receptor (FcR) Blocking reagent per 10^8 total cells. Mix well. Then add 100 μl of CD133 micro beads. Mix well then incubate at 2–8°C for 30 min. Repeat steps 3–7 above to obtain a pure cell suspension of CD133 progenitor cells. Determine cell number and seed approximately 10^5 cells into 3 ml of Progenitor cell media within 25 ml tissue culture flasks. Progenitor cells can be maintained long term with fresh media added to culture flask once a week (see Note 12).

3.4. Flow Cytometric Phenotype of Retinal Microglia and Progenitors

Following culture of microglia in a variety of conditions to simulate inflammation (see Note 13), cells can be analyzed by flow cytometry. Similarly CD133 cells can be cultured in various media to stimulate a spectrum of cell differentiation (see Note 12) and have their phenotype evaluated using flow cytometry. The following protocol outlines methods utilized to evaluate purity of cell populations isolated by magnetic cell sort of microglia (using CD11b) and retinal precursor cells (using CD133) using flow cytometry (Fig. 1).

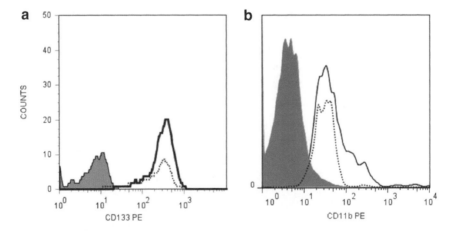

Fig. 1. Magnetic beads used to isolate (**a**) CD133+ and (**b**) CD11b + cells from primary retinal cell suspensions via positive selection was confirmed by flow cytometry and is represented here as histogram to show the increase in cells expressing CD133 cells (**a**) or CD11b (**b**) (*black line*) following magnetic separation from primary suspension (*dotted line*). The *gray* filled peak represents isotype mAb fluorescence expressed for CD133 (**a**) and CD11b (**b**).

1. Obtain cell pellet of cells (microglia/CD133) by centrifuging at 1,500 rpm for 5 min. Remove all supernatant and resuspend in 100 μl of cell isolation buffer.

2. Divide cells into three FACS tubes. Add 20 μl of FC block (see Note 14) and incubate for 15–20 min at room temperature. Do not wash away FC block.

3. Add anti-human conjugated fluorescent antibodies (CD133, CD11b, IgG control which matches the primary antibody isotype) using the manufacturer's recommended concentration to the appropriate tubes (see Note 15) and incubate for 30 min at room temperature in the dark.

4. Wash off excess antibody using isolation buffer by centrifuging at 1,500 rpm for 5 min. Remove supernatant and resuspend cells in 500 μl of isolation buffer.

5. Transfer labeled suspended cells into a labeled FACS tube containing 500 μl of 1% paraformaldehyde FACS wash buffer.

6. Analyze microglia and CD133$^+$ cell populations phenotype using flow cytometer. Positive cells should be identified as cell events fluorescing the appropriate fluorochrome and should be seen as a distinct cell population (Fig. 1).

3.5. Functional Analysis of CD11b + Cells by Real-Time Calcium Imaging

Fura-2, a polyamino carboxylic acid, is a ratiometric fluorescent dye that binds to free intracellular calcium (10). Fura-2 has an emission peak at 505 nM and changes its excitation peak from 340 to 380 nm in response to calcium binding (Fig. 2), thus the ratio of the emissions at these wavelengths (340–380 nm ratio) is directly correlated to the amount of intracellular calcium (Fig. 3b). The advantage of using the ratiometric dyes is that the ratio signal is independent of confounding variables such as dye concentration, illumination intensity, optical path length, and cell thickness that could generate artifacts. Fura-2-acetoxymethyl ester (Fura-2AM) is a membrane-permeable derivative of the ratiometric calcium indicator Fura-2 used to measure cellular calcium concentrations by fluorescence. When added to cells, Fura-2AM crosses cell membranes and once inside the cell, the acetoxymethyl groups are removed by cellular esterases. Removal of the acetoxymethyl esters regenerates "Fura-2," the pentacarboxylate calcium indicator. The following protocol describes the use of Fura-2AM to assess the functional viability of magnetically sorted CD11b+ve human retinal microglia by measuring their ratiometric calcium responses (9, 11 and 12).

1. Magnetically separated CD11b$^+$ retinal microglia cells (see Subheading 3.3) are aliquoted and cultured on uncoated 13 mm diameter glass coverslips within a 24-well plate at a standard density from initial sort (approximately 0.11×10^6 per 2 globes).

2. Following transportation to the calcium imaging facility (see Note 16), CD11b$^+$ microglia are maintained within the 24-well

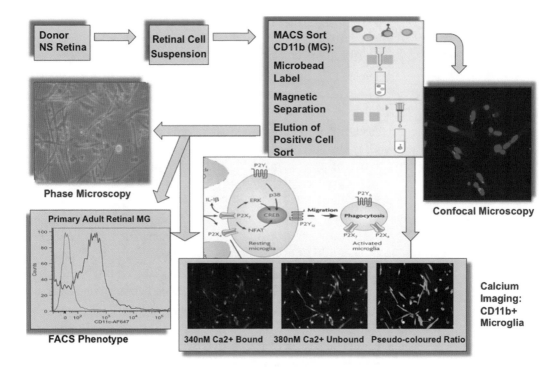

Fig. 2. Calcium imaging of CD11b-(MG) MACS® isolated retinal microglia from cell suspensions generated from dissected donor postmortem adult human retina. Free calcium $(Ca^{2+})_i$ mobilization indicated by conversion of 340–380 nm wavelength ratio (using an equation previously described by Grynkiewicz et al. 1985) recorded using Fura-2AM loaded adult human retinal microglia is shown. Purinergic receptors (P2X4, P2X7, P2Y6, and P2Y12) expressed on retinal microglia are illustrated and may explain one of the mechanisms for microglial cell activation and phagocytic behavior.

plate in a 37°C and 5% CO_2 incubator for at least 24 h before imaging (cells are maintained for a minimum of 1 h prior to imaging following cell transport) being performed (Fig. 3a).

3. CD11b⁺ retinal microglia cells are prepared for functional ratiometric calcium imaging by incubation with 2 μM or 2 μl/1 ml (within 24-well plate) of 4 M fura-2-actoxymethyl-ester (Fura-2AM, 25 μl of 5 μM, Molecular Probes, UK) (see Note 17), dissolved in dimethyl sulfoxide (25 μl of 20% DMSO) with 0.02% or 25 μl of 10% Pluronic F-127 (Molecular Probes, UK) for 30 min at 37°C (Fig. 3c).

4. Fura-2AM loaded coverslips are then removed from the 24-well plate, washed and maintained in a Bath solution (standard HEPES-buffered saline solution (HBSS)) for 30 min at room temperature to allow Fura-2AM to de-esterify (Fig. 3d).

5. The Fura-2AM loaded cells on the glass coverslips are then transferred to a low volume chamber (Warner, RC21) (Fig. 3e) and placed on the stage of the viewing platform of an inverted microscope (Nikon, TE-2000S) (Fig. 3f).

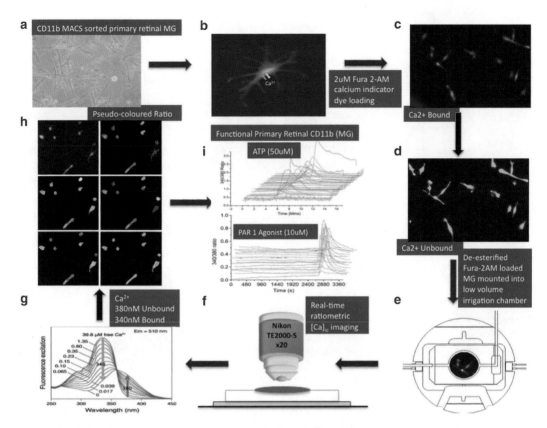

Fig. 3. Protocol for ratiometric calcium imaging of retinal microglia (**a**) isolated by magnetic cell sort using CD11b-MG magnetic beads is illustrated (see Subheading 3.5). Calcium imaging used to measure intracellular calcium (**b**) in real time, involves preloading and incubation of the cells with Fura-2AM (**c**) for 30 min, followed by wash to allow the Fura-2AM to de-esterify (**d**) and continuous perfusion in HBSS using a peristaltic pump attached to a low volume Warner chamber into which the glass coverslip is loaded (**e**). The cells are viewed using a ×40 fluorescence objective lens on an inverted microscope (**f**) and real-time images recorded in on a CCD camera linked to a PC following exposure of the Fura-2AM loaded cells to 200 ms duration pulses of 340 nm wavelength UV light, immediately followed by an identical exposure period of 380 nm from a xenon light source and emissions recorded at 505 nm (**g**). Qualitative and quantitative data generated maybe analyzed using velocity (**h**) and charted graphically using Origin software (**i**). *This figure includes illustrations by Subanthini Balasubramaniam (**e**) and Parantha Narendran (**f**).*

6. Continuous flow irrigation at a rate of approximately 1 ml/min is attached to the Warner Chamber that permits cell perfusion of the Bath solution (see Fig. 3e) and application of stimulant treatments via the peristaltic pump.

7. All images are acquired using the ×40 fluorescence objective and recorded in time-lapse every 5 s as the Fura-2AM loaded microglia are exposed to 200 ms duration pulses of 340 nm wavelength UV light, immediately followed by an identical exposure period of 380 nm wavelength light (from a Xenon light source) (Fig. 3f).

8. Calcium mobilization within microglia cells is reflected as Fura-2AM is excited at wavelengths of 340 nm (calcium bound) and 380 nm (calcium unbound) (Fig. 3g).

9. Fluorescence emitted by both excitation wavelengths passes through the objective, followed by a dichroic mirror that transmit wavelengths above 420 nm and finally through a barrier filter (Chroma, D510/40 (510 nm) emission filter) passing 480–540 nm (Nikon).

10. Fluorescence light emitted is captured using a CCD camera (Hamamatsu, ORCA 12AG, Japan). Images are evaluated and recorded using "Velocity 5" software (Improvision, UK) (Fig. 3h) and stored on a personal computer (PC) for further quantitative and qualitative analysis.

11. Microglial cells of interest may be evaluated following selection by drawing around each microglia to generate quantitative data for individual cell responses to stimulants (e.g., ATP or PAR1). Further quantitative data analysis can then be performed and data illustrated graphically using origin software (Fig. 3i).

4. Notes

1. Sometimes the iris will not be attached following removal of the cornea. This will lead to the lens floating in the vitreous. It is not necessary to remove at this stage unless it gets in the way when trying to remove the vitreous.

2. To get a firm grip of the vitreous use the eyecup as a wall. Push the vitreous toward the eyecup and grab hold of the thick jelly part, which has a larger volume structure, rather than try to grasp near the edge that may result in increased sliding and loss of tissue hold.

3. When removing the vitreous from the eyecup you will find that depending on the age and condition of the eyes the ease of the retina sliding off will vary. Young aged eyes tend to have very pinky/gray sticky retinas that are more delicate and adhere more to the vitreous. You may find that the central area will slide off while leaving the surrounding edge area still attached. This will require you to remove these left on parts with the sharp pointed forceps. Gently stroke the vitreous with the pointed edge and grab. It is a little technical but take your time and you will be able to pull off the remaining retina. The older eyes tend to have thicker retinas with a yellowish tinge. They are very easy to remove and slide off the vitreous with no problem.

4. Depending on the condition of the eye, the degree of digestion will vary. Sometimes the enzymes cause the retina to clog into one ball. On these occasions you can either try to flick into semi-suspension and return to rotator for another 10–15 min or following centrifugation when you add the trypsin inhibitor, you

can use your pipette to force the retinal pieces into suspension by sucking and dispersing with a little force.

5. When passing the cell suspension through the needles occasionally you will get some clogging due to pieces of undigested retina. Gently force the liquid out of the syringe and use a new needle. Pieces of retina will be removed completely in the next step.

6. When passing the cell suspension through the sieve you will occasionally get clogging of the mesh through small undigested pieces of retina. When this happens take a new sieve and continue with sieving the rest of the suspension.

7. Use the isolation buffer at room temperature. When used direct from the fridge, the buffer seems to cause clumping of the cells and makes it difficult to maintain a single cell suspension which is important for micro bead incubation and isolation.

8. For magnetic separation of CD11b/CD133 cells, the protocol supplied with Miltenyi Biotec Magnetic Micro beads Set was followed and adapted to suit separation of cells from human retina.

9. Once you have added the beads make sure you mix thoroughly by flicking the tube. For the CD11b isolation the suspension will have a pinky/gray color, and for the CD133 isolation the suspension will be as above but with a brown tinge (due to the micro beads).

10. If the cell suspension discontinues dripping through the column, you likely have a clog. Remove the remaining cell suspension and pass through a new tube. Remember to remove the cells that have already been isolated and remain in the column.

11. Cultured microglia will adhere to the flask within around 3 days and around 5–7 days the majority will have an elongated appearance. When viewed under the microscope in high-resolution magnification (minimum 40× objective) you can see they are granular in appearance.

12. Cultured CD133+ cells will after approximately 2 weeks in culture develop into neurospheres. Longer cultures (approximately 2 months) will see the neurospheres begin to differentiate. To feed the cells it is recommended not to spin cells down and then remove supernatant but rather to add 1–2 ml of fresh medium to the flask once a week. Continue feeding cells this way until neurospheres are throughout flask then change to feeding cells in a normal way by spinning medium down, removing supernatant, and resuspending neurospheres in fresh medium.

13. To simulate inflammatory conditions 5 ng/ml of lipopolysaccharide (LPS)/100 U/ml of interferon (IFNγ) or 5 ng/ml of tumor necrosis factor (TNFα) can be added. To look for gene upregulation using qPCR, microglia can be cultured in these

conditions for 4–6 h. To evaluate cytokine production or intracellular cytokine expression, microglia cells require culture for a minimum of approximately 12 h, post-micro bead assisted magnetic sort.

14. Human FcR block that prevents FcR region ligation can be purchased from Miltenyi Biotec in a ready to use sterile composition however if you do not have this, an alternative is to use human serum at 10%.

15. It is recommended to predetermine the optimum concentration of your conjugated fluorescent antibodies. Analyze your cells by incubating with a range of concentrations in increasing volumes around the manufacturer's recommendation.

16. Sorted CD11b microglia cells cultured either overnight or over longer periods of 3–5 days (dendriform appearance with long thin and rod-like processes) are transported in sealed packaging to the calcium imaging facility, ensuring minimal alteration in temperature.

17. The advantages of Fura-2-AM ratiometric dye over single wavelength include its ability to overcome photobleaching, variations of intracellular concentration of indicator and variations in cellular volume.

Acknowledgments

This work was supported by grants from Guide Dogs for the Blind (Dr Debra Carter) and The Dr Hans and Mrs Gertrude Hirsch Studentship via the National Eye Research Council (NERC), UK (Balini Balasubramaniam). We are grateful to the Bristol Eye bank team, and most of all to the tissue donors and their families.

References

1. Ahmad I, Tang L, Pham H (2000) Identification of neural progenitors in the adult mammalian eye. Biochem Biophys Res Commun 270: 517–521

2. Tropepe V, Coles BL, Chiasson BJ, Horsford DJ, Elia AJ, McInnes RR, van der Kooy D (2000) Retinal stem cells in the adult mammalian eye. Science 287:2032–2036

3. Coles BL, Angenieux B, Inoue T, Del Rio-Tsonis K, Spence JR, McInnes RR, Arsenijevic Y, van der Kooy D (2004) Facile isolation and the characterization of human retinal stem cells. Proc Natl Acad Sci U S A 101:15772–15777

4. Mayer EJ, Carter DA, Ren Y, Hughes EH, Rice CM, Halfpenny CA, Scolding NJ, Dick AD (2005) Neural progenitor cells from postmortem adult human retina. Br J Ophthalmol 89: 102–106

5. Mayer EJ, Balasubramaniam B, Carter DA, Dick AD (2009) Retinal progenitor cells in regeneration and repair highlight new therapeutic targets. Eur Ophthalmol Rev 3:75–80

6. Dick AD (2009) Influence of microglia on retinal progenitor cell turnover and cell replacement. Eye 23:1939–1945

7. Corti S, Nizzardo M, Nardini M, Donadoni C, Locatelli F, Papadimitriou D et al (2007) Isolation and characterization of murine neural stem/progenitor cells based on Prominin-1 expression. Exp Neurol 205:547–562

8. Carter DA, Dick AD, Mayer EJ (2009) CD133+ adult human retinal cells remain undifferentiated in leukaemia inhibitory factor (LIF). BMC Ophthalmol 9:1

9. Balasubramaniam B, Carter DA, Mayer EJ, Dick AD (2009) Microglia derived IL-6 suppresses neurosphere generation from adult human retinal cell suspensions. Exp Eye Res 89:757–766

10. Grynkiewicz G, Poenie M, Tsien RY (1985) A new generation of Ca2+ indicators with greatly improved fluorescence properties. J Biol Chem 260:3440–3450

11. Barreto-Chang OL, Dolmetsch RE (2009) Calcium imaging of cortical neurons using Fura-2AM. J Vis Exp 23:1067. doi:10.3791/1067, http://www.jove.com/details.stp?id=1067

12. Nicholson E, Balasubramaniam B, Carrick T, Miller S, Kouranova E, Saraf K, von Schack D, Ring R, Whiteside G, Dick AD, Randall AD (2011) Histamine H1 receptors activate human microglia. AJP Cell Phys

Chapter 20

Analysis of Photoreceptor Outer Segment Phagocytosis by RPE Cells in Culture

Yingyu Mao and Silvia C. Finnemann

Abstract

Retinal pigment epithelial (RPE) cells are among the most actively phagocytic cells in nature. Primary RPE and stable RPE cell lines provide experimental model systems that possess the same phagocytic machinery as RPE in situ. Upon experimental challenge with isolated photoreceptor outer segment fragments (POS), these cells promptly and efficiently recognize, bind, internalize, and digest POS. Here, we describe experimental procedures to isolate POS from porcine eyes and to feed POS to RPE cells in culture. Furthermore, we describe three different and complementary methods to quantify total POS uptake by RPE cells and to discriminate surface-bound from engulfed POS.

Key words: Retinal pigment epithelium, Cell culture, Photoreceptor outer segments, Phagocytosis, Cell receptors, Engulfment, Recognition, Quantification, Immunofluorescence microscopy, Immunoblotting, Fluorescence scanning

1. Introduction

The retinal pigment epithelium (RPE) performs numerous functions in support of photoreceptor rod and cone neurons in the retina (1). Among them, the prompt and efficient clearance by receptor-mediated phagocytosis of photoreceptor outer segment fragments (POS) shed daily by photoreceptors in a diurnal rhythm is essential both for long-term viability and functionality of photoreceptors (2, 3). Although the role of the RPE in POS recognition and engulfment has long been recognized, the underlying molecular mechanisms are not fully understood. Comparison of POS phagosome load in RPE in experimental animals such as mice with different mutations is an important step towards identification of proteins that play a role in POS renewal (for methodology see Chapter 17 by Sethna and Finnemann). However, in situ POS

Bernhard H.F. Weber and Thomas Langmann (eds.), *Retinal Degeneration: Methods and Protocols*, Methods in Molecular Biology, vol. 935, DOI 10.1007/978-1-62703-080-9_20, © Springer Science+Business Media, LLC 2013

phagocytosis analysis cannot pinpoint the specific contribution of an individual protein to the phagocytic process: (1) a candidate protein may act in photoreceptors or in the RPE or in both; (2) a candidate protein may promote a specific step of the phagocytic process, such as POS recognition, engulfment, or POS digestion. Analysis of POS uptake by RPE cells in culture allows discrimination of specific roles of proteins in the phagocytic process. Primary RPE cells as well as immortalized RPE cell lines have been shown to retain avid phagocytic activity toward isolated POS particles (4–8). Here, we present methodology to induce and quantify POS phagocytosis by RPE cells in culture. We discuss isolating POS particles from porcine eyes, challenging RPE cells in culture with purified POS, and three different methods for analysis of POS uptake by the RPE, each one of which discriminates surface-bound from engulfed POS particles.

2. Materials

Prepare all solutions using double-distilled water or similar quality water and analytical grade reagents. Prepare and store all reagents at room temperature unless indicated otherwise.

2.1. Solutions

2.1.1. POS Isolation Stock Solutions

1. 100 mM glucose: Dissolve 1.8 g glucose in ddH_2O; fill up to 100 mL in graduated cylinder. Store at 4°C.

2. 200 mM Tris/Acetate pH 7.2: Dissolve 12.1 g Tris Base in 400 mL ddH_2O; adjust pH to 7.2 with glacial acetic acid; fill up to 500 mL in graduated cylinder with ddH_2O.

3. 70% sucrose: Dissolve 175 g sucrose by gradually adding ddH_2O, be careful not to exceed final volume of 250 mL. Transfer to graduated cylinder and fill up to 250 mL with H_2O, rinsing original beaker. Store at 4°C.

4. 0.1 M Na_2CO_3 pH 11.5: Dissolve 1.06 g Na_2CO_3 in final volume of 100 mL ddH_2O.

5. 0.1 M $NaHCO_3$ pH 8.4: Dissolve 0.840 g $NaHCO_3$ in final volume of 100 mL ddH_2O.

2.1.2. POS Isolation Working Solutions

Prepare the following working solutions fresh on the day of the POS isolation using the stock solutions. Suggested volumes of all working solutions allow POS isolation from 75 fresh pig eyes.

1. Homogenization solution (40 mL): 20% w/v sucrose, 20 mM Tris/Acetate pH 7.2, 2 mM $MgCl_2$, 10 mM glucose, 5 mM taurine.

2. 25% sucrose solution (80 mL): 25% sucrose, 20 mM Tris/Acetate pH 7.2, 10 mM glucose, 5 mM taurine.

3. 60% sucrose solution (80 mL): Dissolve 48 g sucrose in a solution with final concentration of 20 mM Tris–Acetate pH 7.2, 10 mM glucose, 5 mM taurine.

4. WASH 1 (100 mL): 20 mM Tris–Acetate pH 7.2, 5 mM taurine.

5. WASH 2 (50 mL): 10% sucrose, 20 mM Tris–Acetate pH 7.2, 5 mM taurine.

6. WASH 3 (100 mL): 10% sucrose, 20 mM phosphate buffer pH 7.2, 5 mM taurine.

7. DMEM: Use DMEM, 4.5 g/L glucose.

8. FITC stock solution: Dissolve 10 mg FITC isomer I (Invitrogen) in 5 mL 0.1 M Na-carbonate buffer, pH 9.5. Spin solution to remove any undissolved small particles before using supernatant solution to label POS.

2.1.3. Solutions for POS Phagocytosis Assays

1. PBS-CM: PBS supplemented with 1 mM $MgCl_2$, 0.2 mM $CaCl_2$.

2. PBS/EDTA: Add 1/500 v/v 0.5 M EDTA, pH 8.0, to PBS to yield PBS, 2 mM EDTA.

3. FITC-quenching solution: 0.4% trypan blue in PBS.

4. HNTG lysis buffer: 50 mM HEPES, pH 7.4, 150 mM NaCl, 10% glycerol, 1.5 mM $MgCl_2$, 1% Triton X-100.

5. Antibodies to opsin and to protein serving as loading control, e.g., porin.

6. DAPI nuclei staining solution: 10 μg/mL 4′,6-diamidino-2-phenylindole DAPI in PBS.

7. Fluoromount G.

2.2. Equipment

1. Ultracentrifuge with swing-out rotor for tubes containing up to 30 mL that reaches $112,398 \times g$ (e.g., Beckman ultracentrifuge with rotor SW28); Refrigerated centrifuge that reaches $3,000 \times g$ for 30 mL tubes (e.g., Sorvall RC-2B with rotor SS-34); refrigerated microtube centrifuge.

2. Sensitive, fluorescence flatbed imager, (e.g., Typhoon Trio™, GE Healthcare).

3. Conventional setup for SDS-PAGE and immunoblotting.

4. Conventional epifluorescence or laser scanning confocal fluorescence microscopy system.

3. Methods

3.1. Isolation of POS from Porcine Eyes

This protocol was developed based on a published procedure by Molday and colleagues (9). Obtain 75 pig eyes from a slaughterhouse and process them as fresh as possible (see Note 1). Do not use frozen eyes. Chill eyes and keep them in the dark. Prechill all solutions on ice. Keep all materials ice-cold at all times.

1. Dissect pig eyes one by one under dim red light (see Notes 2 and 3): Take one eye firmly into your left hand. Poke front with edge of razor blade while holding eye away from you, to avoid splashing into your face. Use razor blade to cut anterior segment of eyeball into two halves. Remove lens. Flip the eyecup inside out. Use side of razor blade to gently dislodge retina, a pinkish layer, off the tapetum.

2. Collect the retina in 50 mL plastic tube containing 15 mL homogenization solution on ice.

3. Repeat until all 75 retinas are collected in the same tube.

4. Shake suspension gently for 2 min. Filter 3× through 1 layer gauze to remove large tissue fragments.

5. Use a gradient maker to prepare three 24 mL linear gradients of 25–60% sucrose, 20 mM Tris/Acetate pH 7.2, 10 mM glucose, 5 mM taurine in 30 mL ultracentrifuge tubes. Keep on ice until use. Use within 30 min of preparation.

6. In dim red light, use a 10 mL plastic pipet to gently overlay equal volumes of the crude retina isolate from step 4 over the three gradients. Balance tubes precisely using extra homogenization solution to equalize weights.

7. Spin immediately in a swing-out ultracentrifuge rotor at $112,398 \times g$ (i.e. 25,000 rpm in a Beckman SW-28 rotor) for 48 min at 4°C.

8. Collect sharp, single pink band in upper third of gradient (see Note 4). Discard the tube and the remaining tissue.

9. Dilute with 5 volumes of ice-cold WASH 1.

10. Separate into as many tubes as needed for centrifugation in 30 mL tubes at $3,000 \times g$ for 10 min.

11. Resuspend pellets in 10 mL WASH 2 each, combine pellets and spin 10 min at $3,000 \times g$.

12. Resuspend pellet in 15 mL WASH 3, spin 10 min at $3,000 \times g$.

    (12a) Unlabeled POS stock: Resuspend POS in 10 mL 2.5% sucrose in DMEM. Dilute 10 μL plus 490 μL DMEM (=1/50) and mix well by pipetting. Count diluted POS in cell counting chamber. Calculate yield and concentration. Dilute to $\sim 1 \times 10^8$ POS/mL with 2.5% sucrose in

DMEM. Store POS at −80°C in aliquots appropriate for single phagocytosis assays.

(12b) FITC-labeled POS stock: Resuspend POS in 5 mL WASH 3, and add 1.5 mL FITC stock solution. Rotate 1 h at RT in the dark. Wash labeled POS twice in WASH 3, twice in 2.5% sucrose in DMEM (spin at $3,000 \times g$ for each wash), then resuspend in 2.5% sucrose in DMEM. Count and store POS as described in (12a).

3.2. Plating of RPE Cells for Phagocytosis Assays

Seed RPE cells on multi-well culture plates depending on the method chosen for POS quantification. Use 96-well clear bottom black plates for fluorescence imaging; seed cells on 5 mm or 1.2 cm coverslips in 96- or 24-well plates, respectively, for POS analysis by immunofluorescence microscopy; seed cells on regular 96-well flat bottom low evaporation culture plates for POS quantification by immunoblotting. In each assay, test samples in triplicate. For POS quantification by fluorescence scanning or immunoblotting, set up two sets of triplicate samples for separate detection of total and internalized POS quantification. Grow RPE cells in culture until desired density and differentiation (see Note 5).

3.3. POS Phagocytosis Assay

1. Calculate the amount of POS needed based on the number of RPE cells per well and number of samples. Confluent, polarized RPE cells should be challenged with ten POS particles per cell (see Note 6).

2. Thaw POS aliquots from −80°C in your hand. Spin POS for 5 min at $2,400 \times g$ at RT in a microcentrifuge. Resuspend pellet immediately in serum free DMEM by gently pipetting up and down. Add pharmacological agents, recombinant proteins, or heat-inactivated FBS (no more than 10% (4)) to the POS suspension as desired. Mix well by pipetting gently.

3. Aspirate medium from RPE cells completely and add POS suspension immediately. Avoid introducing air bubbles. Incubate RPE cells in the tissue culture incubator with POS for the appropriate time depending on your experiment and on your choice of RPE cells (see Note 7).

4. Proceed to one of three methods to quantify phagocytosed POS as outlined below.

3.4. Quantification of Phagocytosed POS

There are three ways to detect and quantify opsin.

3.4.1. Fluorescence Scanning

1. Use FITC-POS for the phagocytosis assay. To terminate POS challenge aspirate POS completely. Wash cells 3×1 min with PBS-CM at room temperature. For multi-well plates, use a plastic squirt bottle to quickly dispense PBS-CM. Avoid damage to the RPE cell layer by adding PBS-CM to the side of wells (see Note 8).

2. Divide wells into two sets: One for detection of total (bound plus internal) POS, the other one for detection of internalized POS. Both sets should allow testing samples in triplicate.

3. To detect internalized POS only, aspirate PBS-CM and incubate cells with FITC-quenching solution for 10 min at room temperature. The other set of wells for total POS quantification remains in PBS-CM during this time. After FITC-quenching, aspirate solution and rinse 2× with PBS-CM. No wait is required between washes.

4. Aspirate solutions from all wells. Fix cells by filling wells with ice-cold methanol. Let sit for 5 min at room temperature.

5. Aspirate methanol and immediately rehydrate cells by filling wells with PBS-CM and incubating overnight at 4°C (see Note 9).

6. Scan the plate with a fluorescence flatbed scanner using setting appropriate for FITC detection (for a Typhoon Trio™ use excitation 488 nm, detection 520 nm, medium sensitivity). A representative image of the resulting scan is shown in Fig. 1.

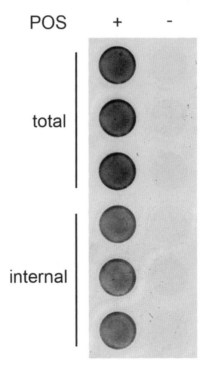

Fig. 1. Fluorescence scanning analysis of POS phagocytosis. Confluent, polarized RPE-J cells were challenged with FITC-POS for 5 h before processing as described in Subheading 3.4.1. The fluorescence scan was obtained using a Trio™ Scanner. Triplicate wells of a 96-well plate were used to detect total (bound plus internal) and internal (trypan blue-quenched) FITC signal (+POS, as indicated). Wells with cells but not fed with POS (−POS) were used to subtract background fluorescence. Cells in these wells were washed and fixed exactly like POS-treated cells.

7. Quantify the intensity of fluorescence signals in representative areas of each well using ImageQuant™ TL software (GE Healthcare). Calculate relative bound POS by subtracting average internal POS values from average total POS values for each sample.

3.4.2. Opsin
Immunoblotting

1. Use unlabeled POS or FITC-POS for the assay. Terminate phagocytosis by washing 3× with PBS-CM and designating triplicate samples as described in Subheading 3.4.1, steps 1 and 2.

2. To detect internalized POS only, rinse washed cells 1× with PBS, then incubate cells with PBS-EDTA for 5–10 min. Samples designated for total POS detection remain in PBS-CM.

3. Aspirate PBS-EDTA and wash wells 3× with PBS. No wait required between washes.

4. Aspirate PBS-CM from all wells and lyse cells with HNTG buffer freshly supplemented with protease inhibitor cocktail. Analyze phagocytosed POS content of samples by SDS-PAGE and opsin immunoblotting (see Notes 10 and 11). Numerous opsin antibodies are commercially available and will work well. Analyze triplicates on the same blot membrane to determine sample-to-sample variability.

5. Re-probe the same membranes for proteins unrelated to the phagocytic pathway to control for equal cell load in each sample (see Note 12). Figure 2 shows an example immunoblot

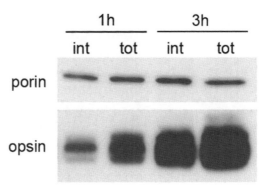

Fig. 2. Immunoblotting analysis of POS phagocytosis. Confluent, polarized RPE-J cells were challenged with unlabeled POS for 1 or 3 h before processing as described in Subheading 3.4.2. The same blot membrane was probed for porin as loading control and for opsin to indicate POS content as indicated. *int* cells treated with EDTA before lysis, samples show internalized POS opsin, *tot* cells lysed without EDTA treatment, samples show total (bound plus internal) POS opsin. As expected, cells bind and internalize increased numbers of POS with time.

detection of phagocytosed POS opsin and of the mitochondrial protein porin as a loading control.

6. Quantify bands representing internal or total POS and normalize POS content of individual samples for cell load as indicated by the loading control protein blot. Average triplicates.

3.4.3. Fluorescence Microscopy

Carry out all steps at room temperature.

1. Use FITC-OS for the phagocytosis assay. Terminate phagocytosis by washing 3× with PBS-CM as described in Subheading 3.4.1.

2. Fix cells with 4% PFA in PBS-CM for 20 min.

3. Quench remaining fixative by incubating cells in 50 mM NH_4Cl in PBS-CM for 20 min.

4. Block with 1% BSA in PBS-CM at RT for 10 min.

5. Incubate cells with opsin antibody diluted in 1% BSA in PBS-CM for 25 min (see Note 13).

6. Wash wells 2× with PBS-CM and 1× with 1% BSA in PBS-CM for 5 min each.

7. Incubate cells with appropriate secondary antibody conjugated with a fluorophore that does not conflict with FITC (e.g., AlexaFluor 568, 596, 647).

8. Wash wells 2× with PBS-CM for 5 min each, 1× with DAPI nuclei stain for 10 min (optional), and 1× with PBS-CM for 5 min.

9. Mount coverslips on microscopy slides with Fluoromount G.

10. Image FITC- and secondary antibody-derived fluorescence signals. Internalized POS will appear in the FITC image only. Surface-bound POS will appear both in the FITC image and in the secondary antibody image. In a color overlay of FITC (green) with secondary antibody (red), internal POS will appear green and surface-bound POS will appear yellow. The example in Fig. 3 shows images of the same field showing surface POS (left) and total FITC-POS (right).

11. Count total and surface-bound POS and cell nuclei in representative areas of at least 50 cells in each sample. Calculate bound POS/cell, total POS/cell, and internal POS/cell (by subtracting bound from total POS/cell). Average counts per cell obtained from triplicates.

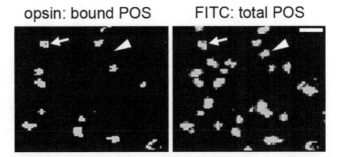

opsin: bound POS   FITC: total POS

Fig. 3. Microscopy analysis of POS phagocytosis. Unpassaged, polarized Long Evans (wild type) rat primary RPE cells were challenged with FITC-POS for 1 h before processing and imaging as described in Subheading 3.4.3. The *left panel* shows immunodetection of surface-bound (external) POS with rhodopsin antibody B6-30 (11) and AlexaFluor594-conjugated donkey anti-mouse IgG. The *right panel* shows the FITC fluorescence signal of total phagocytosed (bound plus internalized) POS in the same field. *Arrow* indicates bound POS, which is visible in both images. *Arrowhead* indicates internalized POS, which are only visible in the FITC image. Scale bar, 10 μm.

4. Notes

1. 25 Cow eyes or 35 calf eyes may be substituted for 75 pig eyes.

2. This is a messy procedure. Cover bench with absorbent pads and prepare 15 cm dishes or plastic trays to collect tissue waste, wear double lab coat and gloves.

3. Handle eyes and crude retinal isolate in dim red light only to avoid bleaching rhodopsin in POS fragments. The pink color of unbleached rhodopsin will allow easy identification of the tissue fraction containing the POS following gradient separation.

4. Depending on the quality of the gradient the band containing the POS particles may be more or less diffuse. Identify the right band by observing the bleaching of rhodopsin, which is visible as a color change from pink to beige. Mark band location on the centrifuge tube using permanent marker while observing the bleaching to ensure collection of the correct tissue fraction.

5. Most if not all RPE cells in culture retain phagocytic activity towards isolated POS. However, phagocytic capacity, pathways and mechanisms used may differ depending on the differentiation state of RPE cells. Different RPE cell lines and primary RPE cells take different periods of time to differentiate into an epithelial phenotype that best resembles RPE in the eye and to reach polarity in culture. Furthermore, RPE cells in culture

may dedifferentiate with time and passage especially if seeded at low confluence after split. We strongly recommend only using post-confluent, mature RPE monolayers for phagocytosis assays that have assembled the known components of the POS phagocytic machinery at their apical surface. It is useful to establish a successful protocol that ensures only high-quality RPE cells with reproducible phagocytic activity are used and to strictly adhere to the protocol for all studies. We also recommend using primary RPE that is unpassaged to maximize their resemblance to the RPE in the eye and to split stable RPE cells at low ratio (e.g., split ARPE-19 cells 1:2 every 2–4 weeks, split RPE-J cells 1:4 exactly 1× per week) to allow the cells to maintain an epithelial phenotype at all times.

6. POS should not be refrozen.

7. Different RPE cell models bind and engulf POS with different kinetics. Furthermore, time of phagocytic challenge may be chosen to represent primarily active POS binding (early phase of uptake), ongoing binding and internalization, or primarily active internalization of bound POS (late phase of uptake). Suggested times of POS challenge based on our work: RPE cell lines, 2–5 h (8); unpassaged primary rat or mouse RPE cells, 30 min to 2 h (3, 10).

8. Aspirate solution completely for every change of solution by holding the plate at a 45° angle. Keep aspirator tip steady, reaching into the bottom of the well and facing the same side of the well for all steps to minimize cell layer damage.

9. After rehydration, cell nuclei may also be stained, e.g., with DAPI. However, note that trypan blue quenching will cause high red background fluorescence emission. This precludes using red fluorescing nuclei counterstains such as propidium iodide for trypan blue treated samples.

10. Apply samples to gels immediately following addition of reducing SDS-sample buffer. Boiling samples cause formation of opsin multimers making opsin quantification ambiguous.

11. It is important to consider stability of epitopes recognized to lysosomal protein degradation when choosing an opsin antibody for the detection of phagocytosed POS. This is particularly relevant when studying late phases of POS phagocytosis during which POS opsin will be degraded.

12. Proteins chosen as loading controls need to be detectable in unboiled samples and must not fluctuate with POS phagocytosis. Examples include VDAC/porin mitochondrial protein and α- or β-tubulins. Actin should not be used because it is directly involved in POS phagocytosis and its level or stability may change during the experiment.

13. Without permeabilization, only external opsin will be detected if incubation with primary antibody is short. After incubation with primary antibody overnight at 4°C some antibody may enter cells causing ambiguous results.

Acknowledgment

This work was supported by NIH grant EY013295.

References

1. Strauss O (2005) The retinal pigment epithelium in visual function. Physiol Rev 85:845–881

2. LaVail MM (1976) Rod outer segment disk shedding in rat retina: relationship to cyclic lighting. Science 194:1071–1074

3. Nandrot EF, Kim Y, Brodie SE, Huang X, Sheppard D, Finnemann SC (2004) Loss of synchronized retinal phagocytosis and age-related blindness in mice lacking αvβ5 integrin. J Exp Med 200:1539–1545

4. Mayerson PL, Hall MO (1986) Rat retinal pigment epithelial cells show specificity of phagocytosis in vitro. J Cell Biol 103:299–308

5. Nabi IR, Mathews AP, Cohen-Gould L, Gundersen D, Rodriguez-Boulan E (1993) Immortalization of polarized rat retinal pigment epithelium. J Cell Sci 104:37–49

6. Davis AA, Bernstein PS, Bok D, Turner J, Nachtigal M, Hunt RC (1995) A human retinal pigment epithelial cell line that retains epithelial characteristics after prolonged culture. Invest Ophthalmol Vis Sci 36:955–964

7. Dunn KC, Aotaki-Keen AE, Putkey FR, Hjelmeland LM (1996) ARPE-19, a human retinal pigment epithelial cell line with differentiated properties. Exp Eye Res 62:155–169

8. Finnemann SC, Bonilha VL, Marmorstein AD, Rodriguez-Boulan E (1997) Phagocytosis of rod outer segments by retinal pigment epithelial cells requires αvβ5 integrin for binding but not for internalization. Proc Natl Acad Sci U S A 94:12932–12937

9. Molday RS, Hicks D, Molday L (1987) Peripherin. A rim-specific membrane protein of rod outer segment discs. Invest Ophthalmol Vis Sci 28:50–61

10. Finnemann SC (2003) Focal adhesion kinase signaling promotes phagocytosis of integrin-bound photoreceptors. EMBO J 22:4143–4154

11. Adamus G, Zam ZS, Arendt A, Palczewski K, McDowell JH, Hargrave PA (1991) Anti-rhodopsin monoclonal antibodies of defined specificity: characterization and application. Vision Res 31:17–31

Chapter 21

Ca²⁺-Imaging Techniques to Analyze Ca²⁺ Signaling in Cells and to Monitor Neuronal Activity in the Retina

Olaf Strauß

Abstract

Ca²⁺ is an important regulator of many cell functions including proliferation, apoptosis, movements, secretion, contraction, excitation, and differentiation. The regulation of these different cell functions is encoded by the specific temporal and spatial distribution of Ca²⁺ signals. In degenerative diseases mutations can lead to changes in cell functions in the worst case to apoptosis. Thus analysis of signals arising as changes in intracellular free Ca²⁺ represent an important step towards the understanding of mutation-dependent or environmental impact into cell function. The classic approach to study changes in intracellular free Ca²⁺ is the measurement of intracellular Ca²⁺ by using Ca²⁺-sensitive fluorescence dyes in conjunction with fluorescence microscopy as a method called Ca²⁺ imaging.

In this chapter the basic method and a short theoretical background will be provided to perform Ca²⁺-imaging experiments. As a model cultured retinal pigment epithelial cells will be used. The basic steps of the method are the loading of the cells with the fluorescence dye by incubation with a membrane permeable ester of the dye. The next step would be the application of an agonist which can be further analyzed by blockers of enzymes or by manipulating the different Ca²⁺-storing compartments which contribute to changes in intracellular free Ca²⁺. At the end of an experiment an on-cell type of calibration will be performed to calculate the underlying concentration of intracellular free Ca²⁺. Furthermore, the successful calibration of an experiment can be used as a measure of a reliable experiment. In addition to that, three examples for basic experiments will be given which can lead to a first insight into the mechanism underlying changes in cytosolic free Ca²⁺ as a second messenger.

Key words: Ca²⁺-imaging fura-2, Retinal pigment epithelium, Thapsigargin, Ca²⁺, Second messenger

1. Introduction

Ca²⁺ is the ion with the highest binding affinity to proteins. Binding of Ca²⁺ to proteins change their three-dimensional structure and lead to a change of their function (1, 2). Therefore, cells keep their intracellular free Ca²⁺ at very small concentrations (basal concentration approximately 100 nM) (3–8). This requires a large amount of energy because cells maintain a transmembranal gradient of Ca²⁺ of

Bernhard H.F. Weber and Thomas Langmann (eds.), *Retinal Degeneration: Methods and Protocols*, Methods in Molecular Biology, vol. 935, DOI 10.1007/978-1-62703-080-9_21, © Springer Science+Business Media, LLC 2013

1:10,000. However, cells can use this Ca^{2+} affinity to proteins for Ca^{2+}-dependent regulation of cellular functions. In fact, nearly every cellular function such as proliferation, movement, secretion, apoptosis, information processing, or regulation of gene expression is depending on changes in intracellular free Ca^{2+}. That cells can regulate so many functions by Ca^{2+} relies on the ability to generate a multitude of different and highly specific Ca^{2+} signals which differ in their spatial and temporal distribution (3–7, 9–11). That is achieved by the use of a specific selection of different types of Ca^{2+} transporting mechanisms such as ion channels, ion transporters, and ATPases in conjunction with different Ca^{2+} pools such as mitochondria, ER Ca^{2+} stores, endosomes, or extracellular Ca^{2+}. Thus, methods to analyze Ca^{2+} signals in cells represent key technologies to understand cell function and the mechanisms underlying their regulation. Furthermore, the detection of Ca^{2+} signals per se enables to monitor neuronal activity and how this activity leads to signal processing in networks. The latter function cannot be monitored by standard electrophysiology techniques in that resolution.

The analysis of Ca^{2+} signals in cells or in networks of cells is based on fluorescence microscopy. The development of Ca^{2+}-sensitive fluorescence dyes represents the first breakthrough of this technology (12–15). The development of new microscope technologies such as two-photon microscopy further enabled to exploit that approach to the analysis of subcellular Ca^{2+} signaling events such as Ca^{2+} puffs or to the understanding of network function such as in the detection of direction-sensitive amacrine cells in the retina. The technique can be applied to cultured cells as well as in situ preparations such as retinal slices. Roger Y. Tsien received 2008 the Nobel Prize for the discovery and development fluorescent dyes and their usage including the detection of Ca^{2+} signals. Among many other tools, he invented the first type of fluorescence dye-based Ca^{2+} signal analysis using the dye fura-2 which is still in use (12).

The basic principle is that a Ca^{2+}-sensitive fluorescence dye in the cytosol is excited by light of a specific wavelength. Ca^{2+}-binding to the dye then leads to changes in the fluorescence intensity which can be used to calculate the intracellular Ca^{2+} concentration in the cell. The fluorescence dyes are either loaded to the cell by incubation with a membrane-permeable ester of the dye which is then trapped inside the cell by activity of esterases or it is present in the cytosol by genetic intervention to produce transgenic animals showing a tissue-specific expression of Ca^{2+}-sensitive fluorescent proteins. Ratiometric measurements allow the calculation of the concentration of intracellular free Ca^{2+} after a calibration procedure (12–15). The selection of the appropriate dyes depends on the microscope technology so that for simple Ca^{2+}-imaging experiments with conventional microscopes fura-2 is preferable. In conjunction with confocal or two-photon microscopy other dyes will be used for which a large selection is available. The ratiometric measurement is based on the usage of two excitation wavelengths

(13, 15). Their emission is recorded separately. The ratio of the fluorescence intensity of these two wavelengths is used to calculate the concentration of intracellular free Ca^{2+}.

Based on this principle a large variety of technologies has been developed with different approaches to study Ca^{2+} signaling. Examples of these technologies are recovery after bleach measurements or detection of Ca^{2+} signals in organelles or in submembranal areas (13, 14, 16–18). Furthermore, even other types of ions can be measured such as Cl^-. In this chapter the simplest of these methods will be explained because it is a basis also to learn and perform other applications. The chapter is organized into the description of the basic method, data analysis, and three examples of experimental procedures to identify Ca^{2+} pools involved in generation of Ca^{2+} signals. The method is described for retinal pigment epithelial cells.

2. Materials

2.1. Equipment

Central part of the technique is a conventional fluorescence microscope equipped with a long distance fluorescence ocular and 40× magnification. The stage is equipped with a perfusion chamber which allows the constant superfusion of the cells and fast exchange between different types of bath solutions (see Note 1). Attached to the microscope is a polychromator which can provide light of different freely selectable wavelengths. The light source is a Xenon lamp. To excite fluorescence and to measure emission at the same time light is conducted to the cells through a dichroitic filter system and an appropriate emission filter. Excitation wavelengths for fura-2 are 340 and 380 nm, emission wavelength is 520 nm. The signal is digitalized by an ultra-sensitive camera. The microscope and polychromator is controlled in conjunction with specialized software for data acquisition and analysis.

2.2. Solutions and Cells

1. Ringer bath solution (see Note 2): 130 mM NaCl, 5 mM KCl, 2 mM $MgCl_2$, 2 mM $CaCl_2$, 10 mM HEPES, 5 mM glucose; pH adjusted to 7.3 with NaOH.

2. Ca^{2+}-free solution for calibration: 130 mM NaCl, 5 mM KCl, 2 mM $MgCl_2$, 1 mM EGTA, 10 mM HEPES, 5 mM glucose; pH adjusted to 7.3 with NaOH plus 1 μM ionomycin.

3. Stock solution ionomycin: 1–4 mM in DMSO.

4. Stock solution fura-2-AM: 1–2 mM in DMSO.

5. Human RPE cell line or primary cultures of human, rat, mouse, or porcine RPE cells can be used. To prepare freshly isolated cells sheets of RPE cells were removed from Bruch's membrane by gentle trypsination and placed on poly-L-lysine coated coverslips.

3. Methods

1. Loading of cells with fura-2: Cultured or freshly isolated cells (attached to a coverslip) were removed from the cell culture medium and incubated in Ringer solution with 10 µM fura-AM for 40 min at 37°C (see Note 3).

2. Preparation of the cells for measurements: All further experiments will be performed at room temperature. Cells are placed into the perfusion chamber at the stage of the microscope. The superfusion with Ringer should be started immediately. In a first observation under fluorescence conditions the cells must shine brightly. Furthermore, residuals of nonincorporated fura-2-AM are visible. The superfusion should be continued to wash away these residual mounts of fura-2-AM. The experiment can now be started.

3. Experiment: For the experiment the fluorescence of fura-2 is recorded. The fluorescence will intermittedly excited at 340 and 380 nm. The fluorescence of both wavelengths is recorded. The fluorescence excited at 340 nm increases with an increase of cytosolic Ca^{2+}, whereas the fluorescence excited at 380 nm decreases with increases in intracellular free Ca^{2+}. Thus in response to application of an agonist which increases intracellular Ca^{2+} the fluorescence of the two excitation wavelengths behaves antiparallel (see Note 4). The experiment should be monitored by the continuous plotting of the fluorescence ratio of the excitation wavelengths 340 and 380 nm. After starting the computer-based acquisition in many cases the cells show no stable Ca^{2+} signals (fluorescence ratios). Before starting the experiment a stable baseline should be awaited. For an experiment usually an agonist is applied dissolved in Ringer solution (see Note 5).

4. Controls: For further analysis of the agonist-stimulated Ca^{2+} signals usually blockers are applied either before or with the agonist at the same time (see Note 5). In order to monitor differences under these two conditions the exertion of a double application paradigm is useful (Fig. 2). For this paradigm control experiments are required: the agonist is applied two times in consequence; each time for the same duration and the same recovery time between the two applications. When in the next experiment a blocker is used than again the agonist is applied first without blocker to monitor how the individual cells responds to that agonist and now in the second application the agonist is applied in the presence of the blocker to monitor the effect of the blocker. With this procedure differences in the individual reaction can be shown in relation to the blocker effect.

5. On cell calibration: Fluorescence ratios can be used to calculate the concentration of intracellular free Ca^{2+} using the relation between Ca^{2+} concentration, concentration of fura-2, and the

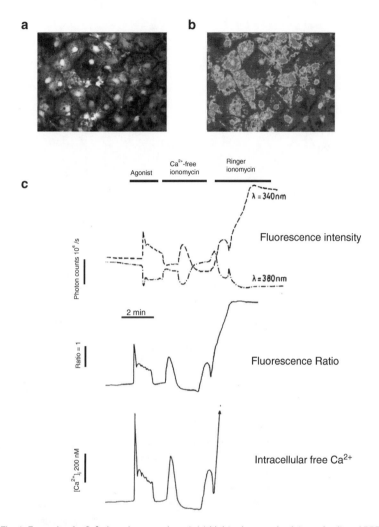

Fig. 1. Example of a Ca²⁺-imaging experiment. (**a**) Light microscopic picture of cultured RPE cells. (**b**) Fura-2 fluorescence in the same cells. Different shades of grey indicate different fluorescence nations and therefore different Ca²⁺ concentrations in individual cells. (**c**) Calculation of the concentration of intracellular free Ca²⁺: *Upper panel* shows the change of the fura-2 fluorescence after application of an agonist and following on cell calibration by depleting fura-2 from Ca²⁺ (Ca²⁺ plus ionomycin) and by saturating fura-2 with Ca²⁺ (Ringer plus ionomycin) for each excitation wavelength 340 and 380 nm separately; note that fluorescence at 340 nm excitation increases with increase in intracellular free Ca²⁺ and that fluorescence at 380 nm decreases with increase in intracellular free Ca²⁺. *Middle panel* shows the ratio of the fluorescence excited at 340 and 380 nm from the same experiment. *Lower panel* shows the calculated concentration of intracellular free Ca²⁺ from this experiment.

fluorescence intensity. As will be described below the usage of the fluorescence ratios enables the calculation of Ca²⁺ concentration independently from the concentration of fura-2 in the cells. For this equation the fluorescence of the fura-2 which is free of Ca²⁺ and the fluorescence of fura-2 which saturated with

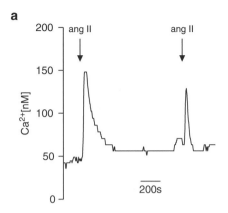

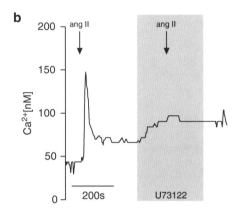

Fig. 2. Example: Analysis of Ca²⁺-signaling pathway using a double application paradigm.
(**a**) Control experiment: The figure shows biphasic Ca²⁺ transients which were stimulated
by AngII application. Note that the Ca²⁺ transient during the second application is a little
bit smaller. (**b**) Check for the contribution of phospholipase C: The same experiment was
performed after an initial AngII application under control conditions a second AngII application was performed in the presence of the phospholipase C blocker U73122. The first
AngII-induced Ca²⁺ peak can be used as internal control of that experiment.

Ca²⁺ are required. These fluorescence values will be obtained by
on cell calibration. After finishing the experiment the fluorescence
will be measured under Ca²⁺-depletion of fura-2 (see Note 6).
For this purpose cells will be superfused by the Ca²⁺-free solution which contains 1 μM ionomycin (see Note 7). Ionomycin
should be freshly added from stock solution which is kept at
4°C. Under these conditions the fluorescence ratio which indicates the concentration of intracellular free Ca²⁺ decreases to
values much smaller than resting levels of the cells. Once the
ratio has reached a new steady state, the bath solution is switched
back to Ringer solution with 1 μM ionomycin. Now the
fluorescence ratio increases to values far above the peak of the
agonist-stimulated signal (see Note 8). Also this value should
reach a steady state. With this the experiment is terminated.

3.2. Data Analysis

Basics: For the data analysis the concentration of the cytosolic free Ca^{2+} is calculated from the calibration procedure (12, 13, 15). The equation to do this uses the ratio of the equilibrium equation of fura-2 and Ca^{2+} for both wavelengths:

$$[Ca^{2+}] = K_d * (R - R_{min}) / (R_{max} - R) * S_f / S_b.$$

In this equation, R is the fluorescence intensity ratio $(F(340)/F(380))$, R_{min} the value where R is minimal (with EGTA and ionomycin) and R_{max} the value when R is maximal (with saturating Ca^{2+} and ionomycin). K_d represents the dissociation constant of Fura-2 (224 nM) (12), and S_f and S_b are the maximum and the minimum fluorescence, respectively, after excitation with 380 nm.

The equation is normally installed in most of the software packages for data analysis of Ca^{2+}-imaging experiments. Usually the procedure of data analysis requires the following steps:

1. From the fluorescence images areas of interests will be defined. These can be entire cells or subcellular areas. From these areas the fluorescence values will be loaded from the data files.

2. Data are plotted as the fluorescence excited at 340 and 380 nm and the corresponding fluorescence ratio against the time of the experiment. Basic parameters from calibration will be loaded from the data and put into the equation. The software will calculate the Ca^{2+} concentration over the area for each of the selected areas.

3. For statistic analysis many cells from one experiment can be used for calculation of Ca^{2+} concentration. However data from at least five individual independent experiments should be used. This would result in for example 30 cells from five experiments. For statistical testing all cells of one group can be used.

3.3. Examples for Strategies to Identify a Source of Ca²⁺ Contributing to Rises in Intracellular Free Ca²⁺

As mentioned above, the specific effect of a Ca^{2+} signal depends on the spatial and temporal distribution of the signal. This pattern is achieved by recruitment of different Ca^{2+} stores, Ca^{2+} channels or Ca^{2+} transporters involved the reaction (3–7, 9–11, 19, 20). Thus the understanding of the functional relevance of Ca^{2+} signal depends on the analysis of the mechanisms contributing to the Ca^{2+} signal. Basically two major sources can be involved the generation of Ca^{2+} signals: cytosolic Ca^{2+} stores or influx of Ca^{2+} from extracellular space. Ca^{2+} signals can arise from either only store depletion, only Ca^{2+}-influx or the combination of both. So usually the first step in the analysis of Ca^{2+} signals would be to clarify which parts of the signal are generated from cytosolic Ca^{2+} stores and which parts arise from influx of Ca^{2+} from extracellular space. In the following, examples for methods will be described to perform this preliminary analysis.

3.3.1. Example 1, Contribution of Extracellular Ca²⁺

1. After reaching a stable baseline the agonist of interest is applied.

2. Wash-out of the agonist and waiting for the complete recovery.

3. Changing from a control ringer solution to a extracellular Ca^{2+} free solution (same solution as Ringer with no Ca^{2+} but contains additional 1 mM EGTA).

4. Application of the agonist under extracellular Ca^{2+}-free conditions.

5. Two possible results can be expected. One is that there is no Ca^{2+} increase by application of the agonist under extracellular Ca^{2+}-free conditions. This means that the whole signal depends on an influx of extracellular Ca^{2+} into the cell. A second possibility can be seen in biphasic Ca^{2+} signals. Here it is possible that only one part, mostly the initial peak phase, is unchanged and the following plateau phase is lacking. Thus the second phase of the biphasic Ca^{2+} signal is depending on a Ca^{2+} influx into the cell (see Note 9).

3.3.2. Example 2, Contribution of Cytosolic Ca²⁺ Stores

1. After reaching a stable baseline the agonist of interest is applied.

2. Wash-out of the agonist and waiting for the complete recovery.

3. Application of thapsigargin (1 µM) an inhibitor of the endoplasmic reticulum Ca^{2+}-ATPase (SERCA), wait until the transient Ca^{2+} has recovered back to the baseline.

4. Application of the agonist again in the presence of thapsigargin. If the agonist now fails to increase intracellular free Ca^{2+} than the release of Ca^{2+} from endoplasmic reticulum is required to initialize the agonist-dependent Ca^{2+} transients.

3.3.3. Example 3, Activation of Store-Operated Ca²⁺ Channels (Fig. 3)

1. After reaching a stable baseline change to extracellular Ca^{2+}-free solution and apply thapsigargin (1 µM).

2. After the transient Ca^{2+} increases due to the application of thapsigargin the base line usually returns to steady-state which is below the resting Ca^{2+} level thapsigargin is washed out. Under these conditions now the cytosolic Ca^{2+} stores are emptied.

3. Return back to the normal Ca^{2+} containing Ringer solution. Under these conditions the concentration of intracellular free Ca^{2+} should increase to levels which are far above the resting Ca^{2+}. The amplitude of this Ca^{2+} increase reflects the activation of store-operated Ca^{2+} channels such as Orai (see Note 10) (7, 9, 11, 20–25).

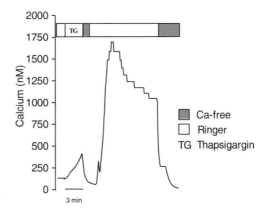

Fig. 3. Induction of store-operated Ca²⁺ entry. After reaching a baseline thapsigargin was applied which inhibits the cytosolic Ca²⁺ store Ca²⁺-ATPase (SERCA). In consequence Ca²⁺ leaks out of cytosolic Ca²⁺ stores leading to an increase in intracellular free Ca²⁺. In the presence of thapsigargin cells were exposed to extracellular Ca²-free solutions to completely empty the Ca²⁺ stores leading to an intracellular Ca²⁺ concentration which is below the base line under resting conditions. Now extracellular Ca²⁺ is re-added to the bath solution in the absence of thapsigargin and a strong increase in intracellular free Ca²⁺ can be observed. That this increase is dependent on extracellular Ca²⁺ can be shown by removing extracellular Ca²⁺ which results in a decrease back to the resting level.

4. Notes

1. There are quite a lot of different companies who offer systems to perform these experiments. Mostly these companies deliver conventional microscopes in conjunction with polychromators, adapted optics (mirrors and filters), camera and hard- and software for data acquisition and analysis. However, some of the items such as perfusion chamber to be mounted on stage of the microscope and the adequate perfusion system need to be produced according to the needs of the projects. These items should be produced custom made, probably by the work shop of the Institute.

2. Here only an example for an extracellular solution is given. It should be adapted to the cell type and species. HEPES buffering is of advantage but HCO_3/CO_2 buffering works as well.

3. The loading of fura-2 should be adapted to each individual cell type. Variations are mostly in the incubation temperature and time. Since fura-2 is a Ca²⁺ buffer as well, too high intracellular concentrations of fura-2 are toxic. Also too long durations for incubation are of disadvantage. Cells tend to eliminate fura-2 from intracellular space. Fluorescence signals can be enhanced by avoiding fura-2 micelle formation using a detergent such as pluronic-F127 or by inhibiting the ATPase which transport fura-2 out of the cell probenicid. For this purpose the incubation

solution contains for example 5 μM fura-2 together with 0.02 % pluronic-F127. However, it should be noted that some of these substances might disturb the intracellular Ca^{2+} signaling as well (26).

4. Before calculating the ratio or the Ca^{2+} concentration, the behavior of the two excitation wavelengths should be controlled. Only courses of the fluorescence ratio from the two excitation wavelengths which result from an antiparallel progression of the fluorescence intensities can be regarded to result from changes in intracellular free Ca^{2+}. In the case of fluorescence intensity changes at only one wavelength the overall fluorescence is too weak. In the case that the fluorescence of the two excitation wavelengths increases or decreases in parallel then the calculated ratio does not reflect changes in intracellular free Ca^{2+}. This can happen when a substance which shows fluorescence by itself is added to the bath solution or when the cells are undergoing damage and the fura-2 is lost.

5. Care has to be taken when certain agonists or blockers were used which are not freely dissolvable in water. Usually these substances are dissolved in hydrophobic solvents such as DMSO or ethanol. When preparing the test solutions one should take care that the final concentration of the hydrophobic solvent does not increase above 0.1 %. Furthermore, another problem arises from light-sensitive properties of substances. One problem can be that the substance itself has fluorescence properties. In this case the agonist or blocker would increase the fluorescence in an unspecific way resulting in false positive or negative effects (see Note 4). Usually this can be seen in parallel shifts in fluorescence intensity of the two excitations wavelengths. These substances should be avoided. The other problem is that the substance is unstable in intense light. The fluorescence of fura-2 is excited at the UV spectrum of light. This has a large energy and can lead to destruction of the substance and reduction of its active concentration. Examples are dihydropyridine derivates used as Ca^{2+} channel blockers.

6. It is of advantage to start the calibration procedure with Ca^{2+}-depletion of fura-2. The second the step, the saturation of fura-2 by Ca^{2+} requires high concentrations of intracellular free Ca^{2+} which can be toxic for cells. Thus in the case when starting the calibration procedure with fura-2 Ca^{2+} saturation then the cell will probably die before there is time to perform the Ca^{2+}-depletion of fura-2.

7. Ionomycin is a Ca^{2+} ionophore which is used to permeabilize the cell membrane for Ca^{2+} ions. The substance is rather unstable and the ability to increase the Ca^{2+} permeability is quickly reduced so that the substance cannot be longer used. Therefore, if possible, the solution for calibration should be freshly prepared.

8. To achieve the fluorescence signal of the Ca²⁺-depleted fura-2 and the Ca²⁺saturated fura-2 it is required that for both situations a steady-state level in intracellular free Ca²⁺ is achieved. Especially when waiting for the Ca²⁺-saturated fluorescence the cell can die and the according fluorescence maximum cannot be measured. In this case the calibration would lead to wrong results. Furthermore, a successful calibration after an experiment can be used as a marker for reliable experiments. Therefore, if desired, only experiments with successful calibrations will be used for data analysis and statistical testing.

9. As for all example experiments the expected results can strongly vary. Most of the time, this depends on the nature of the signaling pathway which is addressed by the analysis. The described experiments give only initial hints to the analysis and further experiments are required to confirm these initial conclusions. However these experiments are useful to obtain a direction for further analysis.

10. The experiments in which intracellular Ca²⁺ stores are depleted must be taken with great care. In some cell types it is sufficient to only apply extracellular Ca²⁺-free solution which also leads to store depletion due to the change of the Ca²⁺ gradient. These cells usually have a large basic Ca²⁺ conductance and this high Ca²⁺ permeability would lead to this effect (8). In these cells store-operated Ca²⁺ channels can simply be activated by switching from extracellular Ca²⁺ solution and then back normal control Ringer solution. This can lead to problems in the interpretation of the data and the experiment type shown in example is not useful to explore the role of intracellular Ca²⁺ stores in a Ca²⁺ signal.

References

1. Carafoli E (2005) Calcium—a universal carrier of biological signals. Delivered on 3 July 2003 at the Special FEBS Meeting in Brussels. FEBS J 272:1073–1089

2. Williams RJ (1974) Calcium ions: their ligands and their functions. Biochem Soc Symp 39: 133–138

3. Berridge MJ (2005) Unlocking the secrets of cell signaling. Annu Rev Physiol 67:1–21

4. Berridge MJ (2009) Inositol trisphosphate and calcium signalling mechanisms. Biochim Biophys Acta 1793:933–940

5. Camello C, Lomax R, Petersen OH, Tepikin AV (2002) Calcium leak from intracellular stores—the enigma of calcium signalling. Cell Calcium 32:355–361

6. Petersen OH, Michalak M, Verkhratsky A (2005) Calcium signalling: past, present and future. Cell Calcium 38:161–169

7. Petersen OH, Tepikin A, Park MK (2001) The endoplasmic reticulum: one continuous or several separate Ca(2+) stores? Trends Neurosci 24:271–276

8. Wimmers S, Strauss O (2007) Basal calcium entry in retinal pigment epithelial cells is mediated by TRPC channels. Invest Ophthalmol Vis Sci 48:5767–5772

9. Berridge MJ (2006) Calcium microdomains: organization and function. Cell Calcium 40:405–412

10. Berridge MJ (2008) Smooth muscle cell calcium activation mechanisms. J Physiol 586:5047–5061

11. Putney JW (2009) Capacitative calcium entry: from concept to molecules. Immunol Rev 231:10–22

12. Grynkiewicz G, Poenie M, Tsien RY (1985) A new generation of Ca2+ indicators with greatly improved fluorescence properties. J Biol Chem 260:3440–3450

13. Hayashi H, Miyata H (1994) Fluorescence imaging of intracellular Ca2+. J Pharmacol Toxicol Methods 31:1–10

14. Knot HJ, Laher I, Sobie EA, Guatimosim S, Gomez-Viquez L, Hartmann H, Song LS, Lederer WJ, Graier WF, Malli R, Frieden M, Petersen OH (2005) Twenty years of calcium imaging: cell physiology to dye for. Mol Interv 5:112–127

15. O'Connor N, Silver RB (2007) Ratio imaging: practical considerations for measuring intracellular Ca2+ and pH in living cells. Methods Cell Biol 81:415–433

16. Denk W, Delaney KR, Gelperin A, Kleinfeld D, Strowbridge BW, Tank DW, Yuste R (1994) Anatomical and functional imaging of neurons using 2-photon laser scanning microscopy. J Neurosci Methods 54:151–162

17. Schmolze DB, Standley C, Fogarty KE, Fischer AH (2011) Advances in microscopy techniques. Arch Pathol Lab Med 135:255–263

18. Tian GF, Takano T, Lin JH, Wang X, Bekar L, Nedergaard M (2006) Imaging of cortical astrocytes using 2-photon laser scanning microscopy in the intact mouse brain. Adv Drug Deliv Rev 58:773–787

19. Kurosaki T, Baba Y (2010) Ca2+ signaling and STIM1. Prog Biophys Mol Biol 103:51–58

20. Parekh AB (2010) Store-operated CRAC channels: function in health and disease. Nat Rev Drug Discov 9:399–410

21. Cordeiro S, Strauss O (2010) Expression of Orai genes and I(CRAC) activation in the human retinal pigment epithelium. Graefes Arch Clin Exp Ophthalmol 249:47–54

22. Neussert R, Muller C, Milenkovic VM, Strauss O (2010) The presence of bestrophin-1 modulates the Ca2+ recruitment from Ca2+ stores in the ER. Pflugers Arch 460:163–175

23. Roberts-Thomson SJ, Peters AA, Grice DM, Monteith GR (2010) ORAI-mediated calcium entry: mechanism and roles, diseases and pharmacology. Pharmacol Ther 127:121–130

24. Smyth JT, Hwang SY, Tomita T, DeHaven WI, Mercer JC, Putney JW (2010) Activation and regulation of store-operated calcium entry. J Cell Mol Med 14:2337–2349

25. Vaca L (2010) SOCIC: the store-operated calcium influx complex. Cell Calcium 47:199–209

26. Yates SL, Fluhler EN, Lippiello PM (1992) Advances in the use of the fluorescent probe fura-2 for the estimation of intrasynaptosomal calcium. J Neurosci Res 32:255–260

Part VI

Gene Regulation

Double Chromatin Immunoprecipitation: Analysis of Target Co-occupancy of Retinal Transcription Factors

Guang-Hua Peng and Shiming Chen

Abstract

Combinatorial binding of transcription factors (TFs) and cofactors to specific regulatory regions of target genes in vivo is an important mechanism of transcriptional regulation. Chromatin immunoprecipitation (ChIP) is a powerful technique to detect protein binding to specific regions of target genes in vivo. However, conventional ChIP analysis for individual factors (single ChIP) does not provide information on co-occupancy of two interacting TFs on target genes, even if both bind to the same chromatin regions. Double ChIP analysis involves sequential (double) immunoprecipitation of two chromatin-binding proteins and can be used to study co-occupancy of two or more factors on specific regions of the same DNA allele. Furthermore, by including a cell type-specific protein in double-ChIP, target co-occupancy in a specific cell type can be studied even if the other partner is more widely expressed. In this chapter, we describe a detailed protocol for double ChIP analysis in mouse retinas. Using the rod-specific transcription factor NR2E3 and the cone/rod homeobox protein CRX as examples, we show that NR2E3 and CRX are co-enriched on the promoter of active *Rho* and *Rbp3* genes in rods, but are present to a much lesser degree on the promoters of silent cone *opsin* genes. These results suggest a new mechanism by which rod and cone genes are differentially regulated by these transcription factors in rod photoreceptors.

Key words: Double chromatin immunoprecipitation, Transcription factor interactions, Target co-occupancy, Retinal photoreceptors

1. Introduction

Physical and functional interaction among multiple DNA binding proteins on target genes is an important mechanism of transcriptional regulation. However, conventional protein–protein interaction assays such as co-immunoprecipitation and co-localization in the same nuclear compartment do not provide information about whether both proteins interact with the same target gene allele. Thus, a combined in vivo protein–DNA and protein–protein interaction assay is needed to study this transcription regulatory

Bernhard H.F. Weber and Thomas Langmann (eds.), *Retinal Degeneration: Methods and Protocols*, Methods in Molecular Biology, vol. 935, DOI 10.1007/978-1-62703-080-9_22, © Springer Science+Business Media, LLC 2013

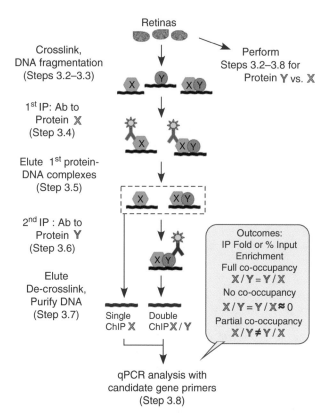

Retinas

Crosslink,
DNA fragmentation
(Steps 3.2–3.3)

Perform
Steps 3.2–3.8 for
Protein $\mathbb{Y}$ vs. $\mathbb{X}$

1st IP: Ab to
Protein $\mathbb{X}$
(Step 3.4)

Elute 1st protein-
DNA complexes
(Step 3.5)

2nd IP : Ab to
Protein $\mathbb{Y}$
(Step 3.6)

Elute
De-crosslink,
Purify DNA
(Step 3.7)

Single
ChIP $\mathbb{X}$

Double
ChIP $\mathbb{X}$ / $\mathbb{Y}$

Outcomes:
IP Fold or % Input
Enrichment
Full co-occupancy
$\mathbb{X}$ / $\mathbb{Y}$ = $\mathbb{Y}$ / $\mathbb{X}$
No co-occupancy
$\mathbb{X}$ / $\mathbb{Y}$ = $\mathbb{Y}$ / $\mathbb{X}$ ≈ 0
Partial co-occupancy
$\mathbb{X}$ / $\mathbb{Y}$ ≠ $\mathbb{Y}$ / $\mathbb{X}$

qPCR analysis with
candidate gene primers
(Step 3.8)

Fig. 1. Diagram of double ChIP protocol, showing major steps described in the text and interpretations based on quantitative double ChIP results.

mechanism. Double chromatin immunoprecipitation (double ChIP) is such an assay for detecting the genomic DNA fragments that co-immunoprecipitate with two DNA-binding proteins (1, 2). Based on regular ChIP (single ChIP), which uses a single round of immunoprecipitation to detect binding of an individual factor to target DNA fragments, double ChIP contains two sequential immunoprecipitation steps as shown in Fig. 1. Following the first immunoprecipitation, enriched protein–DNA complex is eluted and subjected to another round of immunoprecipitation for the second protein. DNA segments enriched by the double immuno-precipitation are then analyzed by quantitative PCR (qChIP). For each protein pair, two parallel double ChIPs are carried out in reverse order for the first and second protein. The results of two reciprocal double qChIPs are then compared with each single qChIP to determine full, partial, or no co-occupancy of the two proteins on the same allele. Interactions among multiple factors can also be studied by analyzing one pair at a time.

The DNA-binding proteins most frequently investigated by double ChIP include specific transcription factors and their co-regulators (3–7), histone modifying enzymes and chromatin remodeling factors (8, 9), modified histones (10), and components of the basal transcription machinery (9). Although the initial double ChIP protocol is based on readout of selected candidate genes, this approach combined with deep sequencing has recently been used to reveal genome-wide target co-occupancy of two DNA-binding proteins (11). We have used double ChIP to study co-occupancy of photoreceptor transcription factors and their co-regulators on candidate rod and cone target genes in mouse retinas. In one study, we showed that, in rods, single chromatin fragments of several rod and cone gene promoters are selectively co-bound by the rod-specific transcription factor NR2E3 and widely expressed PIAS3, a transcription co-regulator and SUMO E3 ligase (12). In another study, we showed that in cones, cone genes, but not rod genes, are co-occupied by the cone-specific transcription factor TRβ2 and PIAS3 (13). These results provided important information on the direct regulatory role of PIAS3 in photoreceptor subtype-specific gene expression. Here we describe a detailed protocol for double ChIP analysis of photoreceptor transcription regulators on selected candidate genes in the mouse retina and discuss critical steps for this assay. In addition, we describe an example of the use of this approach to reveal selective co-enrichment of the rod-specific transcription factor NR2E3 and the cone–rod homeobox protein CRX on the promoter of two rod-expressed genes, *rhodopsin* and *Rbp3*.

2. Materials

2.1. Equipment

1. Rotators: e.g., Rugged rotator (Fisher 14-259-21) or Multi-Function Rotator-30RPM, PTR-30 (VWR, 80076-366).

2. Incubator shaker or shaking water bath: e.g., SWB25 shaking water bath (Thermo Scientific).

3. Real-time PCR machine: e.g., CFX96™ Real-Time PCR System (Bio-Rad).

4. Sonicator: e.g., Model 505 Sonic Dismembrator (Fisher, FB-505-110) with microtip (0.5–15 mL, FB-441-8) for direct sonication, or Cup Horn (eight sample size, FB-462-5) for indirect sonication through water.

5. Centrifuge and microcentrifuge: e.g., Beckman GS-15R refrigerated centrifuge (BECKGS15R) for 15–50 mL tubes and Eppendorf microcentrifuge for 1.5 mL tubes (5418, max. speed $14,000 \times g$).

6. Micro-Grinder (RPI Corp., 299220) and 1.5-mL Pestles (RPI Corp., 199225).

7. Vortex mixer: e.g., Vortex-Genie 2™ (RPI Corp., 155560).

2.2. Mouse Strains

1. *C57BL/6J* mice (Stock number 0664) were purchased from The Jackson Laboratory.

2.3. Reagents and Supplies

2.3.1. Reagents

1. ChIP qualified antibodies specific for the two proteins of interest (e.g., Ab X and Ab Y) and isotype-matched non-specific immunoglobulin control (e.g., normal rabbit or mouse IgG, Santa Cruz).

2. Protease inhibitors.

3. 100 mM phenylmethanesulfonylfluoride (PMSF) (Sigma, P7626) in ethanol—use at 1:100 dilution.

4. 10 mg/mL aprotinin (Sigma, A1153) in 0.01 M HEPES, pH 8.0—use at 1:1,000.

5. 10 mg/mL leupeptin (Roche, 11017101001) in water—use at 1:1,000.

6. Glass beads, 212–300 μm, acid-washed (Sigma, G1277).

7. 10 mg/mL bovine serum albumin (BSA) (Sigma, A2153).

8. 10 mg/mL herring sperm DNA (Sigma, D7290).

9. 11 mg/mL ribonucleic acid, transfer (tRNA) from Baker's Yeast (Sigma, R5636).

10. 10 mg/mL proteinase K (Research Products International Corp., P50220).

11. 10 mg/mL ribonuclease A (RNase A) (Sigma, R6513).

12. 20 mg/mL glycogen (Sigma, G1508).

13. 10% Sodium deoxycholate (Sigma, D5760).

14. 1 M 4-(2-hydroxyethyl) piperazine-1-ethanesulfonic acid (HEPES) (Sigma, H4034).

15. 20% Triton X-100 (Sigma, T8787).

16. 20% Sodium dodecyl sulfate (SDS) (Sigma, L4509).

17. 20% Igepal CA-630 (NP-40) (Sigma, I3021).

18. 37% Formaldehyde (Sigma, F1635).

19. 0.5 M ethylenediaminetetraacetic acid disodium salt solution (EDTA, pH 8.0) (Sigma, E-7889).

20. 1 M piperazine-1,4-bis(2-ethanesulfonic acid) (PIPES) (Sigma, P1851).

21. 1 M lithium chloride (LiCl) (Sigma, L4408).

22. 2.5 M glycine (Fisher, BP381).

23. Phenol:chloroform:isoamyl alcohol 25:24:1 saturated with 10 mM Tris, pH 8.0, 1 mM EDTA (Sigma, P3803).

24. Chloroform (Sigma, C2432).

25. Ethanol, absolute (Pharmco, 111ACS200).

26. 100 mM deoxynucleotide set (Sigma, DNTP100).

27. JumpStart REDTaq DNA polymerase (Sigma, D0563).

28. 10× Taq polymerase buffer (Sigma, P2192).

29. SsoFast™ EvaGreen® Supermix for QPCR (Bio-Rad, 172-5203).

30. 50% (v/v) blocked Protein A beads: see Subheading 3.1.1 for making 50% (v/v) bead slurry from dry beads (Protein A Sepharose CL-4B, GE Health, 17-0780-01) and Subheading 3.1.2 for blocking.

31. 50% (v/v) blocked Protein G beads (50% (v/v) Protein G Sepharose beads, Sigma, P3296). See Subheading 3.1.2 for blocking.

32. 10% *N*-Lauroylsarcosine sodium salt solution (Sarkosyl) (Fisher, BP234).

33. 1 M Tris–HCl, pH 7.4, pH 8.0, and pH 8.1 [Tris base, RPI Corp., T60040; hydrochloric acid (HCl), Fisher, A144s-212].

34. 1 M sodium hydrogen carbonate ($NaHCO_3$) (Fisher, S637).

35. 3 M sodium chloride (NaCl) (Fisher, BP358).

36. 1 M potassium chloride (KCl) (MP Biomedicals, 0219484491).

37. 2-Mercaptoethanol (BME) solution (Sigma, M-6250).

38. Agarose (Bioline, Bio-41025).

2.3.2. Buffers

1. 10× Stock phosphate-buffered saline (PBS): 80 g of NaCl, 2 g of KCl, 14.4 g of Na_2HPO_4, 2.4 g of KH_2PO_4, add H_2O to 800 mL, adjust pH to 7.4 with 1 M HCl, add H_2O to 1 L.

2. Cell lysis buffer: 5 mM PIPES pH 8.0, 85 mM KCl, add 0.5% Igepal CA-630, and protease inhibitors (final: 10 μg/mL aprotinin, 10 μg/mL leupeptin, and 1 mM PMSF) just before use.

3. Nuclei lysis buffer: 50 mM Tris–Cl pH 8.1, 10 mM EDTA, 1% SDS, add protease inhibitors (final: 10 μg/mL aprotinin, 10 μg/mL leupeptin, and 1 mM PMSF) just before use.

4. Immunoprecipitation (IP) dilution buffer: 0.01% SDS, 1.1% Trition X-100, 1.2 mM EDTA, 16.7 mM Tris–Cl pH 8.0, 167 mM NaCl.

5. 1× Dialysis buffer: 2 mM EDTA, 50 mM Tris–Cl pH 8.0, 0.2% Sarkosyl (omit for monoclonal antibody).

6. Immunoprecipitation (IP) elution buffer: 50 mM $NaHCO_3$, 1% SDS (freshly diluted from 1 M $NaHCO_3$ and 20% SDS).

7. 5× Proteinase K buffer: 50 mM Tris–Cl pH 8.0, 25 mM EDTA (pH 8.0), 1.25% SDS.

8. Wash buffer I: 20 mM Tris–Cl pH 8.0, 150 mM NaCl, 2 mM EDTA, 1% Triton X-100, 0.1% SDS.

9. Wash buffer II: 20 mM Tris–Cl pH 8.0, 500 mM NaCl, 2 mM EDTA, 1% Triton X-100, 0.1% SDS.

10. Wash buffer III: 250 mM LiCl, 10 mM Tris–Cl pH 8.0, 1% sodium deoxycholate, 1 mM EDTA, 1% Igepal CA-630.

11. TE buffer: 10 mM Tris–Cl pH 8.0, 1 mM EDTA.

3. Methods

Single chromatin immunoprecipitation (ChIP) assays on mouse retinas were performed based on a detailed protocol described by Farnham Laboratory (http://farnham.genomecenter.ucdavis.edu/protocol.html) with modifications (14). Double chromatin immunoprecipitation assays (double or sequential ChIP) were established on the basis of single ChIP and modified from protocols described by Geisberg and Struhl (15). Major steps and predicted outcomes of double ChIP analysis are illustrated in Fig. 1.

3.1. Preparation of Blocked Protein A/G-Sepharose Beads (See Note 1)

3.1.1. Making 50% (v/v) Slurry of Protein A Beads

For high volume chromatin immunoprecipitation assays, starting from dry Protein A beads is more cost-effective than using presuspended wet beads. This section describes preparation of bead suspension from dry beads. Alternatively, Protein A or G bead slurry (50%, v/v) can be ordered through Sigma, Santa Cruz Biotechnology, or other companies. The wet beads can be used directly in Subheading 3.1.2.

1. Calculate the total volume of beads needed for the entire experiment (see Note 2) and prepare sufficient aliquots of bead slurry.

2. Resuspend each 100 mg of dry Protein A-Sepharose beads (GE Health, 17-0780-01) in 1 mL of 1× PBS pH 7.4, gently rotate (25–30 rpm) for at least 3 h at 4 °C. Centrifuge at $14,000 \times g$ for 5 min at 4 °C.

3. Wash with 1 mL of 1× PBS pH 7.4 with rotation for 5 min at 4 °C. Centrifuge at $14,000 \times g$ for 5 min at 4 °C, and carefully aspirate the supernatant.

4. Resuspend in 1 mL of 1× PBS pH 7.4 plus 3% SDS (final), and 10% 2-mercaptoethanol (BME, final). Boil for 30 min and cool at room temperature for 10 min. Centrifuge at $14,000 \times g$ for 5 min, and aspirate the supernatant.

5. Wash two times with 1 mL of 1× dialysis buffer with rotation for 5 min at 4 °C. Centrifuge at $14,000 \times g$ for 5 min, and aspirate the supernatant.

6. Resuspend Protein A beads with an equal volume of 1× dialysis buffer. Divide into 100 μL aliquots, store in –80 °C for up to 1 year.

3.1.2. Blocking
Protein A/G Beads

1. Add 10 µL of herring sperm DNA (10 mg/mL) and 10 µL of BSA (10 mg/mL) to 100 µL of 50% (v/v) slurry of Protein A or G beads per tube.

2. Incubate on a rotator (25–30 rpm) at 4°C for at least 3 h, overnight is fine.

3. Before using, centrifuge at $14,000 \times g$ for 3 min at 4°C, remove the supernatant, wash three times with 1 mL of 1× dialysis buffer by rotating 5 min (25–30 rpm) at 4°C, followed by centrifugation at $14,000 \times g$ for 3 min and removing the supernatant.

4. Resuspend Protein A or G beads in a volume of 1× dialysis buffer equal to the original starting volume to make 50% (v/v) slurry of blocked Protein A or G beads.

5. Blocked Protein A or G beads can be stored at 4°C for up to 1 week.

3.2. Crosslink
Protein–DNA
Complexes In Vivo

The following steps are designed for a single direction double ChIP (see Figs. 1 and 2 for main steps and sampling). To complete the whole experiment, two reciprocal directions (i.e., X followed by Y and Y followed by X) should be performed in parallel.

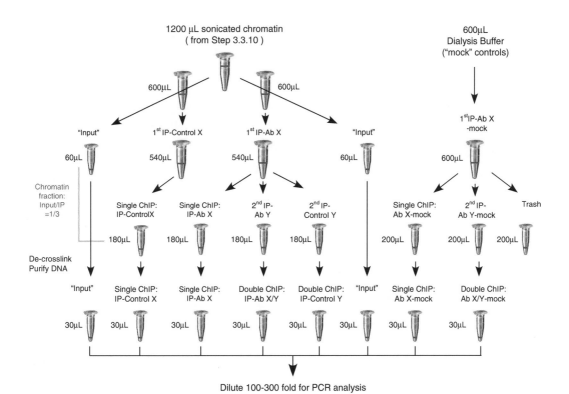

Fig. 2. Flow chart for single and double ChIP sampling, showing initial chromatin volumes at each step.

1. For each single direction double ChIP, dissect 12 mouse retinas (or 30 mg of other tissues) and cut tissues into small pieces using two razor blades.

2. Transfer the retinal tissue into a 14-mL tube (BD Falcon, 352059), add 10 mL of 1× PBS pH 7.4 plus protease inhibitor PMSF (10 μL/mL), add formaldehyde to a final concentration of 1% (see Note 3), and incubate for 15 min at room temperature with rotation (25–30 rpm) to cross-link chromatin binding proteins.

3. Stop the crosslinking reaction by adding fresh glycine to a final concentration of 0.125 M. Continue to rotate at room temperature for 5 min.

3.3. Prepare Chromatin

1. Centrifuge sample at 200×g at 4°C in Beckman GS-15R refrigerated centrifuge and decant the supernatant. Wash once with cold 1× PBS pH 7.4. Centrifuge at 200×g for 5 min at 4°C and decant the supernatant.

2. Add 2 mL of 1× cold PBS pH 7.4 plus protease inhibitors PMSF (10 μL/mL), aprotinin (1 μL/mL), and leupeptin (1 μL/mL). Use a hand-held Micro-Grinder to disaggregate the tissue for 1–2 min on ice.

3. Centrifuge cells at 200×g for 5 min at 4°C, and decant the supernatant.

4. Resuspend the cell pellet in 2 mL of cold cell lysis buffer plus protease inhibitors PMSF (10 μL/mL), aprotinin (1 μL/mL), and leupeptin (1 μL/mL). Lyse cells by incubating on ice for 10–15 min, gently mixing for a few seconds every 5 min on a vortex mixer (the lowest setting) to aid in nuclei release.

5. Centrifuge at 2,500×g for 5 min at 4°C to pellet the nuclei. Discard the supernatant.

6. Resuspend the nuclei in 1.2 mL of nuclei lysis buffer plus the same protease inhibitors as the cell lysis buffer. Incubate on ice for 20 min with periodic (every 5 min) mixing for a few seconds on a vortex mixer (the lowest setting).

7. Add 100 mg of glass beads (Sigma, G1277) to each sample (see Note 4).

8. Sonicate chromatin to an average length between 500 and 1,000 bp (sonicate setting 1.0–2.0, 15 s, stop 15 s, repeat to total work time of 1–3 min). Run 10 μL of chromatin in 0.8% agarose gel (see Fig. 3 for examples) to verify appropriate length of sonicated chromatin (see Note 5).

9. Transfer the sonicated chromatin to a 2-mL microcentrifuge tube (Eppendorf, 022600044). Centrifuge at 14,000×g for 10 min at 4°C.

Sonicated samples

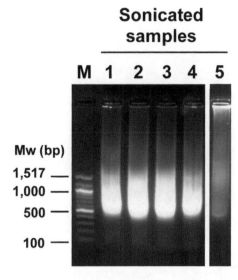

Fig. 3. Agarose gel analysis of the length of genomic DNA fragmented by sonication according to Table 1, derived from four retina samples (*lanes 1–4*) of wild-type mice at postnatal day 14 (step 3.3.8). *Lane 5* shows incomplete sonication of Sample 4 before achieving the desired size (500–1,000 bp) seen in *lane 4* (with additional sonication: 2×15 s).

10. Collect the supernatant and aliquot into two 1.5-mL microcentrifuge tubes (600 μL per tube). The sonicated chromatin can be stored at –80°C for up to 2 months.

3.4. Perform First Immunoprecipitation

1. Take chromatin preparations, preclear chromatin by adding 30 μL of blocked Protein A or G beads to each tube.

2. Incubate on a rotator (25–30 rpm) at 4°C for 15 min. Centrifuge at $14,000 \times g$ for 10 min.

3. Transfer the supernatant to clean 1.5-mL tubes. Remove 60 μL (10% of the amount of total chromatin) from each sample. This is the total "Input" DNA (see Fig. 2). Save it for later.

4. Set up immunoprecipitation (IP) samples on each of the two remaining chromatin preparations (540 μL): one IP uses a specific antibody to Protein X (IP-Ab X) and the other uses a nonspecific immunoglobulin (Ab X isotype matched, e.g., normal rabbit IgG for rabbit polyclonal antibodies or mouse IgG for IgG monoclonal mouse antibodies) as a negative control (IP-Control X) (see Fig. 2). Also, set up a IP-"mock" control sample (i.e., no chromatin DNA negative control) with 600 μL of 1× dialysis buffer in a separate tube. This mock sample receives the antibody to Protein X (labeled as IP-Ab X-mock) and is processed in parallel with the other chromatin IP samples (see Fig. 2). The IP-control and IP-mock samples are critical to control for nonspecific protein–DNA interactions and DNA contamination in the solutions.

5. Adjust the final volume of each sample to 600 μL using IP dilution buffer containing protease inhibitors.

6. Add 2 μg of desired antibody (Ab X or Control X) to each IP sample. Incubate on a rotator (25–30 rpm) at 4°C overnight (see Note 6).

7. Add 30 μL of blocked Protein A or G beads to each sample: IP-Ab X, IP-Control X, and IP-Ab X-mock. Incubate on a rotator (25–30 rpm) at room temperature for 15 min.

8. Wash once each with wash buffer I, II, III, and 1× TE buffer, sequentially (see Note 7). Each time rotate (25–30 rpm) 10 min at room temperature, centrifuge at $14,000 \times g$ for 3 min at room temperature, and discard the supernatant.

3.5. Elute Primary Protein–DNA Complex

1. For each IP sample (IP-Ab X, IP-Control X, or IP-Ab X-mock), elute the first immunoprecipitated protein–DNA complexes from antibody-bound beads by adding 300 μL of IP elution buffer (see Note 8). Rotate (25–30 rpm) for 15 min at room temperature. Centrifuge at $14,000 \times g$ for 3 min. Transfer the supernatant containing immuno-enriched primary protein–DNA complexes to a clean tube.

2. Repeat step 1, and combine both elutes (600 μL total) in one tube.

3. Centrifuge at $14,000 \times g$ for 5 min to remove any traces of primary antibody–Protein A beads. Transfer the supernatant to a clean tube.

4. Take out 200 μL (1/3 volume of total) of eluate into a new tube, labeled as "first IP-Ab X," "first IP-Control X," or "first IP-Ab X-mock." These will serve as single ChIP IP samples in later PCR analysis of enriched DNA fragments (see Fig. 2).

3.6. Perform Second Immunoprecipitation and Elution

1. Perform second immunoprecipitation using the remaining 2/3 (400 μL) of eluate from the first IP-Ab X chromatin sample from step 3.5.3: after being diluted to 600 μL with 1× IP dilution buffer, the first IP sample is split in half (300 μL per tube) and subjected to a second immunoprecipitation using 1.0–1.5 μg of the second specific antibody (e.g., antibody to Y protein, Ab Y), or Y antibody isotype-matched nonspecific control immunoglobulin (Ab-Control Y, e.g., normal rabbit or mouse IgG). Also, process the mock sample in parallel: add 200 μL of 1× IP dilution buffer to 400 μL of the remaining first IP Ab X-mock eluate (final 600 μL). Take out one half volume (300 μL) to a new tube labeled as second IP-Ab Y-mock, and add the second specific antibody (Ab Y). Discard the other half first IP-mock eluate. Incubate all the second IP samples on a rotator (25–30 rpm) at 4°C overnight.

2. Add 15 μL of blocked Protein A or G beads to each second IP sample. Incubate on a rotator (25–30 rpm) at room temperature for 15 min. Centrifuge at 14,000×g for 3 min at room temperature, and discard the supernatant.

3. Wash once each with wash buffer I, II, III, and 1× TE buffer, sequentially. Each time rotate (25–30 rpm) 10 min at room temperature, centrifuge at 14,000×g for 3 min at room temperature, and discard the supernatant.

4. Elute second immunoprecipitated protein–DNA complexes from the beads using 150 μL of IP elution buffer. Gently mix on a vortex machine (low setting, e.g. #3) for 15 min at room temperature. Centrifuge at 14,000×g for 3 min. Transfer supernatants to a clean 1.5 mL tube.

5. Repeat step 4, and combine both elution supernates in the same tube.

6. After the second elution, centrifuge pooled supernatant sample at 14,000×g for 5 min to remove any traces of antibody-Protein A or G beads. Transfer supernatant to a clean tube labeled as "second IP-Ab Y," "second IP-Control Y," or "second IP-Ab Y-mock."

3.7. Reverse Crosslinks and Purify DNA

1. Add 240 μL IP elution buffer to the tubes marked "Input" and add 100 μL IP elution buffer to all the first IP tubes.

2. To all samples, add 1 μL of high concentration RNase A (10 mg/mL) and 5 M NaCl to a final concentration of 0.3 M per tube. Incubate in a 67°C water bath for 4–5 h to reverse formaldehyde crosslinks. Add 2.5× volumes of absolute ethanol and precipitate at –20°C overnight.

3. Centrifuge samples at 14,000×g for 20 min at 4°C, and discard the supernatant. Re-spin and remove residual ethanol. Allow pellets to air dry completely.

4. Dissolve each pellet in 100 μL of TE. Add 25 μL of 5× proteinase K buffer and 1.5 μL of proteinase K (20 mg/mL) to each sample. Incubate in 45°C water bath for 2 h.

5. Add 175 μL of TE to each sample. Extract once with 300 μL of phenol/chloroform/isoamyl alcohol and once with 300 μL chloroform.

6. Add 30 μL of 5 M NaCl, 5 μg of tRNA, and 5 μg of glycogen to each sample and mix well, then add 750 μL of ethanol. Precipitate in –20°C overnight.

7. Centrifuge samples at 14,000×g for 20 min at 4 °C. Allow pellets to air dry. Resuspend DNA in 30 μL of TE buffer and perform PCR analysis for the presence of candidate gene segments.

3.8. Regular and Quantitative Real-Time PCR Analysis of ChIP Results

3.8.1. Agarose Gel Analysis

1. Dilute the samples 100–300 fold with water.

2. Regular PCR: Run four samples per group, including IP-Ab (e.g., X, Y, X/Y, or Y/X), IP-Control (e.g., X or Y), Mock (X, Y, X/Y, or Y/X), and Input with candidate gene-specific primers and JumpStart REDTaq DNA polymerase (Sigma).

3. Run the PCR products on 0.8–1.2% agarose gel.

3.8.2. Quantitative Real-Time PCR

1. Make serial dilutions in water of all samples from step 3.7.7 (e.g. 10-, 20-, 30, 50-, 100-, and 200-fold dilution).

2. Perform quantitative double chromatin immunoprecipitation (12, 13). Briefly, quantitative real-time PCR analysis of regulatory sequences in input samples and immunoprecipitates was performed using SsoFast™ EvaGreen® Supermix and CFX96 real-time PCR system (Bio-Rad).

3. Report ChIP-qPCR results either as "% Input Enrichment" or "IP Fold Enrichment." In general, qPCR calculation is based on the ΔCt method as described by Chakrabarti et al. (16).

4. Normalize each ChIP DNA fractions' Ct value to the input DNA fraction Ct value: ΔCt (normalized ChIP) = Ct (IP) – [Ct (Input) – Log2 (input dilution factor)], where input dilution factor (DF) = (fraction of the input chromatin saved)$^{-1}$. For example, for this study, saved input is 1/3 of the chromatin used for IP (Fig. 2). Thus, DF = 3; Log2 (DF) = 1.5850. Average normalized ChIP Ct values for replicate samples (typically $n = 3$).

5. Calculated % input enrichment: Calculate the % input for each ChIP fraction, including specific and control antibodies and "mock": % input = $2^{[-\Delta Ct \text{ (normalized ChIP)}]}$. Adjust for the background (nonspecific control antibody and "mock"): % input enrichment = % input (specific) – % input (controls).

6. Calculate IP fold enrichment: Adjust the normalized ChIP fraction Ct value for the normalized control fraction Ct values ($\Delta\Delta Ct$): $\Delta\Delta Ct$ (ChIP/controls) = ΔCt (normalized ChIP) – ΔCt (normalized controls), where the controls include the IP control antibody and "mock." Specific IP fold enrichment = $2^{[-\Delta\Delta Ct \text{ (ChIP/controls)}]}$.

7. An Excel-based ChIP-qPCR data analysis template with detailed instruction can be found on the SABiosciences/ Qiagen website: http://www.sabiosciences.com/chippcrarray_data_analysis.php.

3.8.3. Interpretations of Double ChIP Results

Compare quantitative single and double ChIP results to determine full, partial, or no co-occupancy of X and Y proteins.

1. Full co-occupancy: The enrichment of double ChIPs is often higher than individual ChIPs and is not affected by the order

of the individual ChIPs, i.e., X followed by Y (X/Y) or Y followed by X (Y/X) give near identical results (X/Y = Y/X).

2. No co-occupancy: The enrichment of double ChIPs is minimal, within the experimental error of the first IP: X/Y = Y/X = 0.

3. Partial co-occupancy: The enrichment of double ChIPs is above the background, but two reciprocal double ChIPs do not produce same enrichment. In other words, the order of the individual ChIPs makes a difference in the enrichment, i.e., X/Y ≠ Y/X ≠ 0. Note that partial co-occupancy often depends on the IP order. If X/Y is much higher than Y/X, it would suggest that Y is sometimes but not always present with X but not the reverse.

3.9. Example of Single and Double ChIP Analysis

We previously showed that the rod-specific transcription factor NR2E3 acts as an activator for rod genes, such as *rhodopsin* (*Rho*), by interacting with the cone–rod homeobox protein CRX (17). At the same time, NR2E3 also acts as a repressor for cone genes, such as *Opn1sw* (*Sop*) and *Opn1mw* (*Mop*). Thus, we predict that, in rods, NR2E3 and CRX should co-occupy the promoter of rod-specific genes. NR2E3 should also bind the promoter of cone genes, although it may or may not co-occupy these genes with CRX. We carried out quantitative single and double ChIP analysis of NR2E3 and CRX on both rod and cone genes using 24 retinas of wild-type C57BL/6J mice at postnatal day 14 (P14). Because NR2E3 is only expressed in rods, double ChIP results should reflect the situation in rods, while the single ChIP result for CRX may represent the situation in rods or both rods and cones. Figure 4a, b show that, in single ChIP analysis, either CRX (green bars in Fig. 4b) or NR2E3 (red bars in Fig. 4b) binds well to the promoter of *Rho* and *Rbp3* genes as well as the cone *opsin* genes, *Sop* and *Mop*. In double ChIP analysis, CRX and NR2E3 are co-enriched on the promoter of *Rho* and *Rbp3* genes; higher levels of enrichment than those of single ChIP are seen regardless of the order of performance of the two immunoprecipitations (Fig. 4b, blue and purple bars). Thus, we conclude that CRX and NR2E3 fully co-occupy the promoter of *Rho* and *Rbp3* in rods, consistent with the active role of CRX and NR2E3 on these genes. In contrast, much lower levels of co-enrichment of CRX and NR2E3 are seen on the *Sop* promoter. Furthermore, the enrichment on *Sop* is different between the two double ChIPs (blue vs. purple bar). These results suggest that CRX and NR2E3 only partially co-occupy the *Sop* promoter. Interestingly, a higher level of enrichment is seen with CRX/NR2E3 double ChIP (blue) than NR2E3/CRX (purple), suggesting that NR2E3 often co-binds with CRX to the *Sop* promoter, but CRX does not co-bind with NR2E3 in most cases. Finally, no co-occupancy of CRX and NR2E3 on the *Mop* promoter is detected. Our interpretation of these double

a

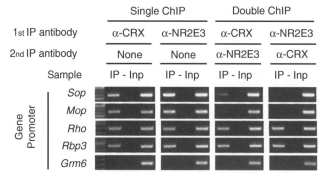

b

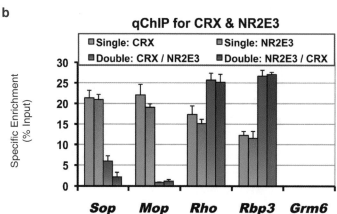

c

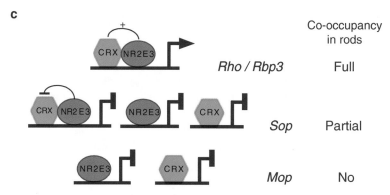

Fig. 4. CRX and NR2E3 co-occupy *rhodopsin* (*Rho*) and *Rbp3* promoters in rod photoreceptors. Double ChIP analysis was performed using 24 retinas of P14 mice and affinity purified rabbit antibodies specific to CRX (p119) (20) and NR2E3 (p183) (17) following the protocol described in the text. (**a**) Agarose gel analysis of regular ChIP-PCR results using 1:100 dilutions of DNA from single and double ChIP samples with the indicated antibodies. "IP" represents specific antibody immunoprecipitation-enriched DNA sample, "−" represents IgG control antibody immunoprecipitated genomic DNA, "Inp" represents input genomic DNA without immunoprecipitation. Five indicated candidate gene promoters were analyzed, including two rod-expressed genes *Rho* and *Rbp3*, two cone *opsin* genes silenced in rods, *Sop* and *Mop*, as well as a bipolar expressed gene, *Grm6*. Primer pairs used to generate these PCR products were published previously (14). Note that double ChIP columns show high-intensity bands for *Rho* and *Rbp* but no or low-intensity bands for *Sop* and *Mop*. No CRX or NR2E3 binding was found on *Grm6* promoter. (**b**) Quantitative real-time PCR analysis of single and double ChIP results, presented as % input enrichment calculated as described in the text. (**c**) A diagram to summarize the hypothesized mechanism behind these results, showing full co-occupancy of CRX and NR2E3 on the promoter of *Rho* and *Rpb3*, but only partial co-occupancy on *Sop* and no co-occupancy on *Mop* in rod photoreceptors.

ChIP results is summarized in Fig. 4c. These results have helped us to understand the molecular mechanisms by which rod and cone genes are differentially repressed in rod photoreceptors. For example, silencing of *Sop* and *Mop* genes in rods may involve different mechanisms, including the lack of specific activator(s) for each gene. Also, NR2E3-mediated repression may target other transcription activators besides CRX.

4. Notes

1. Choice of Protein A or G beads: Various types of Sepharose beads have different affinity for specific antibody isotypes. In general, Protein A beads should be used for polyclonal antibodies made in rabbits. Protein G beads are used for antibodies made in goats or most of the mouse monoclonal antibodies. For more detailed information about the affinity of different bead types for specific antibody isotypes, please go to the website: http://www.scbt.com/support-table-immunoprecipitation_reagents.html. If the isotype of a specific antibody does not have a good affinity to either Protein A or G beads (e.g., mouse IgM), please see Note 6 for alternatives. Also, this protocol is optimized for Sepharose beads. We have not yet tested magnetic beads for ChIP applications.

2. Total volume of blocked beads needed for the entire experiment: 300 μL of blocked beads is sufficient for one protein pair: 90 μL for the first IP (30 μL per tube × 3 tubes) + 45 μL for the second IP (15 μL per tube × 3 tubes) = 135 μL for each double ChIP (see Fig. 2 for sampling) × 2 (two reciprocal directions) = 270 μL total. The blocking procedure is based on one aliquot of beads (100 μL). Thus, for each protein pair, prepare three aliquots (100 μL each) of beads, which can be processed individually or pooled together.

3. Crosslink: It is important to use formaldehyde freshly diluted to 1% in 1× PBS pH 7.4.

4. Choice of glass beads: Diameter = 212–300 μm. Omit this step if Cup Horn-indirect sonication will be used (see Note 5).

5. Fragment chromatin DNA by sonication: Microtip is recommended for direct sonication of samples one-at-a-time in sample tubes. The optimal setting and time for sonication depend on the individual machine, the age of the retinas and sample volume. Table 1 lists suggested ranges for samples consisting of 12 mouse retinas at different ages in 1.2 mL nuclei lysis buffer. For multiple samples, indirect sonication through water in a Cup Horn (e.g., Fisher, FB-462-5) is recommended.

Table 1
Conditions for fragmenting chromatin DNA from 12 mouse retinas in 1.2 mL nuclei lysis buffer using Fisher Model 505 Sonic Dismembrator with microtip

Retina	Sonication time	Setting
E12.5	1.0	1.0
E14.5	1.0	1.0
E16.5	1.2	1.0
E18.5	1.2	1.0
P0	1.5	1.2
P1	1.5	1.2
P3	2.0	1.5
P5	2.0	1.5
P7	2.5	2.0
P10	2.5	2.0
P14	3.0	2.0

The optimal conditions for indirect sonication should be established empirically by each user. In general, indirect sonication takes a longer time (e.g., 6–10 min) than direct sonication through a microtip (1–3 min), but gives less sample-to-sample variation. Furthermore, eight samples can be done at once without concerns about contamination between samples and protein denaturation by the vigorous direct sonication. For indirect sonication in Cup Horn, samples should be transferred into 2 mL microcentrifuge tubes (Microcentrifuge Safe-Lock tube, Eppendorf, 022600044), and there is no need to add the glass beads.

6. If the isotype of a specific antibody used has a low affinity to either Protein A or G beads (e.g., mouse IgM), the next day you should add 2 μg of an appropriate secondary antibody that recognizes the specific immunoglobulin isotype and is capable of binding to Protein A or G beads (e.g., rabbit anti-mouse IgM). Incubate for an additional 1 h before adding blocked beads.

7. Wash buffer: For best results, use freshly made buffer.

8. A key step in double ChIP analysis is to optimize wash conditions to achieve complete dissociation of the immunoprecipitated protein–DNA complexes from the first antibody bound to Protein A or G beads, but the sample is still capable of re-precipitation with the second antibody. There are three ways to

elute target proteins without dissociating the antibody from Sepharose beads: (1) elute with a specific isotope peptide used for generating the antibody (18). (2) Crosslink the primary antibody to the beads (1). (3) Use wash conditions that will only elute immunoprecipitated protein complexes but not the primary antibody from beads. We have successfully used the third method for a number of rabbit polyclonal antibodies (12, 13). For both rounds of immunoprecipitation, we verify the wash conditions using an isotype control antibody (e.g., normal rabbit IgG) as a negative control. Ideally, following the second immunoprecipitation, there should be no enrichment for a specific DNA fragment with the isotype control antibody, but full enrichment with the corresponding specific antibody. We have used the same stringent wash conditions described in this protocol for all the rabbit polyclonal antibodies in our studies with Protein A beads. Others have used 10 mM dithiothreitol (DTT) (in either wash buffer I or IP elution buffer) to facilitate the elution (3, 5, 19). Nonetheless, the optimal wash conditions depend on individual antibodies and should be determined experimentally.

Acknowledgment

We thank Hui Wang for technical assistance and Anne Hennig for critical reading of the manuscript. This work was supported by NIH EY012543 (to SC), NIH EY02687 (to WU-DOVS), Lew Wasserman Merit Award (to SC), and unrestricted fund from Research to Prevent Blindness (to WU-DOVS).

References

1. Chaya D, Zaret KS (2004) Sequential chromatin immunoprecipitation from animal tissues. Methods Enzymol 376:361–372

2. Geisberg JV, Struhl K (2004) Quantitative sequential chromatin immunoprecipitation, a method for analyzing co-occupancy of proteins at genomic regions in vivo. Nucleic Acid Res 32:e151

3. Brunelli L, Cieslik KA, Alcorn JL et al (2007) Peroxisome proliferator-activated receptor-delta upregulates 14-3-3 epsilon in human endothelial cells via CCAAT/enhancer binding protein-beta. Circ Res 100:e59–e71

4. Chaya D, Hayamizu T, Bustin M et al (2001) Transcription factor FoxA (HNF3) on a nucleosome at an enhancer complex in liver chromatin. J Biol Chem 276:44385–44389

5. Heitzer MD, DeFranco DB (2006) Mechanism of action of Hic-5/androgen receptor activator 55, a LIM domain-containing nuclear receptor coactivator. Mol Endocrinol 20:56–64

6. Kajiyama Y, Tian J, Locker J (2006) Characterization of distant enhancers and promoters in the albumin-alpha-fetoprotein locus during active and silenced expression. J Biol Chem 281:30122–30131

7. Wilkinson DS, Tsai WW, Schumacher MA et al (2008) Chromatin-bound p53 anchors activated Smads and the mSin3A corepressor to confer transforming-growth-factor-beta-mediated transcription repression. Mol Cell Biol 28:1988–1998

8. Kobrossy L, Rastegar M, Featherstone M (2006) Interplay between chromatin and

trans-acting factors regulating the Hoxd4 promoter during neural differentiation. J Biol Chem 281:25926–25939

9. Metivier R, Penot G, Hubner MR et al (2003) Estrogen receptor-alpha directs ordered, cyclical, and combinatorial recruitment of cofactors on a natural target promoter. Cell 115:751–763

10. Bernstein BE, Mikkelsen TS, Xie X et al (2006) A bivalent chromatin structure marks key developmental genes in embryonic stem cells. Cell 125:315–326

11. Jin C, Zang C, Wei G et al (2009) H3.3/H2A.Z double variant-containing nucleosomes mark 'nucleosome-free regions' of active promoters and other regulatory regions. Nat Genet 41:941–945

12. Onishi A, Peng GH, Hsu C et al (2009) Pias3-dependent SUMOylation directs rod photoreceptor development. Neuron 61:234–246

13. Onishi A, Peng GH, Chen S et al (2010) Pias3-dependent SUMOylation controls mammalian cone photoreceptor differentiation. Nat Neurosci 13:1059–1065

14. Peng GH, Chen S (2005) Chromatin immunoprecipitation identifies photoreceptor transcription factor targets in mouse models of retinal degeneration: new findings and challenges. Vis Neurosci 22:575–586

15. Geisberg JV, Struhl K (2005) Analysis of protein co-occupancy by quantitative sequential chromatin immunoprecipitation. Curr Protoc Mol Biol 70:21.8.1–21.8.7

16. Chakrabarti SK, James JC, Mirmira RG (2002) Quantitative assessment of gene targeting in vitro and in vivo by the pancreatic transcription factor, Pdx1. Importance of chromatin structure in directing promoter binding. J Biol Chem 277:13286–13293

17. Peng GH, Ahmad O, Ahmad F et al (2005) The photoreceptor-specific nuclear receptor Nr2e3 interacts with Crx and exerts opposing effects on the transcription of rod versus cone genes. Hum Mol Genet 14:747–764

18. Jin C, Felsenfeld G (2007) Nucleosome stability mediated by histone variants H3.3 and H2A.Z. Genes Dev 21:1519–1529

19. Hatzis P, Talianidis I (2002) Dynamics of enhancer–promoter communication during differentiation-induced gene activation. Mol Cell 10:1467–1477

20. Peng GH, Chen S (2007) Crx activates opsin transcription by recruiting HAT-containing co-activators and promoting histone acetylation. Hum Mol Genet 16:3433–3452

Chapter 23

Quantifying the Activity of *cis*-Regulatory Elements in the Mouse Retina by Explant Electroporation

Cynthia L. Montana, Connie A. Myers, and Joseph C. Corbo

Abstract

Transcription factors control gene expression by binding to noncoding regions of DNA known as *cis*-regulatory elements (CREs; i.e., enhancer/promoters). Traditionally, *cis*-regulatory analysis has been carried out via mouse transgenesis which is time-consuming and nonquantitative. Electroporation of DNA reporter constructs into living mouse tissue is a rapid and effective alternative to transgenesis which permits quantitative assessment of *cis*-regulatory activity. Here, we present a simple technique for quantifying the activity of photoreceptor-specific CREs in living explanted mouse retinas.

Key words: Retina, Photoreceptor, *cis*-Regulatory element, Quantification, Electroporation, Mouse

1. Introduction

Transcription factors within cellular gene networks control the spatiotemporal pattern and levels of expression of their target genes by binding to *cis*-regulatory elements (CREs), short (~300–600 bp) stretches of genomic DNA which can lie upstream, downstream, or within the introns of the genes they control. CREs (i.e., enhancers/promoters) typically consist of multiple clustered binding sites for both transcriptional activators and repressors (1–3). They serve as logical integrators of transcriptional input giving a unitary output in the form of spatiotemporally precise and quantitatively exact promoter activity. Most studies of mammalian *cis*-regulation to date have relied on mouse transgenesis as a means of assaying the enhancer function of CREs in vivo (4, 5). This technique is time-consuming, costly and, on account of insertion site effects, largely nonquantitative. Quantitative assays for mammalian CRE function have also been developed in tissue culture systems (e.g., dual luciferase assays), but the in vivo relevance of these results is often uncertain.

Bernhard H.F. Weber and Thomas Langmann (eds.), *Retinal Degeneration: Methods and Protocols*, Methods in Molecular Biology, vol. 935, DOI 10.1007/978-1-62703-080-9_23, © Springer Science+Business Media, LLC 2013

Electroporation offers an excellent alternative to traditional mouse transgenesis in that it permits both spatiotemporal and quantitative assessment of *cis*-regulatory activity in living mammalian tissue. This technique has been particularly useful in the analysis of *cis*-regulation in the central nervous system, especially in the cerebral cortex and the retina (6–8). We recently developed a simple approach to quantify the activity of photoreceptor-specific CREs in electroporated mouse retinas (9). Given that the amount of DNA that is introduced into the retina by electroporation can vary from experiment to experiment, it is necessary to include a co-electroporated "loading control" in all experiments. In this respect, the technique is very similar to the dual luciferase assay used to quantify promoter activity in cultured cells.

When assaying photoreceptor *cis*-regulatory activity, electroporation is usually performed in newborn mice (postnatal day 0, P0) which is the time of peak rod production (10, 11). Once retinal cell types become post-mitotic, electroporation is much less efficient. Given the high rate of rod birth in newborn mice and the fact that rods constitute more than 70% of the cells in the adult mouse retina, the majority of cells that are electroporated at P0 are rods. For this reason, rod photoreceptors are the easiest retinal cell type to study via electroporation. The technique we describe here is primarily useful for quantifying the activity of photoreceptor CREs. Cell-type specific *cis*-regulatory activity can also be quantified in rarer retinal cell types such as bipolar cells (12), but this usually requires selection of areas of interest in vertical cross-sections rather than in flatmount preparations.

2. Materials

2.1. Electroporation Chamber

1. Electroporation microslide model 453 (BTX Harvard Apparatus, catalog #45-0105).
2. 100% Silicone rubber aquarium cement.
3. 3-ml syringe.
4. Plastic microtube rack (Fisher Scientific, catalog #05-541).
5. Dremel tool (for cutting the handle off the plastic microtube rack).
6. Binder clips.
7. Square metal bar, 3–5 mm diameter and about 100 mm long.

2.2. DNA Precipitation

1. 1.5-ml microcentrifuge tubes.
2. DNA, preferably a maxiprep(s) with concentration at least 0.5 µg/µl.

3. 100% Ethanol.

4. 70% Ethanol.

5. 3 M sodium acetate, pH 5.2.

6. Sterile water.

7. Sterile 10× PBS, pH 7.4.

8. Refrigerated microcentrifuge.

2.3. Retinal Dissection and Culture

1. Sterile dissection medium: 1:1 ratio of DMEM:F12 (Gibco #11965 and 11765), 100 U/ml penicillin, 100 µg/ml streptomycin, 0.29 mg/ml L-glutamine, 5 µg/ml insulin. The penicillin, streptomycin, and L-glutamine may be purchased as a 100× premixed solution (Gibo #10378-016). Insulin (Sigma-Aldrich) should be reconstituted as a 5 mg/ml solution (1,000×) in 5 mM HCl, filter-sterilized, and stored at –20°C.

2. Sterile culture medium: Dissection medium (see above) plus 10% FBS (Gibco #26140-079).

3. Sterile 1× PBS, pH 7.4.

4. Post-natal day 0 (P0) mouse pups.

5. 70% Ethanol.

6. Dissecting microscope.

7. Dissection instruments: Large scissors, iris scissors, curved forceps, fine forceps.

8. Sterile, disposable transfer pipettes.

9. Sterile Petri dishes: 35, 60, and 100 mm.

10. ECM 830 square-wave electroporator (BTX Harvard Apparatus) with cables and micrograbber adaptors.

11. Sterile 6-well tissue culture plates.

12. Nuclepore filters (25 mm, 0.2 µm) (Whatman #110606).

13. Tissue culture incubator: 37°C, 5% CO_2.

2.4. Retinal Fixation, Imaging, and Quantitation

1. 4% Paraformaldehyde in 1× PBS: Dissolve 2 g paraformaldehyde in 45 ml distilled water. Apply heat and add 1 drop 5 M sodium hydroxide to facilitate the dissolution. Add 5 ml 10× PBS. Filter the final solution through Whatman filter paper. Allow the solution to cool to room temperature prior to use.

2. 1× PBS, pH 7.4.

3. Glass slides.

4. Glass coverslips: 0.16 mm thick, #1.5 (Fisher Scientific #12-544E).

5. Crushed glass coverslips, fragments 3–5 mm in diameter.

6. Fluorescent dissecting microscope.

7. Fluorescent compound microscope equipped with a camera, preferably monochromatic (e.g., ORCA-ER camera by Hamamatsu).

8. ImageJ software: Download from the NIH website http://rsbweb.nih.gov/ij/.

9. 30% Sucrose in 1× PBS, filter-sterilized (store at 4°C) (see Note 8).

10. Tissue-Tek OCT compound (see Note 8).

11. Tissue molds (see Note 8).

3. Methods

Perform all steps at room temperature unless otherwise indicated. Dissection and culture medium should be stored at 4°C but brought to room temperature prior to the beginning of the procedure.

3.1. Construction of the Electroporation Chamber

1. Order a microslide, BTX Model 453 with a 3.2 mm gap (Harvard Apparatus #45-0105) (Fig. 1a). The metal rails should be completely sealed to the bottom of the slide.

2. Use a Dremel tool to cut a handle off a plastic microcentrifuge tube rack. Cut the handle into five small rectangular pieces each with the following dimensions: length 0.8 cm, height 0.6 cm, width 0.3 cm (Fig. 1b). These plastic pieces are reusable spacers that will be used to mold individual wells in the microslide chamber.

3. Insert the plastic spacers between the metal rails of the microslide at even intervals. The spacers should fit snugly (Fig. 1c).

4. Cut the tip off a P200 pipette tip, fit the tip to a 3 ml syringe, and fill the syringe with 100% silicone rubber aquarium sealant. Fill the gaps between the plastic spacers with sealant. Be sure to fill the gaps from the bottom up so that no bubbles form between the sealant plug and the base of the microslide.

5. Place a metal rod atop the plastic spacers and fasten it with binder clips, so that the spacers are held in place while the sealant dries (Fig. 1d, e). Let the sealant dry overnight.

6. Remove the binder clips, metal rod, and plastic spacers (Fig. 1f). Use a scalpel blade to clean the sealant off the top of the metal rails. Use a dissecting microscope to examine the microslide and ensure that no bubbles are present at the bottom of the silicone dams. Remove any sealant film that may have formed in the wells such that bare metal is exposed inside wells. Fill one well with water and make sure that the water does not leak into the adjacent well(s). Repeat for all wells.

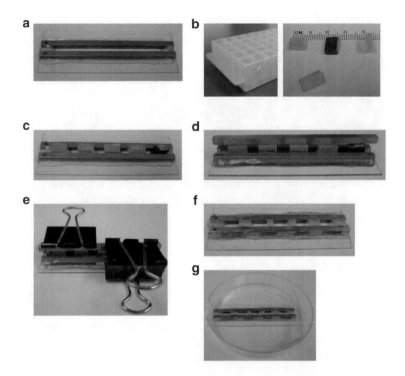

Fig. 1. Construction of the electroporation dish. (**a**) Unmodified microslide chamber from Harvard Apparatus, BTX model 453 (catalog #45-0105). (**b**) A Dremel tool is used to cut the handle off a plastic tube rack. The handle is cut into rectangular spacers with the following dimensions: length 0.8 cm, height 0.6 cm, width 0.3 cm. (**c**) The plastic spacers are fitted into the microslide chamber at equal intervals. Aquarium sealant is injected into the gaps between the spacers (not shown). (**d**) A *metal bar* is placed over the spacers. (**e**) The bar and spacers are clamped onto the slide with binder clips to hold everything in place as the sealant dries overnight. (**f**) The spacers are removed and the wells are tested to ensure that they are watertight. (**g**) The finished slide fits into the plastic dish with the metal bars adjacent to the window in the side of the dish.

7. The finished microslide fits in the plastic dish with the metal poles adjacent to the window in the side of the dish (Fig. 1g); the electrodes will eventually be attached to the metal poles.

3.2. DNA Preparation

1. Add plasmid DNA to a 1.5-ml microcentrifuge tube on ice and bring the volume up to 150 μl with distilled water. Multiple plasmid species may be combined for co-electroporation (see Note 1).

2. Precipitate the DNA by adding 15 μl 3 M sodium acetate (pH 5.2) and 450 μl 100% ethanol. Invert the tube several times to mix.

3. Spin down the DNA at 4°C, $16,000 \times g$, for 30 min. Wash the pellet with 70% ethanol, then spin it down again at 4°C, $16,000 \times g$, for 15 min. Air-dry the pellet until semitranslucent, about 7 min, then resuspend in 54 μl sterile water (vortex well

to mix). Add 6 μl sterile 10× PBS (pH 7.4) and mix by vortexing. The DNA aliquots may be stored at −20°C but should be brought to room temperature prior to electroporation.

3.3. Eye Collection

1. Sterilize the electroporation chamber and all instruments with 70% ethanol (see Note 2).

2. Prepare sterile Petri dishes with dissection medium: Two 35 mm dishes each with 3 ml medium and one 60 mm dish with 6 ml medium.

3. Disinfect the head and neck of a postnatal day 0 (P0) mouse pup with a Kimwipe soaked in 70% ethanol. Quickly decapitate with scissors and transfer the head to a 100 mm dish.

4. Cut away the scalp with small scissors to expose the eyes. Use curved forceps to gently scoop the eye out of the orbit, and place the eye in a 35 mm dish containing dissection medium. It may be helpful to remove the eyes under a dissecting microscope at low power.

5. Repeat steps 3 and 4 until all eyes have been collected. Keep eyes at room temperature while dissecting. You will need 3–4 eyes per DNA aliquot.

3.4. Retinal Dissection

1. Use 70% ethanol to disinfect a razor blade and the plastic wrapper of a sterile transfer pipette. Cut the tip off the pipette with the blade so that it can suck up a whole eye. Store the pipette in the plastic wrapper when not in use.

2. Transfer one eye from the 35 mm dish to the 60 mm dish. Under the dissecting microscope at high power, use fine forceps to remove any tissue from the surface of the eye.

3. Carefully remove the optic nerve, sclera, cornea, and retinal pigmented epithelium. Leave the lens in place (see Note 3).

4. Use the transfer pipette to move the dissected retina into the other 35 mm dish with medium.

5. Repeat steps 2–4 until all eyes have been dissected.

6. Store the retinas in a 37°C tissue culture incubator until ready to electroporate, no longer than 1 h.

3.5. Preparation for Electroporation

1. Prepare 35 mm dishes of medium. For each DNA aliquot, you will need one dish of dissection medium and one dish of culture medium. Label the dishes appropriately.

2. Use a P200 pipette and sterile 1× PBS to wash out the chambers in the electroporation dish. Each chamber holds a volume of 60–100 μl. Wash out each chamber three times.

3. Fill the chambers with the DNA aliquots. Any unused chambers should be filled with 60 μl 1× PBS. Connect the electrodes to the electroporation dish.

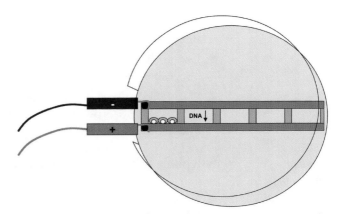

Fig. 2. Diagram of the electroporation dish with retinas. The chambers are filled with DNA solutions (up to five different solutions at a time). Retinas are placed in the chambers and oriented so that the lens is leaning against the metal bar connected to the positive electrode; three or four retinas will fit in each of the five chambers. The electrical current will cause the negatively charged DNA molecules to move into the retinal cells.

4. Use the following settings on the electroporator: Mode, LV; voltage, 30 V; pulse length, 50 ms; number of pulses, 5; interval, 950 ms; polarity, unipolar.

3.6. Electroporation

1. Use fine forceps to grasp the retinas by the lens and transfer them into the electroporation chambers. Each chamber holds up to four mouse retinas (Fig. 2).

2. Use forceps to line up the retinas such that the lens leans against the metal rail attached to the positive electrode. Clean the forceps with a Kimwipe after each transfer to avoid DNA cross-contamination between chambers.

3. Once all retinas are aligned, press "Start" on the electroporator. Tiny bubbles should form on the metal rail attached to the negative electrode.

4. Disconnect the electrodes and turn off the electroporator.

5. Use forceps to gently move the retinas away from the chamber walls.

6. Use a sterile transfer pipette to transfer the retinas from the chambers into the 35 mm dishes containing dissection medium.

7. Wash out each chamber three times with sterile 1× PBS, then rinse with sterile water. Spray dish with 70% ethanol.

3.7. Placing Retinas on Filters for Culture

1. Use a transfer pipette to transfer the retinas into the 35 mm dishes containing culture medium.

2. Label the wells of a sterile 6-well culture plate and fill each well with 3 ml culture medium.

3. Use sterile forceps to place round Whatman Nuclepore filters, shiny side up, atop the medium in each well.

4. Use a sterile transfer pipette to transfer the retinas onto the filter, lens-side-down (see Note 4).

5. Place the culture plate in a 37°C tissue culture incubator (5% CO_2) and grow for the desired amount of time, typically 8 days (see Notes 5–7).

3.8. Harvesting and Flatmounting Fluorescent Retinal Explants

1. Replace the culture medium in each well with 4% paraformaldehyde/1× PBS. If the retinas remain stuck to the filters, use forceps to flip the filters over and gently peel the retinas off the filter. Incubate in paraformaldehyde for 30 min at room temperature. Protect the retinas from light to avoid bleaching the fluorescence.

2. Rinse the retinas twice for 10 min in 1× PBS.

3. Use a disposable pipette to transfer the retinas onto a glass slide in a small drop of PBS. Under a fluorescent dissecting microscope, use forceps to flip the retinas so that they are electroporated-side-up (i.e., lens-side-down).

4. Place glass "feet" made from crushed coverslips at the corners of the slide; these feet prevent flattening of the retina by the coverslip. Place an intact glass coverslip over the slide so that it covers the retinas and rests on the feet. If necessary, use a pipette to add more PBS between the slide and the coverslip.

3.9. Imaging and Quantification of Fluorescence in Flat-Mounted Retinas

1. Use a fluorescent compound microscope to image the flatmounted retina at low power (4× objective) in the red and green channels. All retinas must be imaged with the same exposure time for a given fluorescent channel to enable comparison of fluorescence intensities. In other words, DsRed must be imaged with exposure time "A" in all retinas, and GFP must be imaged with exposure time "B" in all retinas. Make sure that the pixels are not saturated in any image, or else accurate quantification will be impossible. Export images in grayscale TIFF format. The retinal explants may be saved for sectioning (see Note 8).

2. Open the image set for one retina (i.e., red channel and green channel) in ImageJ software (http://rsbweb.nih.gov/ij/). For the sake of this tutorial, the green fluorescent channel (GFP protein) is the control construct that is constant across all retinas in the experiment. The red fluorescent channel (DsRed protein) is the experimental construct that varies for each set of retinas. The images should be in grayscale.

3. In ImageJ, select the control green image and specify a circle of interest with diameter 100 units (Analyze/Tools/ROI manager/More/Specify). Duplicate this circle (ROI manager/

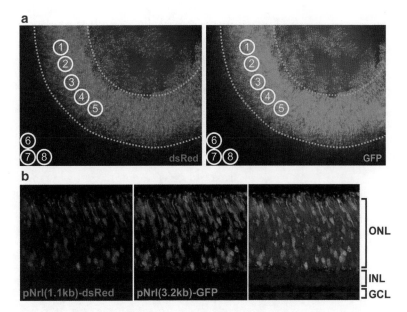

Fig. 3. (**a**) ImageJ measurement of retinal fluorescence levels in flatmount. Grayscale flatmount images in the DsRed (experimental) and GFP (control) channels are opened in ImageJ software. Five measurement circles (1–5) are placed over uniformly electroporated regions, avoiding the edges and lens (*dotted lines*). Three measurement circles (6–8) are placed outside the retina to determine background fluorescence levels. (**b**) Cross-sectional images of an electroporated retinal explant at high power. The explant was fixed at postnatal day 8, cryoprotected in 30% sucrose/1× PBS overnight at 4°C, embedded in OCT, and cryosectioned at 12 μm. The fluorescent constructs pNrl (1.1 kb)-DsRed and pNrl (3.2 kb)-GFP are expressed in photoreceptor cells in the outer nuclear layer (ONL). *INL* inner nuclear layer, *GCL* ganglion cell layer.

Add) to create eight circles total. Move circles 1–5 to select five regions that are uniformly electroporated, avoiding the outer edges of the retina and the region overlying the lens (Fig. 3a). Also, select three regions (circles 6–8) outside the retina/lens to measure background fluorescence. Select the red image, uncheck the "Show all" box in ROI manager, and recheck the box. All eight circles should appear on the red image. Deselect all circle coordinates in ROI manager.

4. With the red image selected, record the mean pixel value for all circles of interest (ROI manager/Measure); measurements 1–8 should appear, where 1–5 are the red retinal measurements and 6–8 are the red background measurements. Select the green image and record the mean pixel value; measurements 9–16 should appear, where 9–13 are the green retinal measurements, and 14–16 are the green background measurements. Copy the measurement data into Excel for analysis.

5. Average the three background measurements in both the red and the green channels. Subtract the red background average

from each of the five retinal measurements in the red channel; repeat for the green channel. For each retinal region-of-interest, divide the background-subtracted red measurement by the background-subtracted green measurement in order to normalize the experimental red level to the control green level.

6. Determine the average and standard deviation of all normalized measurements for a given DsRed construct (e.g., five measurements per retina times three separate retinas). In order to quantitatively compare the results of electroporations carried out on different days, always include a "standard" DsRed/GFP precipitation in each electroporation set. Relative expression values across experiments can be compared by normalizing to the expression level of this "standard."

4. Notes

1. In a typical promoter analysis experiment, two fluorescent constructs are co-electroporated: an experimental promoter driving the fluorescent protein DsRed and a control promoter driving GFP (or vice versa). Ideally, the control construct should be expressed in the same cell type as the experimental construct (e.g., for photoreceptor expression, a good control is the *Nrl* promoter (7) driving GFP which is available through Addgene [http://www.addgene.org/13764/]). When calculating the amount of DNA to add to the tube, keep in mind that the final volume of the DNA aliquot will be 60 µl. Typically, each construct is used at a final concentration of 0.5 µg/µl.

2. It is important to be as sterile as possible throughout the entire procedure, from eye collection and retinal dissection to the placement of electroporated retinas in the culture dish. If sterile conditions are not maintained, fungus and/or bacteria may contaminate the explants as they grow in culture. Be especially vigilant about spraying gloves, surfaces, and dissection instruments with 70% ethanol. Subheading 3.5–3.7 (electroporation and culture prep) should be performed in a sterile laminar flow hood if possible.

3. One dissecting strategy is to poke a small hole in the sclera at the limbus with one pair of forceps. Then, insert one prong from both pairs of forceps into the hole (tangential to the retinal surface) and gently tear open the sclera/RPE. In albino mice, the sclera and RPE appear shiny relative to the retinal tissue, which is a homogeneous matte tan color. It is worthwhile to perform careful dissections, because any gashes in the retinal tissue will cause contortion of the explant as it grows in culture. This will result in nonuniform fluorescence across the

retinal surface in a flat-mount view. It may be impossible to quantify fluorescence levels if the retina is severely distorted. It is not necessary to leave the lens in place, but we have found that it helps to maintain the shape of the retina throughout the procedure and results in more uniform flatmount preparations. In addition, the lens can be utilized as a "handle" for moving the retinas.

4. If the retina lands lens-side-up, pick it up with the pipette and attempt to place it again. It is important to place the retina lens-side-down (i.e., electroporated-side-up) since having the electroporated side of the retina in contact with the filter can adversely affect fluorescence. Do not place more than four retinas on one filter and make sure that the droplets of medium surrounding each retina remain separate from the other droplets. If the filter becomes submerged, remove the retinas from that well, replace the sunken filter with a fresh one, and attempt to place the retinas again.

5. For routine analysis of photoreceptor-specific CREs, 8 days in culture is usually sufficient to detect activity. If desired, retinas may be grown in culture for longer periods. The medium should be changed every 8 days; more frequent medium changes are discouraged because of the increased risk for culture contamination. To change the medium, open the plate in a sterile laminar flow hood, tilt the plate, and remove most—but not all—the medium with a sterile P1000 pipette tip. Do not touch the filter or allow liquid to drip onto the filter. Next, draw up 3 ml fresh medium with a sterile serological pipette and slowly inject the medium into the corner of the well. The filter should slowly lift away from the bottom of the well and float on the surface.

6. If desired, small molecules may be added directly to the culture medium, such as doxycycline and 4-hydroxytamoxifen.

7. The culture plates may be removed from the incubator and examined with a fluorescent dissecting microscope for short periods every day (do not remove the plate lid).

8. To save the retinal explants for histological analysis (e.g., frozen cross-sections) carefully lift off the coverslip and add a few drops 1× PBS to the slide. Use forceps to gently loosen the explants from the slide and transfer them to a vial of sterile 30% sucrose/1× PBS with a disposable transfer pipette. Light-protect the vial with aluminum foil and incubate overnight at 4°C; the retinas should eventually sink when they become permeated by the cryoprotectant. The next day, add an equal volume of Tissue-Tek OCT compound to the vial and gently rock at room temperature for 2–4 h. Remove the sucrose/PBS/OCT solution and replace with 100% OCT, then rock again at

room temperature for 2–4 h. Transfer the retinas and OCT to a plastic tissue mold. Under a fluorescent dissecting microscope, orient the retinas so that they rest on their sides at the bottom of the mold with the fluorescence down. Freeze quickly on dry ice and store at –80°C. Section the blocks with a cryostat at 8–15 μm thickness. The frozen sections may be processed by standard histological techniques including DAPI staining. Figure 3b shows a fluorescent retinal explant that was sectioned, DAPI-stained, and imaged under high power.

References

1. Carroll SB, Grenier JK, Weatherbee SD (2005) From DNA to diversity: molecular genetics and the evolution of animal design, 2nd edn. Blackwell Pub., Malden, MA

2. Davidson EH (2001) Genomic regulatory systems: development and evolution. Academic Press, San Diego, CA

3. Ptashne M, Gann A (2002) Genes & signals. Cold Spring Harbor Laboratory Press, Cold Spring Harbor, NY

4. Blow MJ, McCulley DJ, Li Z, Zhang T, Akiyama JA, Holt A, Plajzer-Frick I, Shoukry M, Wright C, Chen F, Afzal V, Bristow J, Ren B, Black BL, Rubin EM, Visel A, Pennacchio LA (2010) ChIP-Seq identification of weakly conserved heart enhancers. Nat Genet 42:806–810

5. Visel A, Blow MJ, Li Z, Zhang T, Akiyama JA, Holt A, Plajzer-Frick I, Shoukry M, Wright C, Chen F, Afzal V, Ren B, Rubin EM, Pennacchio LA (2009) ChIP-seq accurately predicts tissue-specific activity of enhancers. Nature 457: 854–858

6. Matsuda T, Cepko CL (2004) Electroporation and RNA interference in the rodent retina in vivo and in vitro. Proc Natl Acad Sci U S A 101:16–22

7. Matsuda T, Cepko CL (2007) Controlled expression of transgenes introduced by in vivo electroporation. Proc Natl Acad Sci U S A 104:1027–1032

8. LoTurco J, Manent JB, Sidiqi F (2009) New and improved tools for in utero electroporation studies of developing cerebral cortex. Cereb Cortex 19(Suppl 1):i120–i125

9. Lee J, Myers CA, Williams N, Abdelaziz M, Corbo JC (2010) Quantitative fine-tuning of photoreceptor cis-regulatory elements through affinity modulation of transcription factor binding sites. Gene Ther 17:1390–1399

10. Carter-Dawson LD, LaVail MM (1979) Rods and cones in the mouse retina. II. Autoradiographic analysis of cell generation using tritiated thymidine. J Comp Neurol 188: 263–272

11. Young RW (1985) Cell differentiation in the retina of the mouse. Anat Rec 212:199–205

12. Kim DS, Matsuda T, Cepko CL (2008) A core paired-type and POU homeodomain-containing transcription factor program drives retinal bipolar cell gene expression. J Neurosci 28: 7748–7764

Part VII

Therapy

Chapter 24

Optimized Technique for Subretinal Injections in Mice

Regine Mühlfriedel, Stylianos Michalakis, Marina Garcia Garrido, Martin Biel, and Mathias W. Seeliger

Abstract

Subretinal injections in mice become increasingly important. Currently, the most prominent application is in gene therapy of inherited eye diseases by means of viral vector delivery to photoreceptors or the retinal pigment epithelium (RPE). Since there are no large animal models for most of these diseases, genetically modified mouse models are commonly used in preclinical proof-of-concept studies. However, because of the relatively small mouse eye, adverse effects of the subretinal delivery procedure itself may interfere with the therapeutic outcome. The protocol described here concerns a transscleral *pars plana* subretinal injection in small eyes, and may be used for but not limited to virus-mediated gene transfer.

Key words: Recombinant adeno-associated virus, Gene delivery, Subretinal injection, Transscleral *pars plana* injection, Retina, Mouse eye, Ablation, Bleb formation, Photoreceptor cell

1. Introduction

Recombinant, replication-deficient adeno-associated viral (rAAV) vectors are increasingly used in gene therapy trials in the central nervous system (1–3) and are a promising tool for human gene therapy of hereditary retinal diseases (4–6). As many such vision-threatening disorders are caused by mutations in photoreceptor and/or retinal pigment epithelium (RPE) genes, the currently best strategy for gene therapy is by local viral vector delivery via subretinal injection. The subretinal space is particularly well suited for transfection because injected material gets in direct contact with both photoreceptors (PhR) and RPE cells. Up to now, different routes of injection were described: (a) subretinal injections via a transcorneal route passing lens and vitreous (7–9) as well as (b) transscleral route entering *pars plana* at the limbus or *ora serrata* (10, 11). Recently, rAAVs have been successfully applied in experimental studies for the treatment of retinal dysfunctions or retinal

Bernhard H.F. Weber and Thomas Langmann (eds.), *Retinal Degeneration: Methods and Protocols*, Methods in Molecular Biology, vol. 935, DOI 10.1007/978-1-62703-080-9_24, © Springer Science+Business Media, LLC 2013

degenerative diseases (12–17). However, there are studies that have not succeeded to restore function in other cases (18, 19). Apart from disease model-specific causes, an important factor that may influence the outcome is the quality of vector administration. Despite recent improvements in the development of specific promoters and viral capsids, little efforts have been made so far to study and potentially optimize the procedures for subretinal delivery (20, 21). The injection technique described here bases on our experience with successfully treated gene-deficient mouse lines (22).

2. Materials

2.1. Anesthesia, Solutions, and Agents

1. Purified virus stored at −80 °C (vector titer: 3×10^8 to 8×10^9 vector genomes/μl).

2. Mixture of ketamine (working solution: 66.7 mg/kg) and xylazine (working solution: 11.7 mg/kg).

3. Tropicamide eye drops (Mydriaticum Stulln, Pharma Stulln GmbH, Germany).

4. Carbomer hydrogel (Vidisic®, Dr. Mann Pharma, Berlin).

5. Dexamethason and Gentamicin ointment (Dexamytrex®, Bausch & Lomb, Berlin).

6. Acetone.

2.2. Surgical Instruments and Supplies

1. Operating microscope (Zeiss, Germany).

2. Glass syringe (WPI Nanofil syringe 10 μl, World Precision Instruments, Berlin).

3. Sterile needles (34-gauges with 25° beveled tip, WPI).

4. Sterile curved surgical forceps.

5. Glass cover slips (7–10 mm in diameter).

6. Warming blanket.

3. Methods

3.1. Preparation of the Virus Suspension

1. Centrifuge the purified virus suspension shortly and store the collecting tube on ice.

3.2. Anesthesia and Preparation of Mice

1. Before starting the experiment, sterilize surgical instruments, needles, and syringes by incubating with 70 % ethanol for 10–15 min. Rinse needles three times with sterile water.

2. Anesthetize the mouse by subcutaneous injection of the prepared mixture of ketamin and xylazin. The mouse will develop adequate anesthesia in approximately 5 min.

3. For pupillary mydriasis apply tropic amide eye drops. The pupil is fully dilated within 2–3 min. If necessary, another drop of tropic amide has to be placed on the cornea when the pupil is not adequately dilated up to that point in time. After dilation, it should take <5 min to complete the surgery.

3.3. Injection Procedure

Subretinal injection is performed under direct visualization using an operating microscope.

1. Fill the syringe with 1–2 µl vector suspension. Prevent air bubbles in the solution (see Note 1).

2. Position the mouse with its nose pointing away from the surgeon and its right eye facing up toward the ring light and the microscope.

3. Drop the hydrogel on the cornea and cover it with a glass cover slip. Visualize the fundus in such a way that its blood vessels and the optic nerve head can be clearly seen (see Note 2). This serves as a means to assess the condition of the eye before injection and as a control for the postoperative condition of the retina (Fig. 1a). The cover slip is not removed during the surgery.

4. Grasp the *tunica conjunctiva* with the forceps at favored site as desired (e.g., dorsal part) and place the sterile needle at the inferior site of the *ora serrata*. The tip of the needle should be positioned with the aperture turned up (Fig. 1a).

5. Advance the needle *ab externo* transsclerally into the subretinal space. Under manual control, inject the suspension slowly with low pressure as soon as the tip of the needle becomes visible after its passage through the sclera/RPE (more easily in pigmented mice). The injection in the subretinal space results in a visible retinal detachment due to the bleb formation (Fig. 1b, see Notes 3 and 4). A 34-gauge needle may be reused about ten times before replacement.

6. Withdraw the needle slowly. Rinse the needle two times with sterile water and acetone. Sterilize the needle with 70 % ethanol by rinsing several times and wash again with sterile, desalinated water.

7. Optional: Monitoring and assessment of the quality of subretinal injection, retinal morphology, size of ablation as well as injection site using the in vivo imaging techniques (e.g., cSLO and SD-OCT, Fig. 2).

8. Place the animal on a warming blanket. Apply ointment to the corneas to prevent drying eyes while the animal recovers from anesthesia.

9. Note injection site, volume, virus titre, bleb formation as well as any side effects.

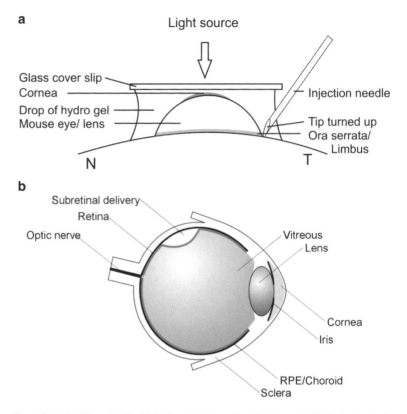

Fig. 1. Sketch of the subretinal injection technique described here. (**a**) Technical setup for the intraocular injection. The fundus is visualized by means of a "contact lens" consisting of a drop of a hydrogel on the cornea, covered with a glass cover slip. The tangential position of the 34-gauge beveled needle is shown just before transscleral passage at the site of the *ora serrata*. N = nasal, T = temporal. (**b**) Schematic view of the cavity following a transscleral injection to the subretinal space, which has formed between the retina and the RPE at the dorsal part of the eye.

3.4. Postoperative Treatment

1. Provide antibiotic ointment two times daily for 48 h. Opacity of the eye is mostly due to injuries of the lens and/or cornea via the needle tip. Animals should be excluded from further studies (see Notes 5 and 6).

4. Notes

1. Air bubbles in the vector solution can be avoided by rinsing (slowly) the needle several times with sterile water and replacing the water with the vector suspension before starting the experiment.

2. Because of the small size of the mouse eye, the success of a subretinal injection is not easy to evaluate, particularly for less experienced investigators. A surgery microscope offers the best

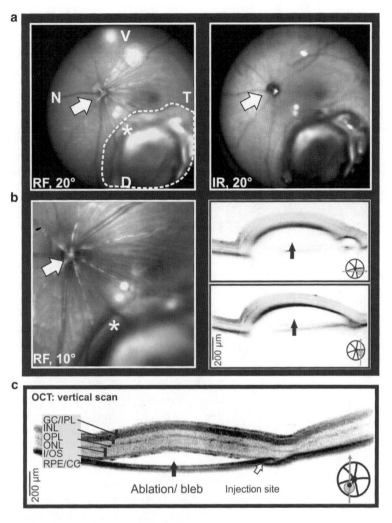

Fig. 2. Quality control of the retinal detachment immediately after subretinal injection by a combination of cSLO and SD-OCT. (a) Fundus images of the injection site in relation to landmarks of the murine retinal morphology (vessels, optic nerve head (*open arrows*)). *Left*: Surface-enhanced view at 514 nm laser wavelength (*green*, labeled RF). The *broken line* indicates the position of the subretinal injection cavity. *Asterisks* indicate a site where retinal vessels are pushed apart by the bleb. Also, their continuation on top of the bleb is well visible. *Right*: Depth-enhanced view at 830 nm laser wavelength (infrared, labeled IR). (b) *Left*: Higher magnification detail (10°) of the 514 nm image in (a). *Right*: SD-OCT images reveal the detachment of the retina (*filled arrows*) in the injected area in horizontal and in vertical orientation following the intervention. (c) Detailed in vivo SD-OCT imaging of the retinal architecture of a subretinally injected eye. The detachment (*filled arrow*) is located between the photoreceptor cell layer (IS/OS) and the RPE. Note the injection site (*open arrow*). D = dorsal, V = ventral, T = temporal, N = nasal, RPE/CC = retinal pigment epithelium/choriocapillaris, I/OS = inner/outer segments, ONL = outer nuclear layer, OPL = outer plexiform layer, INL = inner nuclear layer, GC/IPL = ganglion cells and inner plexiform layer.

view and allows for a well-controlled intraocular procedure. Additionally, in vivo imaging immediately postinjection using cSLO and SD-OCT is very helpful to improve quality of the injection and fine tuning of the surgical procedure. There are several causes of incorrect cargo delivery into the subretinal space.

3. By using the transscleral as well the transcorneal route of administration, retinal and choroidal vessels may be injured by the needle tip resulting in hemorrhages. By using a glass cover slip during the injection, the fundus and the retinal vessels may be well visualized. This information is used to select the optimal combination of the fixation site (where the eye is held with the fine forceps) and the entry position (where the needle passes through the RPE).

4. By using the transscleral as well the transcorneal route of administration, injected material may go suprachoroidally or subchoroidally. This can be avoided by strict control of the position of the tip of the needle as well as by generation of a sufficient retinal detachment by bleb formation.

5. By using the transscleral as well as the transcorneal route of administration, material may end up in the vitreous or the lens, resulting in damages and in incorrect administration of the cargo. Transscleral injection: Overly high pressure during the injection results in fine ruptures of the retinal layers. The tip of the needle may easily pass through the inner retina/ganglion cells, resulting in incorrect injections in the lens or vitreous. The difference between a needle tip located either subretinally or intravitreally may be visualized by the properties of reflectance: when located intravitreally, tips appear more clear and bright than those located subretinally. Transcorneal injection: Premature injection by misinterpretation of the tip position before reaching the subretinal space.

6. The postoperative treatment with antibiotic ointment is important to prevent eyes from drying out and infections resulting in neovascularizations of the cornea. These processes lead to irreversible side effects that may prevent further follow-up examinations.

Acknowledgment

This work was supported by Deutsche Forschungsgemeinschaft (Se837/6-1, Se837/7-1).

References

1. McCown TJ (2005) Adeno-associated virus (AAV) vectors in the CNS. Curr Gene Ther 5:333–338 (Review)

2. Marks WJ Jr, Ostrem JL, Verhagen L et al (2008) Safety and tolerability of intraputaminal delivery of CERE-120 (adeno-associated virus serotype 2-neurturin) to patients with idiopathic Parkinson's disease: an open-label, phase I trial. Lancet Neurol 7:400–408

3. den Hollander AI, Black A, Bennett J (2010) Lighting a candle in the dark: advances in genetics and gene therapy of recessive retinal dystrophies. J Clin Invest 120:3042–3053

4. Bainbridge JW, Smith AJ, Barker SS et al (2008) Effect of gene therapy on visual function in Leber's congenital amaurosis. N Engl J Med 358:2231–2239

5. Bennett J, Ashtari M, Wellman J et al (2012) AAV2 gene therapy readministration in three adults with congenital blindness. Sci Transl Med 4, 120ra15

6. Jacobson SG, Cideciyan AV, Ratnakaram R et al (2012) Gene therapy for leber congenital amaurosis caused by RPE65 mutations: safety and efficacy in 15 children and adults followed up to 3 years. Arch Ophthalmol 130:9–24

7. Timmers AM, Zhang H, Squitieri A et al (2001) Subretinal injections in rodent eyes: effects on electrophysiology and histology of rat retina. Mol Vis 7:131–137

8. Johnson CJ, Berglin L, Chrenek MA et al (2008) Technical brief: subretinal injection and electroporation into adult mouse eyes. Mol Vis 14:2211–2226

9. Busskamp V, Duebel J, Balya D et al (2010) Genetic reactivation of cone photoreceptors restores visual responses in retinitis pigmentosa. Science 329:413–417

10. Price J, Turner D, Cepko C et al (1987) Lineage analysis in the vertebrate nervous system by retrovirus-mediated gene transfer. Proc Natl Acad Sci U S A 84:156–160

11. Schlichtenbrede FC, da Cruz L, Stephens C et al (2003) Long-term evaluation of retinal function in Prph2Rd2/Rd2 mice following AAV-mediated gene replacement therapy. J Gene Med 5:757–764

12. Alexander JJ, Umino Y, Everhart D et al (2007) Restoration of cone vision in a mouse model of achromatopsia. Nat Med 13:685–687

13. Janssen A, Min SH, Molday LL et al (2008) Effect of late-stage therapy on disease progression in AAV-mediated rescue of photoreceptor cells in the retinoschisin-deficient mouse. Mol Ther 16:1010–1017

14. Cideciyan AV, Hauswirth WW, Aleman TS et al (2009) Human RPE65 gene therapy for Leber congenital amaurosis: persistence of early visual improvements and safety at 1 year. Hum Gene Ther 20:999–1004

15. Simonelli F, Maguire AM, Testa F et al (2010) Gene therapy for Leber's congenital amaurosis is safe and effective through 1.5 years after vector administration. Mol Ther 18:643–650

16. Palfi A, Millington-Ward S, Chadderton N et al (2010) Adeno-associated virus-mediated rhodopsin replacement provides therapeutic benefit in mice with a targeted disruption of the rhodopsin gene. Hum Gene Ther 21:311–323

17. Sun X, Pawlyk B, Xu X et al (2010) Gene therapy with a promoter targeting both rods and cones rescues retinal degeneration caused by AIPL1 mutations. Gene Ther 17:117–131

18. Towne C, Setola V, Schneider BL et al (2011) Neuroprotection by gene therapy targeting mutant SOD1 in individual pools of motor neurons does not translate into therapeutic benefit in fALS mice. Mol Ther 19:274–283

19. Lhériteau E, Libeau L, Mendes-Madeira A et al (2010) Regulation of retinal function but non-rescue of vision in RPE65-deficient dogs treated with doxycycline-regulatable AAV vectors. Mol Ther 18:1085–1093

20. Bainbridge JW, Mistry A, Schlichtenbrede FC et al (2003) Stable rAAV-mediated transduction of rod and cone photoreceptors in the canine retina. Gene Ther 10:1336–1344

21. Liang FQ, Anand V, Maguire AM et al (2001) Intraocular delivery of recombinant virus. Methods Mol Med 47:125–139

22. Michalakis S, Mühlfriedel R, Tanimoto N et al (2010) Restoration of cone vision in the CNGA3$^{-/-}$ mouse model for congenital complete lack of cone photoreceptor function. Mol Ther 18:2057–2063

Chapter 25

Adeno-Associated Viral Vectors for Gene Therapy of Inherited Retinal Degenerations

John G. Flannery and Meike Visel

Abstract

Adeno-associated virus (AAV) vectors are in wide use for in vivo gene transfer for the treatment of inherited retinal disease. AAV vectors have been tested in many animal models and have demonstrated efficacy with low toxicity. In this chapter we describe some of the recent methods for small-scale production of these vectors for use in a laboratory setting in volumes and purity appropriate for testing in small and large animals.

Key words: Adeno-associated virus, Gene transfer, Retinal degeneration

1. Introduction

Gene transfer to nondividing retinal neurons, epithelia, and glia is an essential technique for basic studies of retinal function as well as development and testing of gene-augmentation, knockdown, and gene replacement therapeutics. Adeno-associated viral (AAV) vectors have emerged as the viral vector of choice for many applications as they provide long-term stable expression of the genetic "payload" and few deleterious side effects.

To date, most of the retinal cell types that have been targeted with therapeutic gene constructs for ocular disease have been neurons (photoreceptors, retinal ganglion cells) and epithelia (RPE). Fortunately, the natural "tropism" for the best-characterized AAV (serotype 1–9) are neurons and epithelia. AAV serotypes 8 and 9 efficiently transduce Muller glia when delivered into the subretinal space. The types of therapeutic cDNA "payloads" that have been transferred to the retina are enzymes and structural proteins to replace recessive null mutations, as well as shRNA and ribozymes to "knock down" a dominant mutation and neurotrophins and

Bernhard H.F. Weber and Thomas Langmann (eds.), *Retinal Degeneration: Methods and Protocols*, Methods in Molecular Biology, vol. 935, DOI 10.1007/978-1-62703-080-9_25, © Springer Science+Business Media, LLC 2013

survival factors. In addition, groups have transferred molecules to suppress retinal neovascularization, such as the soluble VEGF receptor sFLT.

The intraocular use of AAV vectors is expanding with the advent of the field of optogenetics—as genetically encoded optical switches such as channelrhodopsins (1), halorhodopsin (2), LiGluR (3), as well as fluorescent optical reporters such as GCaMP (4, 5) find wider application to circuit analysis in the retina (6). In addition, the use of cre-expressing and cre-dependent expression vectors to achieve mosaic transgene expression is expanding rapidly.

Clearly, AAV vectors have limitations for their use in retinal gene therapies—which primarily are dictated by the structure of the wild-type virus. The recombinant AAV viral particle consists of the icosahedral viral capsid, which encloses the "payload" gene to be transferred and the appropriate promoter. The AAV capsid diameter is approximately 25 nm, which physically limits the amount of DNA that it may accommodate within. The wild-type AAV has a genome of 4,675 nucleotides and the recombinant vectors cannot encapsidate DNA sequences significantly larger than 5 kb. Wild-type AAV is a dependovirus; it is not enveloped and replication incompetent. The recombinant versions as generated in the methods of this chapter are similarly unable to replicate. Wild-type AAV will replicate only in a cell when co-infected by a helper virus, such as adenovirus or herpes simplex.

The laboratory production methods outlined in this chapter are modified from the mechanisms of wild-type replication in vivo. In brief, the approach is termed "triple transfection" as it consists of transfecting a mammalian cell line with three plasmids (7):

1. A therapeutic gene flanked by the viral inverted terminal repeats (ITR).
2. A plasmid encoding the AAV capsid and replication genes.
3. The adenoviral genes (normally supplied by adenoviral coin-fection) that are required for the helper functions.

Two to three days later, the transfected cells and media are harvested and the recombinant AAV particles are purified from the cell lysate.

The primary limitation for the use of AAV in treating retinal disease is the packaging limit imposed by the physical size of the capsid. The naturally occurring serotypes all have a packaging limitation of approximately 4.7 kb. There have been reports of delivery of larger inserts (8); however, upon closer examination the transfer appears to be mediated by transfer of fractional portions of the gene construct and homologous recombination within the target cell rather than encapsidation and transfer of a single, intact gene construct significantly larger than 5 kb (9, 10).

Overall, the initial question is: "Which retinal cell type to transduce?" The AAV vector must transduce the cell class harboring the mutation in gene replacement for recessive diseases and "knockdown" for dominant diseases. However, in the case of neuroprotection or anti-angiogenesis therapy with a secreted molecule it is not necessary to transduce the cell harboring the mutation, and in fact it may be advantageous to secrete the factor from a neighboring "healthy" cell type (11).

In all applications in the eye, targeting of the gene construct to the intended cell type, while minimizing the ectopic expression in neighboring cells, is an essential goal. This may be approached in a rational series of steps, initially choosing the site of injection (Figs. 1, 2, and 3), secondarily by controlling the viral binding to the cell surface (Fig. 4), and finally by the choice of promoter contained within the vector. The initial decision is whether the viral particles will be delivered intraocularly into the vitreous cavity, or the subretinal space. As the diffusion distances of the viral particles are short, and the viral capsids interact with cell surface receptors—this choice of where to introduce the particles largely controls which cell types are exposed to the vector. Most recently, studies have indicated a potential additional route via intravascular gene transfer to the retina with AAV serotype 9 (12, 13).

After the initial selection of injection route, the second factor controlling which cells are transduced is the vector serotype—which plays a major role in the capsid-to-cell surface receptor interaction.

The ability to transfect specific retinal cell classes has increased by the identification and characterization of multiple AAV serotypes, of which serotypes 1–9 are the best characterized to date. It is important to note that although AAV serotype 2 is currently used in most clinical trials for eye disease, that choice is somewhat dictated by the fact that the preclinical data and pathway to IND filing requires many years, and that this process was initiated prior to the in vivo characterization of many of the serotypes. AAV serotype 2 remains a good choice for many applications in the retina, but its clinical use should not be construed that it is the best or only option for many studies.

In addition to the naturally occurring serotypes, study of the AAV capsid structure has progressed to the point where rational modifications to the capsid can be designed to change or increase their infectivity or efficiency. These modifications include insertions of short peptides into precise locations on the capsid surface (14), modifications of the surface tyrosines to reduce ubiquitination (15), or selection of serotypes to minimize interaction with preexisting anti-AAV antibodies. In addition, AAV libraries (16) have been generated with specific targeting properties for application to the retina (17–19).

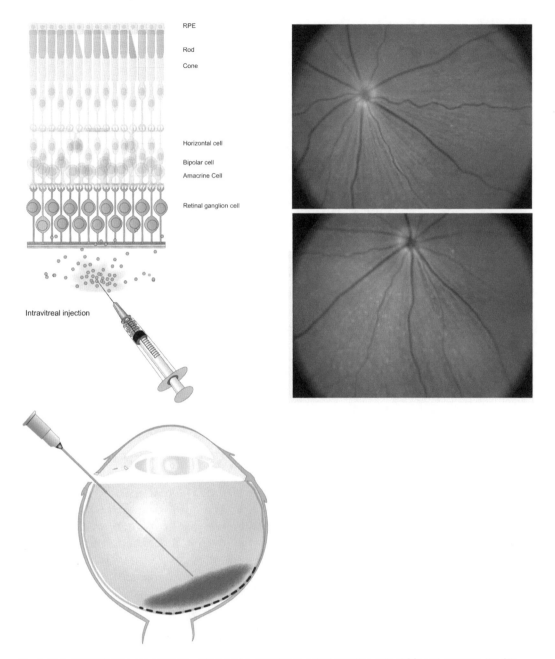

Fig. 1. Intravitreal injection can generate widespread expression in retinal ganglion cells (RGC) and retinal Muller Glia.

Finally, the property that governs whether a particular gene construct is successfully delivered to a cell is the promoter elements included within the construct. This part of the vector design is highly specialized to the particular application, and design feature is beyond the scope of this chapter; however careful consideration must be paid to this, as the packaging limits of 4.7 kb confer

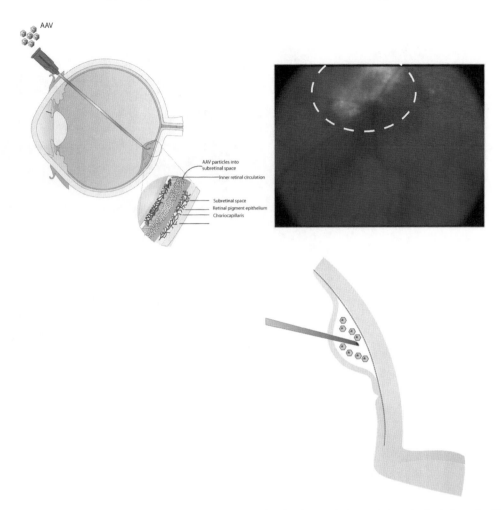

Fig. 2. Subretinal injection can generate efficient transduction of rod and cone photoreceptors and retinal pigment epithelium within a confined region of the injection site or "bleb".

significant constraints on the size of the promoter region that may be included.

Regardless of the serotype and promoter ultimately chosen, the production and packaging goals remain similar—generation of high-titer AAV with minimal impurities. It is important to note that the following methods described are similar to those used in the Standard Operating Procedures for many Academic and commercial vector core facilities. Caution must be taken when using vectors from these multi-application facilities for intraocular use. For most non-ocular applications, AAV vectors are generated using a triple transfection protocol and purified using a sequential process of nuclei isolation, density gradient centrifugation, and heparin sulfate affinity column chromatography. However, for most in vivo applications, such as injection into a large tissue (e.g., muscle or brain)

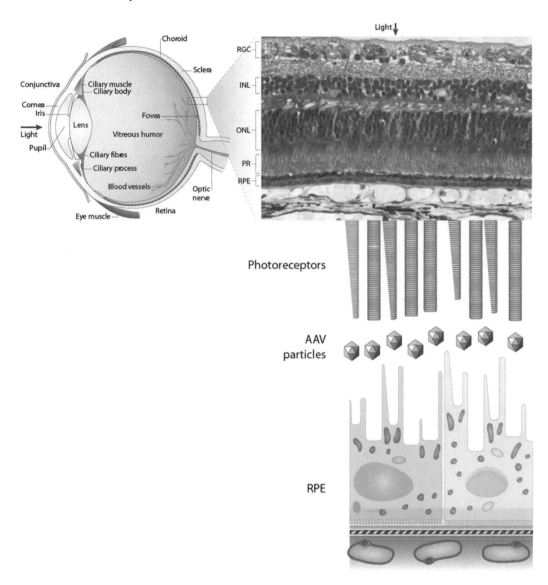

Fig. 3. Subretinal injection of AAV places the viral particles in physical contact with rod and cone photoreceptors, as well as the retinal pigment epithelium.

or systemically, a small amount of protein impurities will generate no significant immune response. In the context of a typical ~1 μl injection of concentrated AAV into the mouse eye, however, this proportion of antigenic protein can generate a substantial uveitis immune response. Similarly, many vectors generated in shared facility are resuspended in high-salt buffer to enhance storage and stability. The introduction of microliter quantities of AAV suspended in these very-high-salt solutions can have a dramatic change in the osmolarity of the subretinal space and induce significant damage to the photoreceptors and RPE.

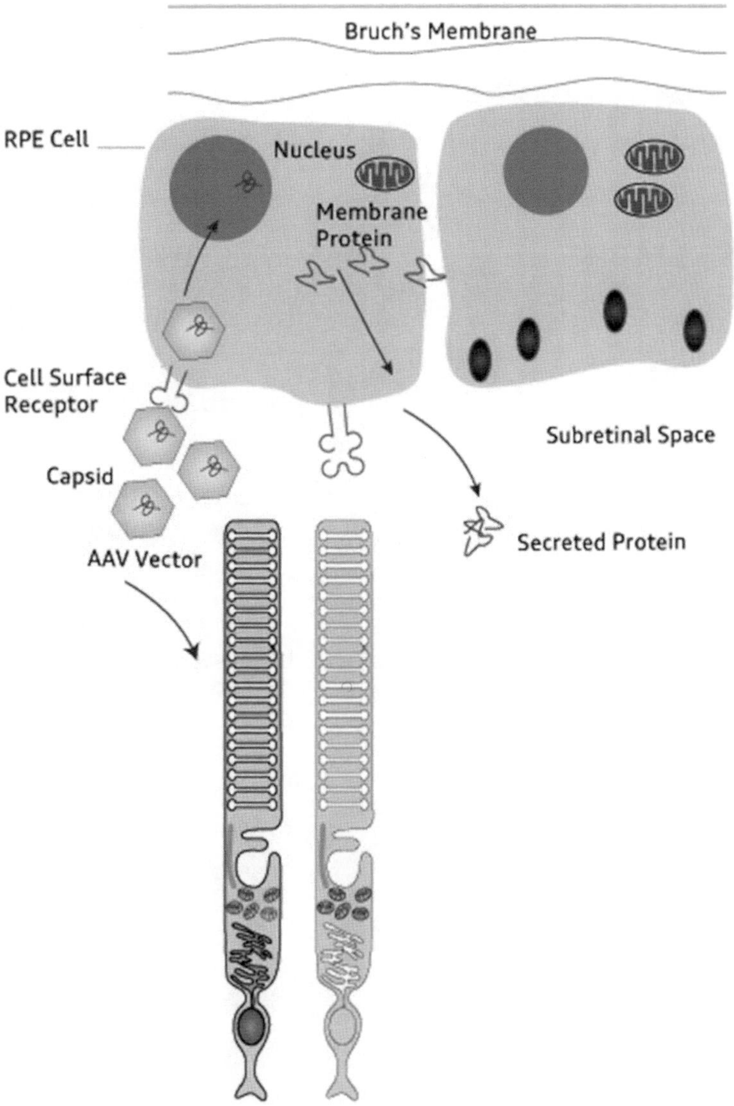

Fig. 4. AAV capsid binding to cell surface receptors mediates the cellular "tropism" of an AAV serotype. The first step of infection is mediated by interactions between the AAV capsid and cell surface receptors. In the case of subretinal injection, the AAV particles encounter the apical RPE, as well as the rods and cones. Only if the AAV particle is successfully endocytosed into the target cell, will the promoter choice have an effect on expression.

In this chapter, we outline a general method for production of small quantities of purified AAV vectors appropriate for use in the eye to transduce the retina (Fig. 5). These are not GMP/GLP methods, but can generate titers above 10^{13} particles/ml if carefully implemented. The described method is not optimized to generate large quantities of vector for systemic use in animals, nor in adequate

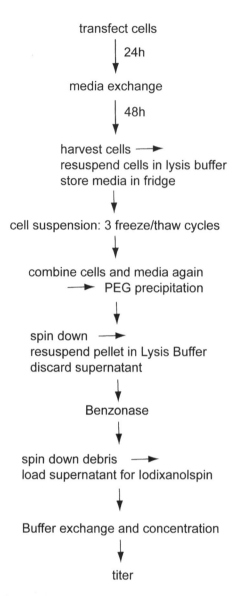

Fig. 5. General outline for production of AAV vectors.

quantities or purity for clinical trials in humans. In general, these methods are appropriate for studies in rodent models, but are scalable to generate larger volumes for larger animals if required.

2. Materials

2.1. Packaging of Vector

1. AAV cis-plasmid (see Notes 1, 4, and 5).
2. AAV trans-plasmid (see Notes 2, 4, and 5).

3. Adenoviral helper (see Notes 3–5).

4. 15 cm cell culture plates.

5. 293 Cells (ATCC #CRL-1573; see Note 6).

6. DMEM high glucose with 10% FBS and 2 mM L-glutamine added.

7. Dulbecco's phosphate-buffered saline (D-PBS).

8. Trypsin.

9. jetPRIME™ and jetPRIME™ buffer (see Note 7).

10. AAV lysis buffer: 50 mM Tris–HCl, 150 mM NaCl, and 0.05% Tween-20 in distilled water; adjust the pH to 8.5 and sterile filter before use.

11. Benzonase 250 U/μl.

12. Precipitation solution: 40% PEG 8000, 2.5 M NaCl in distilled water; sterile filter before use (see Note 9).

2.2. Iodixanol Purification

1. Buffer A (60% Iodixanol): Optiprep media.

2. Buffer B (10× PBS-MK): Dissolve 10 mM $MgCl_2$ and 25 mM KCl in 10× D-PBS and filter.

3. Buffer C (1× PBS-MK): Dilute Buffer B 1:10 with distilled water.

4. Buffer D (1× PBS-MK+2 M NaCl): Dilute Buffer B 1:10 with distilled water, add 2 M NaCl, and filter.

5. Buffer E (54% Iodixanol): Combine 250 ml Buffer A with 27.8 ml Buffer B.

6. 70.1 Ti rotor (Beckman Coulter).

7. Beckman Coulter Quick-Seal tubes (#342413).

8. Beckman Coulter tube topper.

9. 5 ml syringe.

10. Metal cannula to fill Quick-Seal tubes.

11. ~21 g and ~18 g needle.

12. 70% Ethanol.

13. Prepare Iodixanol solutions for layering:

15% Iodixanol: 37.5 ml Buffer E+67.5 ml Buffer D+30 ml Buffer C.

25% Iodixanol: 62.5 ml Buffer E+72.5 Buffer C+337.5 μl Phenol Red (0.5%).

40% Iodixanol: 100 ml Buffer E+35 ml Buffer C.

60% Iodixanol: Add 125 μl Phenol Red to 50 ml Buffer A.

2.3. Concentration and Buffer Exchange

1. Amicon Ultra-4 centrifugal filter unit (100,000 MNWL).
2. D-PBS+ with 0.01% Tween-20.
3. D-PBS+ with 0.001% Tween-20.
4. Sterile syringes.
5. Syringe filter (0.2 μM).

2.4. QPCR Quantification of Viral Titer

1. DNAseI, reaction Buffer, EDTA.
2. Proteinase K.
3. Platinum Taq, 50 mM $MgCl_2$, 10× Platinum Taq Buffer.
4. Forward ITR primer: 5′-GGAACCCCTAGTGATGGAGTT-3′.
5. Reverse ITR primer: 5′-CGGCCTCAGTGAGCGA-3′.
6. AAV2 ITR probe: 5′-FAM-CACTCCCTCTCTGCGCGCT CG-BHQ-3′.
7. QPCR instrument.

3. Methods

3.1. Packaging

1. Before starting the transfection process, make certain that you have adequate quantities of the plasmids on hand.
2. 24 h before the transfection, pass the 293 cells. Plate 1E+7 (or the amount of cells that will result in a 60–80% confluent plate on the transfection day) 293 cells in each of the eight 15 cm plates in 15 ml DMEM high glucose with 10% FBS and 2 mM L-glutamine.
3. The next day check the cells for density and prepare the transfection. It is not recommended to transfect more than five plates at once, since the transfection mix should not incubate for prolonged periods.
4. We recommend preparing two sets of the following (for four plates):
   4 ml jetPRIME buffer.
   + 28.4 μg AAV cis-plasmid.
   + 17.2 μg AAV trans-plasmid.
   + 34.4 μg adenoviral helper plasmid.
5. Vortex briefly. Add 160 μl jetPRIME and vortex the mixture for 10 s.
6. After 10 min of incubation, add 1 ml of the transfection mix drop-wise evenly on each plate (see Notes 7 and 8).

7. Gently rock the plates back and forth from side to side. After 4–12 h of incubation, the medium can be replaced with 20 ml fresh medium.

8. 72 h after transfection, harvest cells by pipetting media up and down and dispense into four 50 ml tubes.

9. Spin at $1,000 \times g$ for 10 min to pellet cells. Decant the supernatant (*maintain in refrigerator or on ice*) and resuspend cells in a total of 20 ml AAV lysis buffer (5 ml lysis buffer in each falcon tube).

10. Freeze/thaw the pellet three times in a dry ice/ethanol slurry and a 37°C water bath.

11. Gently vortex the pellet between cycles. After the freeze/thaw cycles, combine the cell lysate with the supernatant.

12. Add 40% PEG + 2.5 M NaCl to a final concentration of 8% PEG + 0.5 M NaCl and incubate on ice for 2 h (see Note 9).

13. Spin down the precipitate at $3,700 \times g$ for 20 min at 4°C.

14. Aspirate the supernatant and resuspend the pellet by pipetting up and down in a total volume of 21 ml AAV lysis buffer.

15. Let the solution sit overnight in the refrigerator, or alternatively for 1 h at 37°C to assist in resuspension.

16. Add 4.2 μl of Benzonase for a final concentration of 50 U/ml and incubate at 37°C for 30 min.

17. Centrifuge at $3,700 \times g$ for 20 min at 4°C to pellet debris, and keep the supernatant which contains AAV vector.

3.2. Initial Purification with Iodixanol

1. Layer AAV-containing solution and Iodixanol carefully into each of the four quick seal ultracentrifuge tubes using a 5 ml syringe and long metal cannula in the following order:

   (a) 5.25 ml AAV crude lysate.

   (b) 2.4 ml 15% Iodixanol.

   (c) 1.9 ml 25% Iodixanol.

   (d) 1.6 ml 40% Iodixanol.

   (e) 1.6 ml 60% Iodixanol.

2. The cannula should be placed at the bottom of the tube and the plunger needs to be pushed slowly so that the layering is not disturbed. It is also important to avoid air bubbles. We first measure and pipette the solutions in a 15 ml tube and then remove the whole volume.

3. Gently fill up the top of the tube with AAV lysis buffer up to the beginning of the neck of the tube.

4. Seal tubes with tube topper and check for leaks by gently squeezing walls of tube.

5. Centrifuge at 69,000 rpm (437,250×g) for 60 min at 18°C with acceleration and brake on setting #9.

6. After the centrifugation spin has completed, pierce tube at the top with a 21-gauge needle.

7. Hold a tissue between needle and tube to prevent liquid from spraying out.

8. Wipe the outside of the tube with 70% ethanol, 2 mm below the 40–60% interface, and puncture the tube with an 18 gauge needle attached to a 5 ml syringe (approximately at the height of the sealing line in the plastic tube).

9. Turn the bevel of the needle down and slowly remove ~75% (~1.2–1.5 ml) of the clear 40% Iodixanol layer (see Note 10).

3.3. Concentration and Buffer Exchange

1. Pre-incubate Amicon Ultra-4 centrifugal filter unit with 4 ml D-PBS + 0.01% Tween for 10 min and spin at 3,700×g for 5 min.

2. Add 4 ml of the diluted Iodixanol fraction containing the vector to the filter and spin at 3,700×g for 5–10 min at 4°C (or the time it takes to spin down to ~50–100 µl).

3. Discard the flow-through and refill the filter with the Iodixanol fraction until it is gone.

4. Add 4 ml D-PBS + 0.001% Tween-20, and spin at 3,700×g for 5–10 min at 4°C (or the time it takes to spin down to ~50–100 µl).

5. Repeat this two more times for a total of three buffer washes.

6. Remove the final buffer exchanged vector in a volume of 100–250 µl.

7. Wash the filter unit with an additional ~50 µl D-PBS + 0.001% Tween-20 and pool if desired (see Note 11).

3.4. QPCR Quantification of Viral Titer

To determine the viral genome titer we begin with a DNAse I/ Proteinase K digest followed by QPCR (20).

1. Take 5 µl of the AAV-containing solution after PEG precipitation and after the Iodixanol spin, or 1 µl of the concentrated virus.

2. Digest with 1 µL DNAse in 50 µl volume. Incubate for 30 min at 37°C. Add 1 µl EDTA (usually part of the DNAse kit) and inactivate the DNAse for 10 min at 65°C. The DNAse will remove any residual DNA from the sample.

3. To digest the AAV capsid and release the DNA, add 10 µg (0.5 µl) Proteinase K (20 mg/ml) and incubate for 60 min at 50°C. Heat-inactivate the Proteinase K for 20 min at 95°C.

4. Use 5 µl in the QPCR analysis: The forward and reverse primers for the QPCR amplify a 62 bp fragment located in the

AAV2-ITR. The Probe is labeled with FAM and has a black hole quencher (BHQ). The QPCR was carried out in a final volume of 25 µl using 340 nM reverse ITR primer, 100 nM forward ITR primer, 100 nM AAV2 ITR probe, 0.4 mM dNTPs, 2 mM $MgCl_2$, 1× Platinum Taq Buffer, and 1 U Platinum Taq and 5 µl template (standard, sample, and no-template control). For the standard, we use the plasmid used for transfection, in seven, tenfold serial dilutions (5 µl each of 2E+9 to 2E+3 genomes/ml). This results in a final concentration of 1E+10 to 1E+4 genomes/ml. The program is started by an initial denaturation step at 95°C for 15 min followed by 40 cycles of denaturation at 95°C for 1 min and annealing/extension at 60°C for 1 min (21) (see Note 12).

3.5. Timeline and Storage

It is possible to take breaks during the purification process but the interruption should be kept as short as possible (see Note 13). If long-term storage of the final preparation is required, it is a good idea to make single-use aliquots and to store them at –80°C. If the AAV is used within a few weeks, storage in the refrigerator is adequate (see Note 14).

4. Notes

1. The AAV cis plasmid contains the promoter and gene of interest flanked by AAV terminal repeats (Fig. 6). When creating a new construct, keep in mind that the full-length final plasmid flanked by the ITRs should not be larger than 4.7 kb. The ITRs are necessary and account for ~300 bp. If one attempts to package and encapsidate a DNA construct in AAV that is larger than 4.7 kb, the titer will drop significantly. Having a Kozak sequence in front of the gene of interest can help with translation (22). Also adding a woodchuck hepatitis virus post-transcriptional regulatory element (WPRE) often can enhance expression (22, 23). To prevent recombination the plasmid should be grown in Sure cells (Agilent). It is important not to let the cultures grow longer than 12–14 h; there may be an advantage to growing the culture at 30°C instead of 37°C (24). Before using this plasmid for packaging, always verify the plasmid with a SmaI digest. The enzyme cuts in the terminal repeats and the digest will show if the ITRs are still intact or if one or both are missing. Up to 20% recombination is acceptable, but more than this will also result in a lower titer. Sometimes viral preps will be of low final titer, despite the fact that the plasmid appears correct. In many cases, cutting and pasting the construct into a new AAV backbone (containing the ITRs) can improve the outcome.

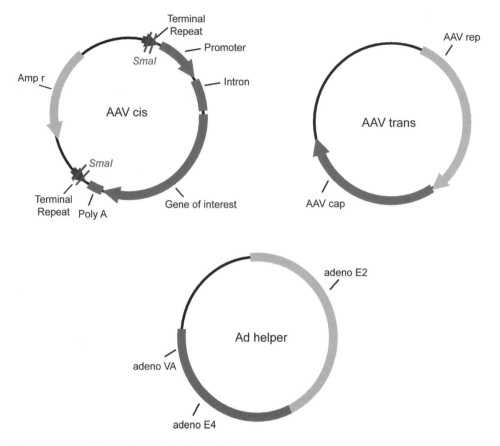

Fig. 6. Typical plasmids used for triple transfection method.

2. The AAV trans-plasmid contains the rep and cap gene. In most cases, the rep gene originates from AAV2 whereas the cap gene encodes for the desired serotype (Fig. 6).

3. The Ad helper plasmid provides the adenoviral proteins required for assembly of the virus E2, E4, and VA. This plasmid should be grown in Sure cells (Agilent) and checked with a restriction digest.

4. When choosing a Maxi prep method keep in mind that the end-product should contain low endotoxin levels and should be free of ethidium, CsCl, and RNA. We use the Endofree Maxi Prep Kit from Qiagen.

5. All plasmids needed for packaging (AAV trans, AAV cis, and Ad helper) can be obtained from the Penn Vector Core at the University of Pennsylvania (http://www.med.upenn.edu/gtp/vectorcore/index.shtml) or the Vector Core at the University of North Carolina at Chapel Hill (http://genetherapy.unc.edu/mta.htm). Agilent offers a kit: the AAV Helper-Free System containing an Ad Helper plasmid and AAV cis

cloning plasmids. There are also various AAV cis plasmids available through Addgene (http://www.addgene.org/).

6. Through the Ad E1 gene, the 293 cells provide another key to the adenoviral helper function.

7. We compared different transfection methods (Lipofectamine 2000, polyethylenimine, Fugene, PolyFect, $CaCl_2$) and found that transfection with jetPRIME gave the highest titer in our hands. Other transfection methods are described elsewhere (24, 25).

8. If you have an AAV cis-plasmid carrying a fluorescent protein and the promoter drives expression in 293 cells, you can check if the transfection was successful by looking for expression under the fluorescence microscope. This does not provide useful information about the viral titer as it only indicates success of the cis-plasmid transfection.

9. Some purification methods only use the lysed cells or the media of the transfected culture, and some use both. When we compared the concentrations in our cell lysate and media after PEG precipitation, we found that there is nearly as much AAV in the media as in the cells. For that reason, we use both the media and the cell lysate for the purification, combining them in the PEG precipitation step. It is important to note that PEG only precipitates part of the contaminating materials and therefore functions as an initial purification step (26, 27). Dissolving 40% PEG 8000, 2.5 M NaCl in water takes some time. You may need to warm up the solution slightly at first and let it stir overnight.

10. The majority of the AAV particles will be within the 40% density step. A denser appearing band between the 40 and 25% layer is typically observed; this band primarily consists of cellular proteins and should be avoided as it can generate an immune response if injected intraocularly (Fig. 7). It is possible to reduce the volume of the last resuspension steps from four tubes in the Iodixanol spin to three or sometimes two. The drawback of this is that using fewer tubes for one preparation can result in higher concentration of contaminating materials (28, 29).

11. During the final concentration/buffer exchange step, it is extremely important to mix well between each centrifugation. Otherwise, the heavier Iodixanol collects at the bottom of the tube and is still present at the end of the concentration. After washing the sides of the filter in the final step, you will combine the concentrated virus and this last wash. When doing this, check closely for a smear, which indicates the presence of the remaining Iodixanol. If this occurs, add additional buffer exchange spin(s) until no further Iodixanol is visible.

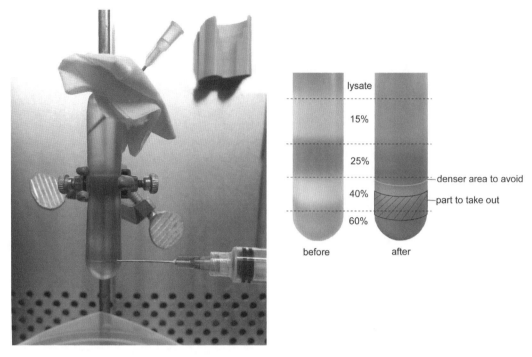

Fig. 7. Iodixanol purification: Pool all four Iodixanol fractions for a total of ~5–6 ml. Dilute with the same amount of D-PBS + 0.001% Tween-20. This solution is now ready for the buffer exchange and concentration steps (see Note 10).

12. An alternative to the use of ITR primers and probe to determine the vector genome titer of an AAV preparation is to design primers and a probe against any other part of the chimeric gene insert. Primers against your gene of interest, for example, can also be used to estimate the infectious titer. Other methods to determine the quantity and quality of the preparation include dot blot, ELISA, electron microscopy, and SDS-PAGE gels stained with silver stain or SYPRO ruby (24, 25, 30) (Fig. 8) (see Note 15). It is also possible to compare AAV2 packaged in the research lab to a reference standard material (30).

13. It is possible to interrupt the purification at some steps in the process: (a) after a freeze step during the freeze/thaw cycles; frozen pellet should be kept at −80°C and culture media containing virus in the refrigerator. (b) Instead of 2 h on ice, the PEG precipitation can be performed overnight in the refrigerator. (c) Resuspending the PEG pellet may be done overnight in the refrigerator. (d) The Iodixanol fraction can be kept in the refrigerator.

14. When troubleshooting an inadequate preparation to determine which step failed in an AAV preparation that did not generate a good result, it is always best to minimize the time that the

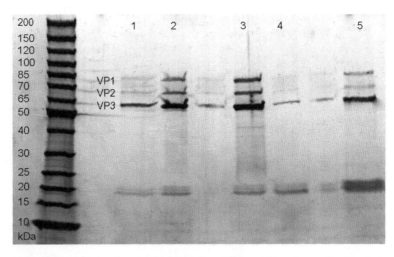

Fig. 8. SYPRO Ruby protein gel. *Lanes 1–5* show different AAV serotypes. Clear bands for VP1 (90 kDa), VP2 (72 kDa), and VP3 (60 kDa) are visible.

samples were stored before examination. Always keep in mind that each freeze/thaw cycle reduces the infectivity of the virus. Using the described method, the final titer in most cases is typically between 1×10^{12} and 1×10^{14} vg/ml (viral genomes per ml) in a final volume of 100–150 µl.

15. When examined on a silver stain or SYPRO Ruby Protein Gel, the AAV purified with the described method generates clean, distinct bands for the three capsid proteins VP1, VP2, and VP3. If a more stringent purification is desired for some serotypes, one may add a column purification step after the Iodixanol spin and before the concentration (31).

References

1. Deisseroth K (2011) Optogenetics. Nat Methods 8(1):26–29

2. Busskamp V, Duebel J, Balya D, Fradot M, Viney TJ, Siegert S, Groner AC, Cabuy E, Forster V, Seeliger M, Biel M, Humphries P, Paques M, Mohand-Said S, Trono D, Deisseroth K, Sahel JA, Picaud S, Roska B (2010) Genetic reactivation of cone photoreceptors restores visual responses in retinitis pigmentosa. Science 329(5990):413–417

3. Caporale N, Kolstad KD, Lee T, Tochitsky I, Dalkara D, Trauner D, Kramer R, Dan Y, Isacoff EY, Flannery JG (2011) LiGluR restores visual responses in rodent models of inherited blindness. Mol Ther 19(7): 1212–1219

4. Tian G, Zhou Y, Hajkova D, Miyagi M, Dinculescu A, Hauswirth WW, Palczewski K, Geng R, Alagramam KN, Isosomppi J, Sankila EM, Flannery JG, Imanishi Y (2009) Clarin-1, encoded by the Usher Syndrome III causative gene, forms a membranous microdomain: possible role of clarin-1 in organizing the actin cytoskeleton. J Biol Chem 284(28): 18980–18993

5. Muto A, Ohkura M, Kotani T, Higashijima S, Nakai J, Kawakami K (2011) Genetic visualization with an improved GCaMP calcium indicator reveals spatiotemporal activation of the spinal motor neurons in zebrafish. Proc Natl Acad Sci U S A 108(13):5425–5430

6. Greenberg KP, Pham A, Werblin FS (2011) Differential targeting of optical neuromodulators to ganglion cell soma and dendrites allows dynamic control of center-surround antagonism. Neuron 69(4):713–720

7. Xiao X, Li J, Samulski RJ (1998) Production of high-titer recombinant adeno-associated virus vectors in the absence of helper adenovirus. J Virol 72(3):2224–2232

8. Allocca M, Doria M, Petrillo M, Colella P, Garcia-Hoyos M, Gibbs D, Kim SR, Maguire A, Rex TS, Di Vicino U, Cutillo L, Sparrow JR, Williams DS, Bennett J, Auricchio A (2008) Serotype-dependent packaging of large genes in adeno-associated viral vectors results in effective gene delivery in mice. J Clin Invest 118(5):1955–1964

9. Wu Z, Yang H, Colosi P (2010) Effect of genome size on AAV vector packaging. Mol Ther 18(1):80–86

10. Dong B, Nakai H, Xiao W (2010) Characterization of genome integrity for over-sized recombinant AAV vector. Mol Ther 18(1):87–92

11. Dalkara D, Kolstad KD, Guerin KI, Hoffmann NV, Visel M, Klimczak RR, Schaffer DV, Flannery JG (2011) AAV mediated GDNF secretion from retinal glia slows down retinal degeneration in a rat model of retinitis pigmentosa. Mol Ther 19(9):1602–1608

12. Foust KD, Nurre E, Montgomery CL, Hernandez A, Chan CM, Kaspar BK (2009) Intravascular AAV9 preferentially targets neonatal neurons and adult astrocytes. Nat Biotechnol 27(1):59–65

13. Bostick B, Ghosh A, Yue Y, Long C, Duan D (2007) Systemic AAV-9 transduction in mice is influenced by animal age but not by the route of administration. Gene Ther 14(22): 1605–1609

14. Girod A, Ried M, Wobus C, Lahm H, Leike K, Kleinschmidt J, Deleage G, Hallek M (1999) Genetic capsid modifications allow efficient retargeting of adeno-associated virus type 2. Nat Med 5(9):1052–1056

15. Petrs-Silva H, Dinculescu A, Li Q, Min SH, Chiodo V, Pang JJ, Zhong L, Zolotukhin S, Srivastava A, Lewin AS, Hauswirth WW (2009) High-efficiency transduction of the mouse retina by tyrosine-mutant AAV serotype vectors. Mol Ther 17(3):463–471

16. Schaffer DV, Maheshri N (2004) Directed evolution of AAV mutants for enhanced gene delivery. Conf Proc IEEE Eng Med Biol Soc 5:3520–3523

17. Klimczak RR, Koerber JT, Dalkara D, Flannery JG, Schaffer DV (2009) A novel adeno-associated viral variant for efficient and selective intravitreal transduction of rat Muller cells. PLoS One 4(10):e7467

18. Dalkara D, Kolstad KD, Caporale N, Visel M, Klimczak RR, Schaffer DV, Flannery JG (2009) Inner limiting membrane barriers to AAV-mediated retinal transduction from the vitreous. Mol Ther 17(12):2096–2102

19. Koerber JT, Klimczak R, Jang JH, Dalkara D, Flannery JG, Schaffer DV (2009) Molecular evolution of adeno-associated virus for enhanced glial gene delivery. Mol Ther 17(12):2088–2095

20. Rohr UP, Wulf MA, Stahn S, Steidl U, Haas R, Kronenwett R (2002) Fast and reliable titration of recombinant adeno-associated virus type-2 using quantitative real-time PCR. J Virol Methods 106(1):81–88

21. Aurnhammer C, Haase M, Muether N, Hausl M, Rauschhuber C, Huber I, Nitschko H, Busch U, Sing A, Ehrhardt A, Baiker AE (2011) An universal real-time PCR for the detection and quantification of adeno-associated virus serotype 2 derived inverted terminal repeat sequences. Hum Gene Ther Med 23(1): 18–28

22. Kozak M (1987) An analysis of 5′-noncoding sequences from 699 vertebrate messenger RNAs. Nucleic Acid Res 15(20):8125–8148

23. Loeb JE, Cordier WS, Harris ME, Weitzman MD, Hope TJ (1999) Enhanced expression of transgenes from adeno-associated virus vectors with the woodchuck hepatitis virus posttranscriptional regulatory element: implications for gene therapy. Hum Gene Ther 10(14): 2295–2305

24. Choi VW, Asokan A, Haberman RA, Samulski RJ (2007) Production of recombinant adeno-associated viral vectors. Curr Protoc Hum Genet Chapter 12: Unit 12.9

25. Grieger JC, Choi VW, Samulski RJ (2006) Production and characterization of adeno-associated viral vectors. Nat Protoc 1(3): 1412–1428

26. Ayuso E, Mingozzi F, Montane J, Leon X, Anguela XM, Haurigot V, Edmonson SA, Africa L, Zhou S, High KA, Bosch F, Wright JF (2010) High AAV vector purity results in serotype- and tissue-independent enhancement of transduction efficiency. Gene Ther 17(4): 503–510

27. Vandenberghe LH, Xiao R, Lock M, Lin J, Korn M, Wilson JM (2010) Efficient serotype-dependent release of functional vector into the culture medium during adeno-associated virus manufacturing. Hum Gene Ther 21(10): 1251–1257

28. Zolotukhin S, Byrne BJ, Mason E, Zolotukhin I, Potter M, Chesnut K, Summerford C, Samulski RJ, Muzyczka N (1999) Recombinant adeno-associated virus purification using novel methods improves infectious titer and yield. Gene Ther 6(6):973–985

29. Hauswirth WW, Lewin AS, Zolotukhin S, Muzyczka N (2000) Production and purification of recombinant adeno-associated virus. Methods Enzymol 316:743–761

30. Lock M, McGorray S, Auricchio A, Ayuso E, Beecham EJ, Blouin-Tavel V, Bosch F, Bose M, Byrne BJ, Caton T, Chiorini JA, Chtarto A, Clark KR, Conlon T, Darmon C, Doria M, Douar A, Flotte TR, Francis JD, Francois A, Giacca M, Korn MT, Korytov I, Leon X, Leuchs B, Lux G, Melas C, Mizukami H, Moullier P, Muller M, Ozawa K, Philipsberg T, Poulard K, Raupp C, Riviere C, Roosendaal SD, Samulski RJ, Soltys SM, Surosky R, Tenenbaum L, Thomas DL, van Montfort B, Veres G, Wright JF, Xu Y, Zelenaia O, Zentilin L, Snyder RO (2010) Characterization of a recombinant adeno-associated virus type 2 Reference Standard Material. Hum Gene Ther 21(10):1273–1285

31. Zolotukhin S, Potter M, Zolotukhin I, Sakai Y, Loiler S, Fraites TJ Jr, Chiodo VA, Phillipsberg T, Muzyczka N, Hauswirth WW, Flotte TR, Byrne BJ, Snyder RO (2002) Production and purification of serotype 1, 2, and 5 recombinant adeno-associated viral vectors. Methods 28(2):158–167

Chapter 26

Barrier Modulation in Drug Delivery to the Retina

Matthew Campbell, Marian M. Humphries, and Peter Humphries

Abstract

The inner blood–retina barrier (iBRB) is essential in restricting the movement of systemic components such as enzymes, anaphylatoxins, or pathogens that could otherwise enter the neural retina and cause extensive damage. The barrier has evolved to confer protection to the delicate microenvironment of the retina, and the tight junctions located between adjacent microvascular endothelial cells can restrict the passage of up to 98% of clinically validated low-molecular-weight therapeutics which could hold significant promise for a range of degenerative retinal conditions. Here, we describe a method for the selective RNAi-mediated targeting of one component of the tight junction, claudin-5. We outline the generation of a doxycycline inducible adeno-associated viral vector for the localized, inducible, and size-selective modulation of the iBRB and describe how this vector can be used in ophthalmology research.

Key words: Inner blood–retina barrier (iBRB), RNAi, Claudin-5, AAV, Drug delivery, Tight junction

1. Introduction

It has been estimated that up to 98% of systemically deliverable low-molecular-weight anti-neovascular or anti-apoptotic drugs, many of which would have significant therapeutic potential in the treatment of degenerative retinal conditions, are prevented from entering the retina via the peripheral circulation because of the presence of the inner blood–retina barrier (iBRB) (1). We recently reported an experimental platform in mice for noninvasive systemic drug delivery to the retina based on transient RNAi-mediated suppression of transcripts encoding claudin-5, a component of the tight junctions of the inner retinal vasculature (2–5). This process allows for passive diffusion of low-molecular-weight compounds from the peripheral circulation into the retina while excluding larger potentially harmful substances, and we have used it to radically improve vision in a model of autosomal recessive retinitis pigmentosa by systemic drug delivery following barrier modulation.

Bernhard H.F. Weber and Thomas Langmann (eds.), *Retinal Degeneration: Methods and Protocols*, Methods in Molecular Biology, vol. 935, DOI 10.1007/978-1-62703-080-9_26, © Springer Science+Business Media, LLC 2013

We have also used the process to enhance the systemic delivery of low-molecular-weight VEGFR2 antagonists in a mouse model of choroidal neovascularization, specifically the laser-induced thermal injury model commonly used for the screening of therapeutic anti-neovascular drugs. The method is based on the incorporation into an adeno-associated viral vector (AAV2/9) of a doxycycline inducible gene that regulates the expression of shRNA targeting claudin-5. AAV9 is a serotype of AAV that was recently described as having strong efficiency in transducing vascular endothelium. The vector can be delivered by a single sub-retinal inoculation, and allows for controlled, localized, and reversible modulation of the iBRB following exposure of mice to the inducing agent doxycycline. Levels of claudin-5 will return to baseline levels following removal of doxycycline from the diet.

This form of noninvasive therapy may well be feasible as a therapeutic option in patients for sustained noninvasive ocular drug delivery. Here, we describe how the vector is generated prior to production of AAV and how these vectors are assayed for efficacy.

2. Materials

It is essential to use molecular biology grade materials at each stage of the inducible AAV vector generation. All solutions must be prepared with deionized water, stored at room temperature unless stated otherwise and autoclaved prior to use.

2.1. Buffers for Vector Construction

1. 1× TE: 10 ml 1 M Tris–HCl (pH 8.0), 400 μl 0.25 M EDTA. Make up to 1 l with distilled H_2O.

2. LB medium: 10.0 g tryptone, 5.0 g yeast extract, 10 g NaCl. Make up to 1 l with H_2O and autoclave.

3. LB agar: 10.0 g tryptone, 5.0 g yeast extract, 10 g NaCl, 15 g agar. Make up to 1 l with H_2O and autoclave. To cooled LB agar (45°C) add 10 ml of filter-sterilized ampicillin at 10 mg/ml.

4. TAE (for 1% agarose): 242 g Tris base, 57.1 ml glacial acetic acid, 18.6 g EDTA. Add H_2O to 1 l.

2.2. Materials for Sub-retinal Injections

1. Domitor and ketamine.

2. 1% Cyclopentolate and 2.5% phenylephrine eye drops.

3. 30 Gauge needles and 1 ml syringes.

4. 34-Gauge blunt-ended micro 10 μl Hamilton syringe, Bonaduz, Switzerland.

5. Atipamezole hydrochloride.

6. Amethocaine eye drops.

2.3. Reagents for Western Blot Analysis of Claudin-5 Expression

Electrophoretic equipment used in this laboratory is from Atto (Japan), but any standard SDS-PAGE electrophoresis and transfer apparatus can be used.

1. Doxycycline hyclate, Tris-base, SDS, bis-acrylamide (30%), APS, TEMED, glycine, dithiothreitol, protease inhibitor cocktail/100 ml (Sigma Aldrich, Ireland), glycerol, mercaptoethanol, bromophenol blue, methanol, NaCl. BCA-assay kit (Pierce). PVDF membrane.

2. Rabbit anti-claudin-5 (Invitrogen), rabbit anti-beta-actin (Abcam), anti rabbit IgG-HRP.

3. SuperSignal Chemiluminescent detection solution (Pierce).

4. Fuji X-ray film and cassette.

3. Methods

The shRNA sequences below are ordered as primer sequences from Sigma Genosys.

3.1. shRNA Oligo Design

shRNA sequences are based on siRNA's targeting claudin-5 and were designed by Dharmacon (4, 6–8). XhoI and HindIII restriction sites are placed at the 5' end of the top and bottom strand respectively. A guanine residue is placed at the beginning of the sense strand (Pol III transcription preferential start site). A 9 bp hairpin loop is inserted between the target sense sequence and the target antisense sequence (9–13). In addition a terminator sequence of six T residues are added in addition to a unique restriction site (Fig. 1a and b). In addition, a non-targeting shRNA must be used as a control vector. The guide sense strand of this non-targeting shRNA targets the nonmammalian gene luciferase.

3.2. Annealing of Oligonucleotides

1. Oligonucleotides are synthesized by Sigma Genosys and re-suspended in TE buffer to a final concentration of 100 μM.

2. Equal quantities of each strand are added to get approximately 50 μM of double-stranded product. Heat to 95°C for 30 s; 72°C for 2 min; 37°C for 2 min; and 25°C for 2 min. Store on ice for immediate use or freeze at –20°C until required (www.clontech.com).

3.3. Cloning Design (Insertion of shRNA into pSingle-tTS-shRNA Vector)

1. Ligation: Annealed oligos are ligated into XhoI/HindIII cut pSingle-tTS-shRNA vector (14–24) in the following reaction: 1 μl XhoI/HindIII cut pSingle-tTS-shRNA DNA vector (75 ng/μl), 1 μl annealed oligonucleotides at 0.5 μM, 3 μl 5× T4 DNA ligase buffer (Invitrogen), 1 μl T4 DNA ligase (1 unit/μl) (Invitrogen), and 9 μl H$_2$O for a final volume of

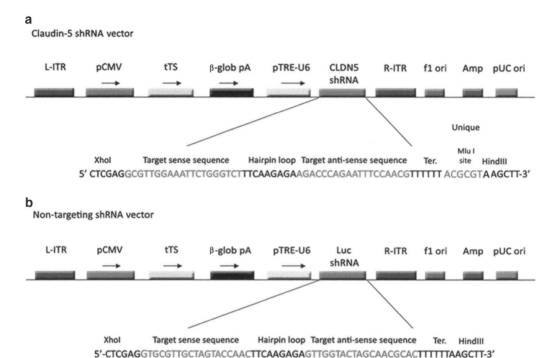

Fig. 1. Inducible claudin-5 vector map. (**a**) Plasmid incorporating the doxycycline inducible system with claudin-5 shRNA or (**b**) a non-targeting (NT) luciferase shRNA: Left and right inverted terminal repeats (L-ITR and R-ITR), CMV promoter/enhancer (pCMV), tTS (tetracycline inducible transcriptional suppressor), *β-glob pA* (beta-globin polyadenylation), *pTRE-U6* (Tet-responsive U6 promoter), f1 ori (f1 origin of replication), Amp (ampicillin selection), pUC (pUC origin of replication).

15 μl. Incubate at 18°C overnight. Set up two additional reactions as controls: (a) without annealed oligonucleotides and (b) without T4 DNA ligase.

2. Transformation: Thaw 100 μl of XL1-Blue competent cells (Agilent Technologies) on ice and add 2 μl of above ligations. Incubate reactions on ice for 30 min. Heat shock at 42°C for 45 s. Incubate on ice for 2 min. Add 898 μl of pre-warmed (42°C) LB medium, mix gently, and incubate at 37°C for 1 h. Plate 100 μl of transformation on LB agar plates (containing ampicillin 50–100 μg/ml) and incubate at 37°C overnight. Pick 10–20 plaque-forming units (pfu), re-streak onto fresh LB agar plates (Amp), and also grow colonies in 5 ml of LB Medium (Amp) overnight. Perform mini-plasmid DNA extractions using QIAprep Spin Miniprep Kit (Qiagen).

3. shRNA construct selection: Select construct for your shRNA of interest by digesting with the unique restriction endonuclease (using manufacturer's conditions) inserted into the synthesized oligonucleotide. Grow up the plasmid of choice in bulk and sequence across the shRNA to confirm insertion/orientation.

3.4. Insertion of the Inducible Fragment of the pSingle-tTS-shRNA Vector into pAAVMCS Vector

1. The inducible fragment of pSingle-tTS containing the claudin-5 shRNA is removed by double-digestion and eluted from a 1% agarose gel using QIAquick Gel Extraction Kit (Qiagen). pAAVMCS vector (Agilent Technologies) is digested with NotI restriction endonuclease, and the fragment containing the inverted terminal repeats (ITRs) eluted as above.

2. Digestion conditions: 10 μg Vector DNA, 4 units of restriction endonuclease/μg of DNA, 10× buffer, BSA × 100 if required, and H$_2$O to 100 μl. Incubate at manufacturer's recommended temperature and heat deactivate if necessary.

3. Klenow filling: 3′ overhangs are blunt ended using DNA polymerase (Klenow) using the manufacturer's conditions (New England Biolabs) before ligation.

4. Calf Intestinal Phosphatase (CIP): The pAAVMCS vector insert is treated with CIP to prevent vector self-ligation using the manufacturer's conditions (Promega).

5. Ligation and selection: Ligation of the inducible fragment of p-Single-tTS containing the claudin-5 shRNA and pAAVMCS fragment (containing the ITRs) is performed as stated above. After transformation using XL1-blue cells and overnight incubation, pfu's are picked and plasmid DNA is extracted as above. Clones containing the claudin-5 shRNA are selected using the original unique restriction endonuclease. In addition the plasmids are digested and sequenced to establish correct orientation.

6. Bulk preparation of plasmids: Plasmids are grown in bulk using Qiagen's EndoFree Plasmid Maxi Kits.

7. AAV preparations: Approximately 530 μg of plasmid DNA is sent to Vector Biolabs (Philadelphia) for AAV 2/9 construction (see Note 1 on synthesis).

3.5. Sub-retinal Inoculation of AAV in Mice

While sub-retinal injections are commonly used in animal research associated with ocular biology, it is a highly specialized and delicate technique that requires a significant amount of practice before reproducible results can be obtained. However, the technique used at this facility is outlined below.

3.5.1. Preparation of Mice for AAV Inoculation

1. Adult mice are anesthetized by intraperitoneal (i.p.) injection of a solution of domitor and ketamine (10 μg and 750 μg/10 g body weight, respectively).

2. Pupils are dilated with 1% cyclopentolate and 2.5% phenylephrine eye drops and left for 5 min.

3. A single drop of local analgesia (Amethocaine) is placed into each eye and a small puncture is administered in the sclera using a 30-guage needle.

4. Under an operating microscope, a 34-gauge blunt-ended micro-needle attached to a 10 μl syringe (Hamilton, Bonaduz, Switzerland) is inserted through the puncture, and a single 3 μl of AAV vector is administered to the sub-retinal space, after a retinal detachment is induced (see Notes 2 and 3 on viral titer).

5. Following surgery, a reversing agent (100 μg/10 g body weight, Atipamezole hydrochloride) is delivered by i.p. injection. Body temperature is constantly maintained using a homeothermic heating device.

3.6. Western Blot Analysis of Claudin-5 Expression to Confirm Suppression Efficacy

Western blot analysis allows for confirmation of AAV efficacy (see Notes 4 and 5 on experimental design and usage of these vectors). This is normally undertaken 2–3 weeks post inoculation of AAV and subsequent supplementation of doxycycline hyclate (Sigma Aldrich, Ireland) in the drinking water (2 mg/ml doxycycline in 5% sucrose diluted in water) or in the chow (Harlan Laboratories). It is an essential step prior to any experimentation with this AAV as the users must identify how effective the viral preparation will be for their own experimental paradigm.

3.6.1. Preparation of SDS-PAGE Gels

1. Electrophoresis plates are washed thoroughly before use, with water and ethanol. 12% Acrylamide resolving gels are made by adding the following components together: 6.6 ml H_2O, 5 ml 1.5 M Tris pH 8.8, 0.2 ml 10% SDS, 8 ml bis-acrylamide (30%), 0.2 ml 10% APS, and 20 μl TEMED.

2. The gels are made up according to the reagents outlined above. Gels are poured into the plates, leaving a space the length of the Teflon comb for the stacking gel, approximately 1 cm. Deionized H_2O is gently pipetted on top of the resolving gel. This prevents bubbles from forming. The gel is allowed to set for approximately 30 min.

3. 4% Acrylamide stacking gels are made by adding the following components together: 6.8 ml H_2O, 2.5 ml 0.5 M Tris pH 6.8, 0.1 ml 10% SDS, 1.33 ml bis-acrylamide (30%), 0.1 ml 10% APS, and 10 μl TEMED.

4. When the resolving gel is set, the stacking gel is poured on top and the Teflon comb is placed into the gel. This is then allowed to set for approximately 20 min.

5. The prepared plates are placed into electrophoretic apparatus. The electrophoretic apparatus is then filled with 1× running buffer prepared from a 10× solution containing 30.3 g Tris, 144.2 g glycine, and 10 g SDS, and made up to 1 l, with a pH of 8.6.

3.6.2. Loading of Protein Samples into Wells

1. Mice are sacrificed using CO_2 and immediately, retinas are dissected from the eyecups, ensuring that all pigmented material is removed prior to preparation of protein lysates. Protein is

isolated from total retinal tissue by homogenizing in lysis buffer containing 62.5 mM Tris, 2% SDS, 10 mM dithiothreitol, and 10 µl protease inhibitor cocktail/100 ml (Sigma Aldrich, Ireland). The homogenate is centrifuged at $10,000 \times g$ for 20 min at 4°C, and the supernatant is then removed for SDS-PAGE.

2. Protein levels are quantified using a BCA-assay kit (Pierce) and 30 µl of protein sample is added to 10 µl of a 4× sample buffer (6.05 g Tris, 16 g SDS, 20 ml glycerol, 16 mg bromophenol blue, 10% mercaptoethanol, pH 6.6, in 100 ml), bringing the final concentration of sample buffer to 1×.

3. Protein samples are then boiled for 2 min, to allow for denaturing.

4. Retinal protein samples are then loaded into separate lanes of the 12% gel, with a pre-stained protein marker on the outermost lane in order to determine the molecular weight of resolved bands.

5. The electrophoretic equipment is then run at ~30 mA per gel for approximately 2 h 20 min.

3.6.3. Semidry Transfer to PVDF Membrane

1. Once the protein front has reached 1 cm from the bottom of the gel, the plates are removed from the electrophoretic apparatus, and the stacking gel removed.

2. A BIO-RAD semidry electroblot apparatus is prepared by cutting eight pieces of blotting paper to the exact size of the resolving gel.

3. Four pieces of blotting paper are soaked in transfer buffer, and placed on the anode of the electroblot apparatus. Transfer buffer contains 3.03 g Tris, 14.42 g glycine, and 200 ml methanol, and is made up to 1 l with deionized water.

4. Polyvinylidene difluoride (PVDF) membrane is cut to the same size as the resolving gel and then placed in methanol for 30 s to activate the membrane. The PVDF is then placed in transfer buffer for 30 s to equilibrate and finally is placed on top of the soaked blotting paper, and the resolving gel is gently placed over this, followed by the remaining four pieces of blotting paper, which are also soaked in transfer buffer.

5. The cathode is placed over this, and the electroblot apparatus is run at 40 mA per gel for approximately 2–3 h.

6. The proteins should move from the gel to the PVDF membrane due to the negative charge induced by SDS, and will be attracted to the positive charge of the anode on which the PVDF membrane is placed.

3.6.4. Processing of Blots and Detection of Claudin-5

1. Following electroblotting to PVDF, the membrane is briefly washed in Tris-buffered saline (TBS, 50 mM Tris, 150 mM NaCl, pH 7.4; i.e., 6.05 g Tris-base, 8.766 g NaCl, adjust the

pH with HCl, and bring the volume to 1 l with dH$_2$O), in order to remove trace amounts of methanol in the transfer buffer which may increase background.

2. The membrane is incubated with 5% blocking solution (i.e., 5 g Marvell nonfat dry skimmed milk in 100 ml TBS). Blocking can be carried out for 1 h at room temperature on a shaker, or overnight at 4°C. This will prevent nonspecific binding of the primary antibody.

3. Following blocking, the membrane is washed with TBS briefly.

4. A primary antibody, specific for claudin-5 (Invitrogen) (1:500 dilution), is added to the membrane in 5% blocking solution.

5. The membrane is incubated with primary antibody overnight at 4°C.

6. The antibody/blocker solution is pipetted off the membrane, and the membrane is washed for 15 min with TBS (3× 15 min with TBS).

7. A secondary anti-rabbit IgG-HRP antibody is then incubated with the membrane at a dilution of 1:2,000 for approximately 3 h at room temperature. HRP-conjugated antibodies can cleave the chemiluminescent substrate luminol to an activated intermediate which decays to the ground state by emitting light.

8. Following incubation with the secondary antibody, the membrane is washed 4× 15 min with TBS/Tween (0.1%), ensuring that the shaker is moving at a high speed.

3.6.5. Chemiluminescent Detection of Proteins

1. Using a PIERCE reagent kit, equal volumes of substrate solution and enhancer solution are added to a SARSTEDT tube.

2. Detection solution is pipetted on the membrane and left for 1 min, after which time it is drained off the membrane using tissue or blotting paper.

3. PVDF membrane is placed on a transparent sheet (acetate film), and a sheet of X-ray film is cut to cover the PVDF membrane.

4. The film is placed over the blot in a film cassette, and exposed to the membrane for 3, 5, 10, and 20 min. Typically claudin-5 signal will need a 5-min development.

5. The film is developed using a film-developing machine.

6. For protein loading normalization, the PVDF is stripped using Pierce stripping solution Pierce and a rabbit anti-β-actin antibody is applied to the membrane overnight (1:2,000 dilution) at 4°C. The protocol for subsequent development of β-actin blot is identical to that described above for claudin-5.

4. Notes

1. Once the inducible vector is cloned, purified plasmid DNA is prepared in high concentration and can be sent to specialist commercial entities for AAV synthesis or the standard triple transfection protocol described elsewhere can be used.

2. It is essential that vector titer is established by the end user whether the AAV is synthesized commercially or "in-house."

3. Once synthesized, the AAV vectors can be aliquoted and stored at −80°C. Once thawed, the vectors should be used immediately. They can be stored at 4°C but it is not recommended to store them in these conditions for longer than 3 months. It is not recommended to freeze–thaw the AAV vectors as efficacy will be compromised.

4. An initial experiment should be undertaken whereby mice, post sub-retinal inoculation, should be dosed with doxycycline for 1, 2, and 3 weeks and subsequently sacrificed at each individual time-point and levels of claudin-5 expression analyzed. This will allow for the determination of vector efficacy.

5. These vectors can be used for a wide variety of experiments involving systemic drug delivery to the retina and indeed the brain. Therefore careful attention should be paid to the choice of low-molecular-weight compound to be studied as the size-selectivity post claudin-5 suppression is to molecules with a molecular weight below approximately 1 kDa.

References

1. Pardridge WM (2005) Molecular biology of the blood–brain barrier. Mol Biotechnol 30(1):57–70

2. Campbell M, Humphries MM, Kiang A-S, Nguyen ATH, Gobbo OL, Tam LCS, Suzuki M, Hanrahan F, Ozaki E, Farrar G-J, Kenna PF, Humphries P (2011) Systemic low molecular weight drug delivery to pre-selected neuronal regions. EMBO Mol Med 3:235–245

3. Campbell M, Nguyen ATH, Kiang AS, Tam LCS, Gobbo OL, Kerskens C, Ni Dhubhghaill S, Humphries MM, Farrar GJ, Kenna PF, Humphries P (2009) An experimental platform for systemic drug delivery to the retina. Proc Natl Acad Sci U S A 106(42):17817–17822

4. Campbell M, Kiang AS, Kenna PF, Kerskens C, Blau C, O'Dwyer L, Tivnan A, Kelly JA, Brankin B, Farrar GJ, Humphries P (2008) RNAi-mediated reversible opening of the blood–brain barrier. J Gene Med 10(8):930–947

5. Tam LC, Kiang AS, Campbell M, Keaney J, Farrar GJ, Humphries MM, Kenna PF, Humphries P (2010) Prevention of autosomal dominant retinitis pigmentosa by systemic drug therapy targeting heat shock protein 90 (Hsp90). Hum Mol Genet 19(22): 4421–4436

6. Hammond SM, Caudy AA, Hammon GJ (2001) Post-transcriptional gene silencing by double-sranded RNA. Nat Rev Genet 2:110–119

7. Sharp PA (2001) RNA interference—2001. Genes Dev 15(5):485–490

8. Hutvangner G, Zamore PD (2002) RNAi: nature abhors a double-strand. Curr Opin Genet Dev 12(2):225–232

9. Paddison PJ, Caudy AA, Bernstein E, Hannon GJ, Conklin DS (2002) Short hairpin RNAs (shRNAs) induce sequence-specific silencing in mammalian cells. Genes Dev 16(8):948–958

10. Paul CP, Good PD, Winer I, Engelke DR (2002) Effective expression of small interfering RNA in human cells. Nat Biotechnol 20(5): 505–508

11. Yu J-Y, DeRuiter SL, Turner DL (2002) RNA interference by expression of short-interfering RNAs and hairpin RNAs in mammalian cells. Proc Natl Acad Sci U S A 99(9):6047–6052

12. Lee NS, Dohjima T, Bauer G, Li H, Li MJ, Ehsani A, Salvaterra P, Rossi J (2002) Expression of small interfering RNAs targeted against HIV-1 rev transcripts in human cells. Nat Biotechnol 20(5):500–505

13. Brummelkamp TR, Bernards R, Agami R (2002) A system for stable expression of short interfering RNAs in mammalian cells. Science 296:550–553

14. Kunkel GR, Pederson T (1989) Transcription of a human U6 small nuclear RNA gene in vivo withstands deletion of intragenic sequences but not of an up-stream TATATA box. Nucleic Acid Res 17:7371–7379

15. Gossen M, Bujard H (1992) Tight control of gene expression in mammalian cells by tetracycline responsive promoters. Proc Natl Acad Sci U S A 89(12):5547–5551

16. Gossen M, Bonin AL, Bujard H (1993) Control of gene activity in higher eukaryotic cells by prokaryotic regulatory elements. Trends Biochem Sci 18:471–475

17. Gossen M, Bonin AL, Freundlieb S, Bujard H (1994) Inducible gene expression systems for higher eukaryotic cells. Curr Opin Biotechnol 5:516–520

18. Wigzgall R, O'Leary E, Leaf A, Onaldi D, Bonventre JV (1994) The Kruppel-associated box-A (KRAB-A) domain of zinc finger proteins mediates transcriptional repression. Proc Natl Acad Sci U S A 91(10):4514–4518

19. Gossen M, Bujard H (1995) Efficacy of tetracycline-controlled gene expression is influenced by cell type. Bio Techniques 19(2):213–215

20. Freundlieb S, Schirra-Muller C, Bujard H (1999) A tetracycline controlled activation/repression system with increased potential for gene transfer into mammalian cells. J Gene Med 1:4–12

21. pTet-tTS Vector (1999) Clontechniques XIV(2):10–11

22. Wiznerowicz M, Trono D (2003) Conditional suppression of cellular genes: lentivirus vector-mediated drug-inducible RNA interference. J Virol 77(16):8957–8961

23. pTRE-Tight Vectors (2003) Clontechniques XVIII(2):10–11

24. Knockout Single Vector System for Inducible RNAi (2006) Clontechniques XXI(3):2–3

INDEX

A

Ad E1 gene...365
Adeno-associated virus (AAV)......................... 5, 351–353,
    355–367, 372, 375–376, 379
Adenosine-5'-triphosphate (ATP) 227, 229,
    236, 260, 263–265, 267, 280
AlexaFluor488...247, 250
Allele-specific primer extension
    (APEX) 6–7, 16, 17, 196
Amacrine cell...99, 102, 108, 187,
    189, 191, 201, 202, 204, 205, 298
Amethocaine 372, 375
Angiography...29, 32–33, 43,
    49–51, 54, 57, 63, 65, 80
APEX. *See* Allele-specific primer extension (APEX)
Apoptosis...93, 99, 101, 103,
    105, 107, 108, 173, 207–213, 298
Aprotinin... 314, 315, 318
Atipamezole hydrochloride 372, 376
ATP. *See* Adenosine-5'-triphosphate (ATP)
ATPases.................................... 166, 189, 190, 298, 304, 305
Automatic tissue processor 246

B

Barrier modulation 371–379
BCA-assay...373, 377
Black hole quencher (BHQ)...363
Bleb formation... 345, 348
Br-dUTP..212

C

Ca²⁺ microfluorimetry...257–270
Capsid 344, 352, 353, 357, 362, 367
Carbomer hydro gel...344
Ca²⁺-sensitive fluorescent dyes.......................................298
Ca²⁺ signaling 297–307
CD133...271, 272, 275–277, 281
CD11b 272, 273, 275–279, 281
293 cells 359, 360, 365
Cell specific markers...185–198
Channel rhodopsin..351
Chemiluminescence...123
Choroidal neovascularization (CNV)............42, 54–61, 372

Chromatin immunoprecipitation............................311–327
cis-regulatory element...329–340
Claudin 5...371–379
CNV. *See* Choroidal neovascularization (CNV)
Complementary RNA (cRNA) 215, 216, 223–225
Compound eye 161–179
Cone rod homeobox (CRX).......................19, 313, 323–325
Confocal scanning laser ophthalmoscopy
    (cSLO) 43, 49, 54, 59, 60, 62, 79, 80, 345, 347, 348
Copy number variant (CNV)-detection.......................... 7, 9
Cornea...34, 36, 44, 47–49, 53,
    63, 65, 70, 72, 76, 82, 84, 85, 90–94, 102, 105,
    161, 163, 165, 173, 175, 178, 193, 195, 220,
    248, 261, 267, 280, 334, 345, 346, 348
cRNA. *See* Complementary RNA (cRNA)
CRX. *See* Cone rod homeobox (CRX)
Cryolabeling 177
cSLO. *See* Confocal scanning laser ophthalmoscopy
    (cSLO)
Cytosolic Ca²⁺ stores...303–305

D

Danio rerio.. 127–136
DAPI staining 340
Davidson's fixative 246, 247, 251
Deep pseudopupil (DPP) 162, 165, 173
Denhardt's solution 217
DIG-dNTPs 216
Dihydropyridine derivates 306
Dissecting microscope 115, 141, 142,
    144–146, 151, 178, 191–193, 225, 248,
    331, 332, 334, 336, 339, 340
DNA-protein cross-linking............................ 212, 228, 318
DNase I 362
DNA variants 6
Doxycycline 339, 372–374, 376, 379
DPP. *See* Deep pseudopupil (DPP)
Drug delivery...371–379
DsRed reporter...336–338

E

ECAR. *See* Extracellular acidification rates ((ECAR)
Electron microscopy...79, 103, 104,
    161–179, 190, 246, 366

Bernhard H.F. Weber and Thomas Langmann (eds.), *Retinal Degeneration: Methods and Protocols*, Methods in Molecular Biology,
vol. 935, DOI 10.1007/978-1-62703-080-9, © Springer Science+Business Media, LLC 2013

Electron transport chain (ETC) 228, 238, 242
Electroporation 329–340
ELISA 366
Enhancer 329, 374, 378
ETC. *See* Electron transport chain (ETC)
Excitotoxic damage 99–108
Extracellular acidification rates
    (ECAR) 230, 236–239, 241, 242
Extracellular flux assay 227–242
Eyecup preparation 220
Eye tracking 139–159

F

FACS. *See* Fluorescence-activated cell sorting (FACS)
FCCP 236–239, 241, 242
FGF2 272
FITC-POS 289–293
Flatmounts 63
Flicker 74, 76
Flow cytometry 207, 208, 211, 272, 276
Fluo-4/AM 259, 262–264, 268
Fluorescein angiography 29, 32–33, 50, 51, 63, 65
Fluorescein isothiocyanate (FITC) 58, 166,
    197, 207, 213, 287, 289–293
Fluorescence-activated cell sorting
    (FACS) 208, 210–213, 277
Formalin 208–210, 212
Forward scatter (FSC) 211
Fragment crystallizable receptor (FcR) 276
Fruitfly, *Drosophila melanogaster* 161–179
FSC. *See* Forward scatter (FSC)
Full-field electroretinography 30, 32–37,
    61, 62, 69–76, 164
Fundus photography 29, 32–33
fura-2/AM 264, 266, 270

G

Ganglion cell 54, 99–108, 186, 187,
    189, 201, 203, 264, 268, 347, 348, 351, 354
Gelvatol 217, 218, 222, 225
Gene therapy 5, 6, 343, 351–367
Genetic heterogeneity 4, 16, 17
GFP. *See* Green fluorescent protein (GFP)
Glass syringe 344
Green fluorescent protein (GFP) 51, 55, 59,
    120, 123, 136, 165, 167, 173, 223, 336–338

H

HEPES buffer 305
Histoclear II 246–249
Histone modification 312, 313
Homozygosity mapping 5, 7, 10, 17, 18

Horizontal cells 187, 189, 191, 201, 202
Horizontally-sliced preparation 201–205

I

IBMX 232, 238, 239
iBRB. *See* Inner blood–retina barrier (iBRB)
Identity-by-descent (IBD)-mapping 5, 7, 8
IFNγ. *See* Interferon gamma (IFNγ)
Image J software 247, 250, 332, 336, 337
Image Quant TL software 291
Immunoblotting 121, 287, 289, 291–292
Indocyanine green angiography 51
Infrared image 49, 50, 53, 54, 63
Inner blood–retina barrier (iBRB) 371, 372
In situ hybridization 215–225
Interferon gamma (IFNγ) 281
Intravitreal injection 99–102, 104, 105, 108, 354
Inverted terminal repeats 352, 374, 375
Iodixanol fraction 362, 366
Ion channels 298
Ionomycin 210, 299, 301–303, 306
Ion transporters 298
IP$_3$ 258

K

K$_D$ value 267
Knockdown 19, 128, 131, 351, 353

L

Laser-scanning microscopy 246, 247,
    253, 265, 287
Leukaemia inhibitory factor (LIF) 272
Light damage 87–96
Linkage analysis 4, 5, 7–8
Lipopolysaccharide (LPS) 281
Long-term culture 276

M

MACS 275, 278
Magnetic microbeads 281, 325
Microarrays 5, 7, 19, 216
Microglia 59, 93, 271–282
Microslide chamber 332, 333
Microtome 133, 177, 219, 247, 249
Mitochondrial DNA Damage 227–242
Molecular diagnostics 5–6, 9, 10
Monochromatic light 88, 90, 94
Mouse models 27–37, 41–65,
    69–76, 79–85, 99–108, 198, 372
M13 primers 218
mRNA metabolism 127
Müller glial cells 202, 257–270

N

Necrosis 93, 212, 281
Next generation sequencing
(NGS)...................................5, 9–12, 14–19, 192, 193
Nitrocellulose filter 259, 260, 263
N-Methyl-d-Aspartate (NMDA) 99–108
NR2E3 .... 313, 323–325
NRL 338

O

OCR. *See* Oxygen consumption rates (OCR)
OCT. *See* Optical coherence tomography (OCT)
OCT compound.. 332, 339
Optical coherence tomography (OCT) 6, 43–45,
50–54, 57, 61–64, 79–85, 197, 332, 337, 339, 340
Optokinetics 139–159
Orai 304
Ora serrata.....................................193, 261, 343, 345, 346
Oregon Green® 259
Outer segment......................................19, 48, 56, 61,
62, 71, 164, 186, 188, 190, 229,
245–253, 285–295, 347
Oxygen consumption rates (OCR)...........230, 236–239, 242

P

Paraffin section 102, 103, 247, 249–251
PEG precipitation 362, 365, 366
Pentacarboxylate calcium indicator....................................277
PFA fixation 132, 178
Phagocytosis.............................207, 229, 245–253, 285–295
Photobleaching.. 266, 269, 282
Photoreceptor..3, 4, 6, 19, 30,
34, 42, 48, 52, 54, 56, 60–62, 74, 88, 94–96, 108,
113, 121, 127–136, 161, 163–165, 168, 175, 178,
186–191, 197, 202–204, 211, 229, 245–253, 262,
263, 268, 269, 285–295, 313, 324, 325, 330, 337,
338, 343, 347, 351, 355, 356
Pico green 231, 234, 235
Poly-L-lysine coated cover slips 299
Porcine retina...288
POS isolation 286–287
POS phagosomes... 246, 250–251
Primary retinal cell suspension
(RCS) 271, 272, 274–276
Probe 9, 36, 197, 215–221,
223–225, 231, 262, 266, 267, 273, 278,
291, 360, 363, 366
Promoter... 9, 58, 113, 123, 165, 167,
218, 223, 313, 323, 324, 329, 330, 338,
344, 352–355, 357, 363, 365, 374
Protease K 217, 218, 220, 224
Protein A/G beads...317
PVDF membrane.. 373, 377, 378

Q

Quantitative polymerase chain reaction...................227–242

R

Recombinant adeno-associated virus (rAAV) 5, 343
Red-free image 45, 49
Retinal cell degeneration 42
Retinal disease genes 3–19
Retinal dissection 331, 334, 338
Retinal explant.....................................210, 272, 274,
336, 337, 339, 340
Retinal ganglion cell (RGC).....................99–108, 351, 354
Retinal neovascularization 42, 53–58, 61, 352
Retinal pigment epithelium (RPE) 4, 5, 28,
41, 42, 48, 52, 54, 55, 58–60, 186, 188–191,
229–233, 237, 245–253, 285–295, 299, 301,
338, 343, 345–348, 351, 355–357
Retinal transcription factors 311–327
Retinal whole mount 188, 192–196
Retinitis pigmentosa (RP)..............................3, 4, 10–12,
14, 18, 19, 88, 113, 127, 189, 190, 371
Reverse crosslink 321
RGC. *See* Retinal ganglion cell (RGC)
Rhabdomere phenotypes 173
Rhodopsine 4, 16, 61, 62, 88,
93, 94, 96, 97, 113, 114, 120, 122, 162, 164,
165, 188–190, 247, 252, 293, 313, 323, 324
Riboprobe..220–221
Ringer solution 300, 302, 304, 307
RNA-polymerase..................................215, 216, 218, 219, 223
RNA-RNA hybrids... 215, 225
Rod and cone photoreceptors 56, 189, 355, 356
Rotenone 236–239, 242
RP. *See* Retinitis pigmentosa (RP)
RPE. *See* Retinal pigment epithelium (RPE)
RPE cell lines 231, 232, 286, 293, 294, 299

S

SAGE...216
Sanger sequencing 6, 9, 14–17
Sclera...101, 194, 195, 220,
261, 267, 334, 338, 345, 375
SD-OCT. *See* Spectral-domain optical coherence
tomography (SD-OCT)
SDS-PAGE...118, 121, 130, 134,
287, 291, 366, 373, 376, 377
shRNA 351, 372–375
Single flash 74, 76
Sodium nitroprusside (SNP) 5, 7–9, 11, 15, 17, 18, 211
Sonication..313, 319, 325, 326
Spectral-domain optical coherence tomography
(SD-OCT) 44, 63, 81, 345, 347, 348
Spliceosome...128

Store-operated Ca²⁺ channels 304–305, 307
Streptavidin 212
Subretinal injection......... 5, 58, 343–348, 355–357, 372, 375
Sucrose gradient 193, 288
SUMO E3 ligase 313
SYPRO ruby 366, 367

T

Terminal dUTP nick end labeling (TUNEL)
    labeling 102–103, 107, 207, 210, 211
Tet-responsive U6 promoter..374
Thapsigargin.. 304, 305
Tight junction 371
TNFα. *See* Tumor necrosis factor (TNFα)
TOPO-TA vector 223
Transfection...343, 352, 355,
    360, 361, 363–365, 379
Transgenics...28, 58, 59, 61, 95,
    113–123, 168, 185, 298
Triton X-100 ....129, 130, 192, 197,
    208–210, 253, 287, 314–316
Tropic amide eye drops..................... 47, 70, 72, 80, 344, 345
Trypsin 210, 233, 272, 274, 275, 280, 299, 359
Tumor necrosis factor (TNFα)..281

V

VEGFR2 antagonists...372
Visual pigment 48, 88, 94, 162, 164
Voltage-dependent calcium channel................................257

W

661W cells..232, 236, 238, 239
Whole exome sequencing..10
Whole mount.. 43, 58, 59, 107, 165,
    178, 188, 192–196, 202, 260, 262,
    264–265, 268
Woodchuck hepatitis virus post-transcriptional regulatory
    element (WPRE) 363

X

Xenopus laevis 113, 116, 122
x-rhod-1/AM 262, 264, 265, 268

Z

Zebrafish, *Danio rerio*.. 127–136
Zeiss LSM Image Examiner 260

Printed by Printforce, the Netherlands